RETINA
THE FUNDAMENTALS

RETINA
THE FUNDAMENTALS

Gloria Wu, M.D.

Assistant Surgeon, Massachusetts Eye and Ear Infirmary
Clinical Instructor, Harvard Medical School
Associate Clinical Professor, Tufts University School of Medicine
Boston, Massachusetts

W.B. Saunders Company
A Division of Harcourt Brace & Company
Philadelphia London Toronto Montreal Sydney Tokyo

W.B. SAUNDERS COMPANY
A Division of
Harcourt Brace & Company

The Curtis Center
Independence Square West
Philadelphia, PA 19106

Library of Congress Cataloging-in-Publicaton Data

Wu, Gloria.
Retina : the fundamentals / Gloria Wu.—Ed. 1.
p. cm.
ISBN 0-7216-6691-4
1. Retina—Diseases. I. Title.
[DNLM: 1. Retinal Diseases—handbooks. WW 39 W959r 1995]
RE551.W8 1995
617.7'3—dc20
DNLM/DLC 95-1647

Retina The Fundamentals ISBN 0-7216-6691-4

Printed in the United States of America

Last digit is the print number: 9 8 7 6 5 4 3 2 1

To my husband, Paul, and my children, Margaret and Catherine

Preface

Over the past decade, there have been numerous remarkable advances in diagnosis and management of retinal diseases. This growth in knowledge and understanding has created a greater challenge for the general ophthalmologist, who seeks to stay current in all ocular disorders. Thus, this book has been written as a concise, up-to-date text that covers all major aspects of retinal diseases. To achieve this purpose, the chapters include the topics of basic embryology, anatomy and physiology of the retina, basic examination techniques for the posterior segment, and congenital disorders of the retina. Common diagnostic questions in retina arise in the areas of diabetic retinopathy and vascular disease of the retina and chapters are devoted to these topics. Inflammatory disease and infectious disease of the retina are reviewed in separate chapters. Acquired retinal disease and tumors are included. Lastly, surgical management is outlined to explain the current approaches to therapy in this era of new vitreous substitutes and new surgical techniques.

This volume began as a series of lectures and courses taught at the American Academy of Ophthalmology and at medical schools and hospitals. I expanded my original notes to take into account many of the questions commonly encountered in ophthalmic practice as well.

In writing the text, I have come to appreciate all of the knowledge and insight that my mentors have provided to me over the years. First and foremost, I wish to thank Drs. D. Jackson Coleman, Harvey A. Lincoff, and Stanley Chang for being my first preceptors in the field of retina when I was a resident. I am particularly indebted to my teachers at the Retina Associates who have provided inspiration, stimulation, and support: Drs. Charles L. Schepens, J. Wallace McMeel, H. MacKenzie Freeman, Ronald C. Pruett, Felipe Tolentino, Tatsuo Hirose, Clement Trempe, Sheldon M. Buzney, John J. Weiter, and Alex Jalkh.

In the actual compilation of the manuscript, I would like to gratefully acknowledge the superb organizational skills of Min Jeong Ra, Alanna Bravman, Carolyn Fredey, Elizabeth Hayes, Nicole Gaeta, Sarah Wilson, Elane Chen, and F. John Wilcox.

During the year that I spent writing the manuscript, I received expert editorial assistance and enthusiastic personal encouragement from Richard Zorab and Kim Kist at W. B. Saunders.

I am also grateful for the privilege of serving my patients. Their questions have continued to inspire all of us, as physicians, to further our quest for solutions.

Lastly, I would like to thank my husband and children for their support and good humor throughout this project.

Gloria Wu

Contents

CHAPTER ONE

Anatomy and Physiology of the Retina

Ocular Embryology

At the 22-day embryo stage, the earliest beginnings of the eye appears with the closure of the neural tube, laterally, grooves occur forming the outpocketings of the forebrain. These become the optic vesicles. Shortly thereafter, the optic vesicles invaginate and form the double-walled optic cup. The inner and outer layers of this cup are initially separated by a lumen, the intraretinal space (the potential space between the future retinal pigment epithelium and the retina), but with further development, this lumen disappears and the two layers are apposed to each other. Along this earlier invagination is the choroid fissure and here, the hyaloid artery extends to reach the inner chamber of the eye. As the lips of the choroid fissure fuse, the mouth of the optic cup becomes the round opening, the pupil.

As these events occur, the cells of the surface ectoderm, initially in contact with the optic vesicle, begin to elongate and form the lens placode. This placode subsequently invaginates and develops into the lens vesicle. During the fifth week, the lens vesicle loses contact with the surface ectoderm and is located at the mouth of the optic cup—the future pupil (Figs. 1–1 to 1–3).[1]

THE RETINA

The development of the outer layer of the optic cup is characterized by the appearance of small pigment granules during the fifth week of development. The outer layer is known as the pigment layer of the retina, the future retinal pigment epithelium.

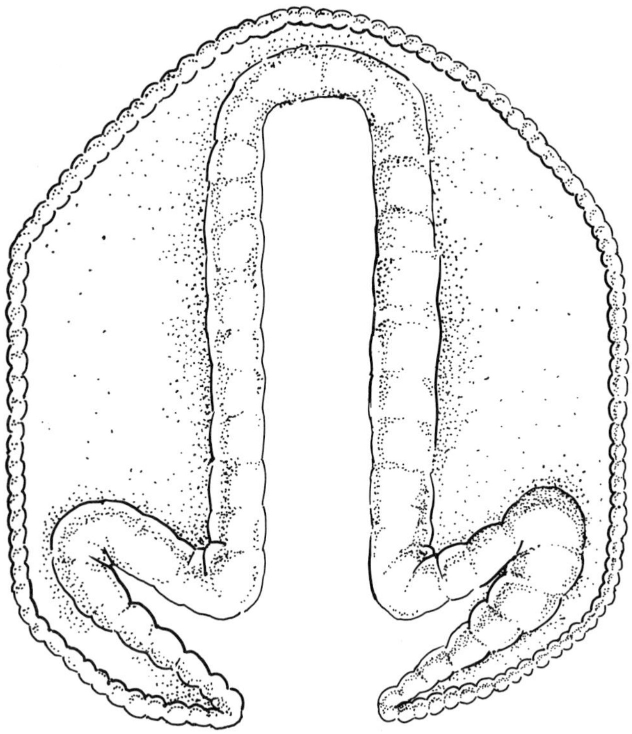

FIGURE 1–1

Twenty-two-day embryo with optic grooves.

The inner layer of the retina will be discussed as its posterior 4/5 (the retina as we know it) and its anterior 1/5 (the iris and ciliary body). Its posterior 4/5, thickens. Bordering the intraretinal space is the ependymal layer, which in the eye, differentiates into the rods and cones. Adjacent to the photoreceptors is the mantle layer, giving rise to neurons and supporting cells, which in the adult, becomes the outer nuclear, the inner nuclear, and the ganglion cell layers. On the surface of the mantle layer is the marginal zone that contains the axons of the nerve cells and is the precursor of the nerve fiber layer. The nerve fibers in this zone converge toward the optic stalk, which develops into the optic nerve.

The anterior 1/5 of the inner layer of the optic cup, the pars ceca retina, remains one cell layer thick. It is later divided into the inner layer of the iris and the ciliary body.

The Ten Layers of the Retina

Anatomically, there are ten layers of the retina and we will from time to time, refer to these in this text. Some of them are particularly important to the understanding of retinal disease states. The layers are, from inside the vitreous, going more posteriorly (Fig. 1–4):

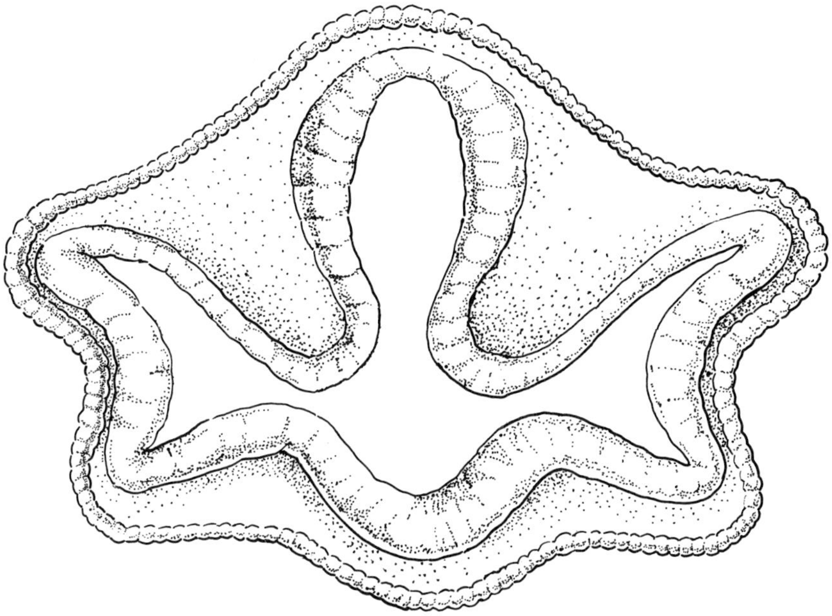

FIGURE 1–2

Five mm embryo-invagination of optic vesicle and lens placode.

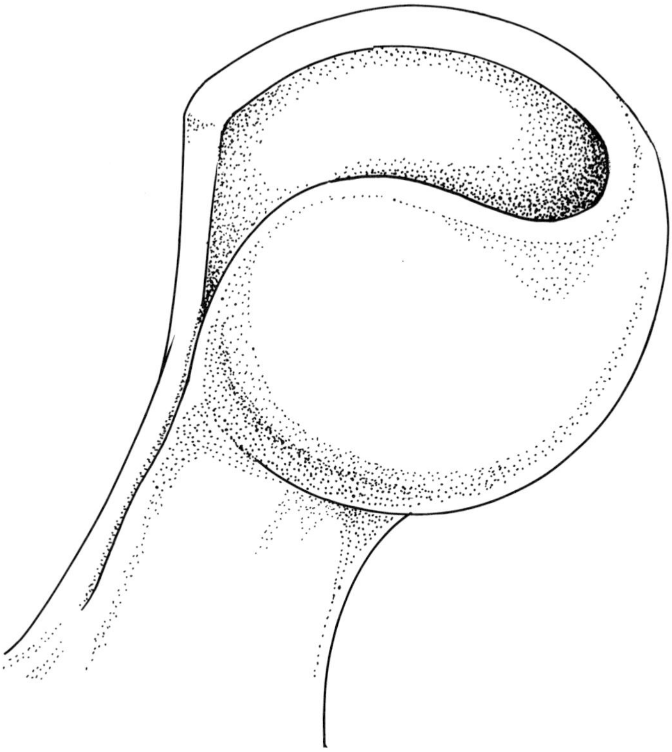

FIGURE 1–3

Six weeks embryo with optic cup and optic stalk.

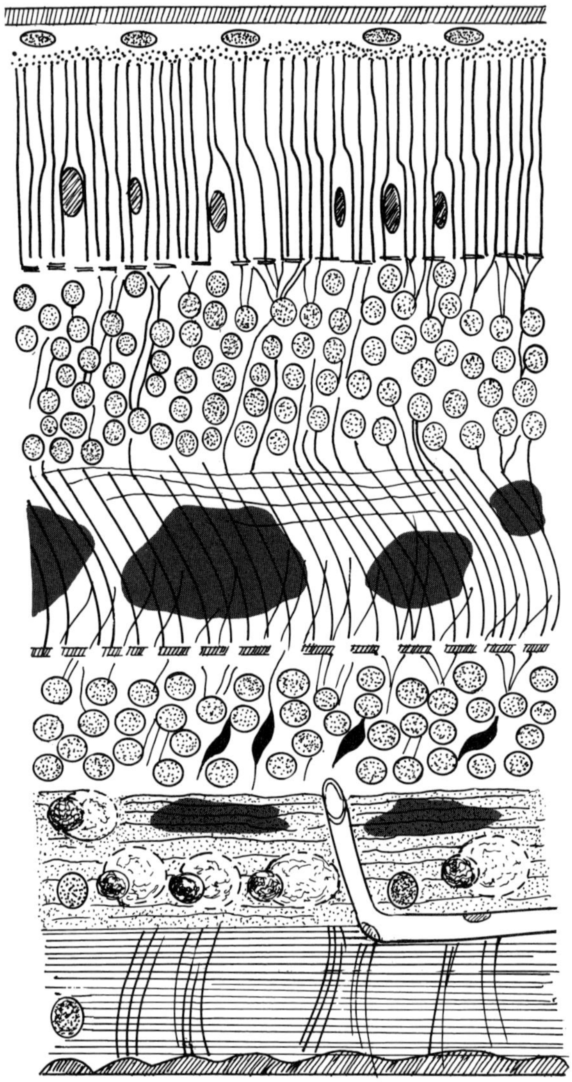

FIGURE 1-4

Ten layers of the retina. *a.* Retinal pigment epithelium; *b.* rods and cones; *c.* external limiting membranes; *d.* outer nuclear layer; *e.* outer plexiform layer; *f.* inner nuclear layer; *g.* inner plexiform layer; *h.* ganglion cell layer; *i.* nerve fiber layer; *j.* internal limiting membrane; A capillary is seen between layers *g* and *h.*

1. Internal limiting membrane
2. Nerve fiber layer
3. Ganglion cell layer
4. Inner plexiform layer
5. Inner nuclear layer
6. Outer plexiform layer
7. Outer nuclear layer
8. External limiting membrane
9. Rods and cones
10. Retinal pigment epithelium

In retina and vitreous disease states, the internal limiting membrane may show changes as the vitreous contracts or changes during trauma or diabetic macular edema. In addition, in diabetic retinopathy, hard exudates may be found in the outer plexiform layer near the macula, diabetic macular edema and its associated microaneurysms are found in the inner plexiform layer where the blood supply comes from the central retinal artery. In rhegmatogenous retinal detachments, the potential space between the retinal pigment epithelium and layers 1 through 9 separate and fluid accumulates. This is the space which existed embryonically and now is filled with subretinal fluid causing a bullous retinal detachment. In age-related macular degeneration, the site of pathologic processes occur between the retinal pigment epithelium and the layer of the rods and cones.

In addition, external to the retinal pigment epithelium is Bruch's membrane and going outwardly, the next layer is the choriocapillaris, the choroid (layer of medium vessels, then the layer of large vessels), the suprachoroid, and lastly, the sclera. Age-related macular degeneration also affects the interaction between the retinal pigment epithelium and Bruch's membrane and choriocapillaris.

The suprachoroidal space contains the long and short posterior ciliary arteries and nerves.

The choroid is divided into the layer of medium-sized vessels (Sattler's layer) and large vessels (Haller's layer). The choriocapillaris nourishes the outer part of the retinal layers.

REFERENCES

1. Langman J: Medical Embryology. Baltimore, Williams & Wilkins, 1975, pp. 368-371.
2. Warwick R: Wolff's Anatomy of the Eye and Orbit. Philadelphia, W.B. Saunders, 1981, pp. 99-108.

CHAPTER TWO

Examination of the Retina and Vitreous

HISTORY

The first step in the history-taking of a retina patient is the documentation of the chief complaint. The most important question to ask is, "Does this affect your vision?" or "Can you see the way you normally see?" or "Do you have total loss of vision?" By these simple questions, you are immediately finding out if this is an emergency, an urgent problem, or a benign problem.

Pertinent Questions to Ask the Patient

1. When did the visual disturbance occur? How many hours ago? In retinal detachments, we are interested if the loss of vision occurred weeks ago or a few hours ago. This type of information tells the ophthalmologist about the acuteness of the problem and hence the emergent nature of the treatment. If there has been associated trauma, the ophthalmologist is concerned about the possibility of bacterial, fungal, or metallic contaminants in cases when the lacerated globe may have been left exposed, uncovered, and untreated for more than 24 hours.
2. How did the loss of vision occur? Was it associated with a headache (differential diagnosis includes migraine headache) or was it associated with tingling sensation of your limbs or one side of your body? (Differential diagnosis includes retinal stroke or embolic phenomena which may affect the patient's vision as well as the neurologic system.)
3. How long did this episode last? For example, did the flashes and floaters last for a few minutes or for the entire day?
4. Is there family history of retinal disease? Is there a family history of retinal detachment surgery?
5. Does the patient have a history of previous retinal disease in the fellow eye?

6. Has the patient had foreign travel?
7. Has the patient eaten raw or poorly cooked pork, beef, or lamb?
8. Does the patient have any pets? In young patients, this is part of the history for *Toxocara canis, Toxoplasmosis,* etc.
9. Has the patient lived in various areas of the country where certain infectious diseases are known to be associated? For example, Lyme disease is found mostly in the New England areas, but now Lyme disease outbreaks have been found all over the continental United States. Has the patient lived in areas where histoplasmosis is common, i.e., Midwestern United States and the Eastern seaboard?
10. Is the patient known to have systemic diseases such as diabetes mellitus or hypertension that may explain the sudden visual loss?
11. What medications does the patient take that may compromise vision gradually or acutely? Is the patient taking coumadin and/or experiencing a new vitreous hemorrhage?

CLINICAL EXAMINATION TECHNIQUES

1. The best corrected visual acuity or pinhole visual acuity provides very useful information. Can the patient see 20/20?
2. Slit-lamp examination: Perform a systematic slit-lamp examination, looking at the cornea for defects, for evidence of trauma, for neovascularization. Look at the anterior chamber for cells, flare. Various inflammatory diseases of the retina present with anterior chamber reaction. Examine the iris for rubeosis iridis: It is important to look for the small red dots at the pupillary margin. These may be very hard to see, but sit in total darkness, dark adapt yourself and you may see fine neovascular twigs there. Using the Zeiss lens allows the ophthalmologist to see if there are neovascular twigs in the angle. The Zeiss lens is useful because gonio solution is not required and, afterward, the dilated funduscopic examination can still be performed with good visualization.
3. Dilated funduscopic examination: With the patient lying down in the examination chair or examination table, look at the retina with indirect ophthalmoscopy first to obtain an overview of the retinal topography. Afterward, the examiner can concentrate on the parts of the retina which are most abnormal.

The next step is the examination of the ora serrata with scleral depression. It is best to have the patient's pupils as well dilated as possible. This may entail several sets of dilating drops such as 2.5% phenylephrine and 1% tropicamide. The maximal dilation allows for the evaluation of the ora serrata with minimal scleral depression and minimal discomfort for the patient. Always use a drop of topical anesthetic to alleviate some of the discomfort for the patient (Fig. 2–1).

Some physicians always examine the right eye first in their patients with floaters. Others always examine the unaffected fellow eye first. It is important to find the way that best suits you so that you will always examine each eye in a systematic manner and record your findings systematically.

For beginners, scleral depression is best accomplished by the use of an applicator stick or a Mira scleral depressor or Storz scleral depressor stick, beginning with the lower lid, at 6:00. The lower lid serves as a cushion for the depressor and the patient gradually becomes introduced to the sensation of scleral depression. It is best to proceed in a clockwise or counterclockwise position to examine each clockhour of the ora serrata. It becomes slightly more difficult to examine the superior quadrants of the retina because of the anatomy of the upper eyelid and the orbital rim. The most difficult point of scleral depression is nasally because the caruncle is sensitive to pressure and the patient's nose is also in the way of the examiner's slight maneuverings and hand movements (Figs. 2–1 and 2–2).

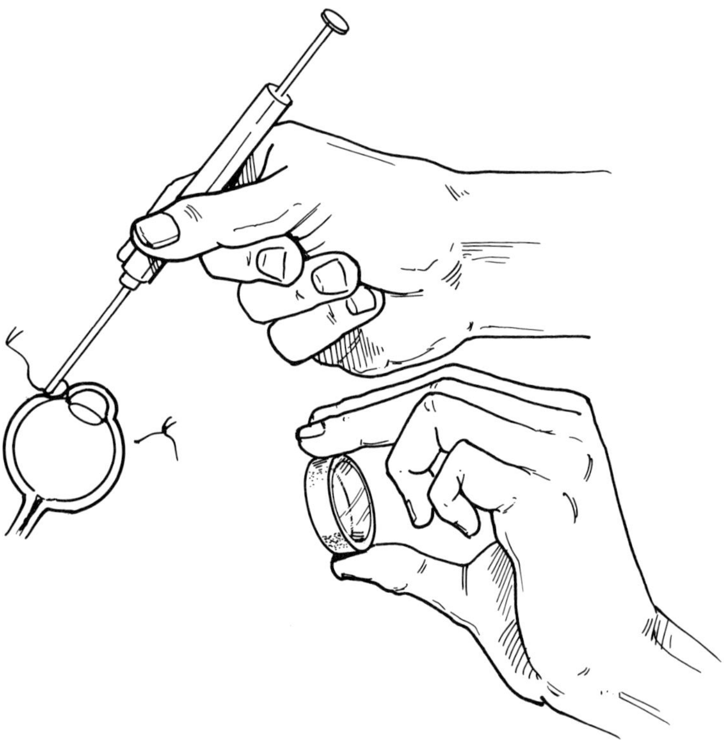

FIGURE 2–1

Diagram of scleral depression using Storz scleral depressor.

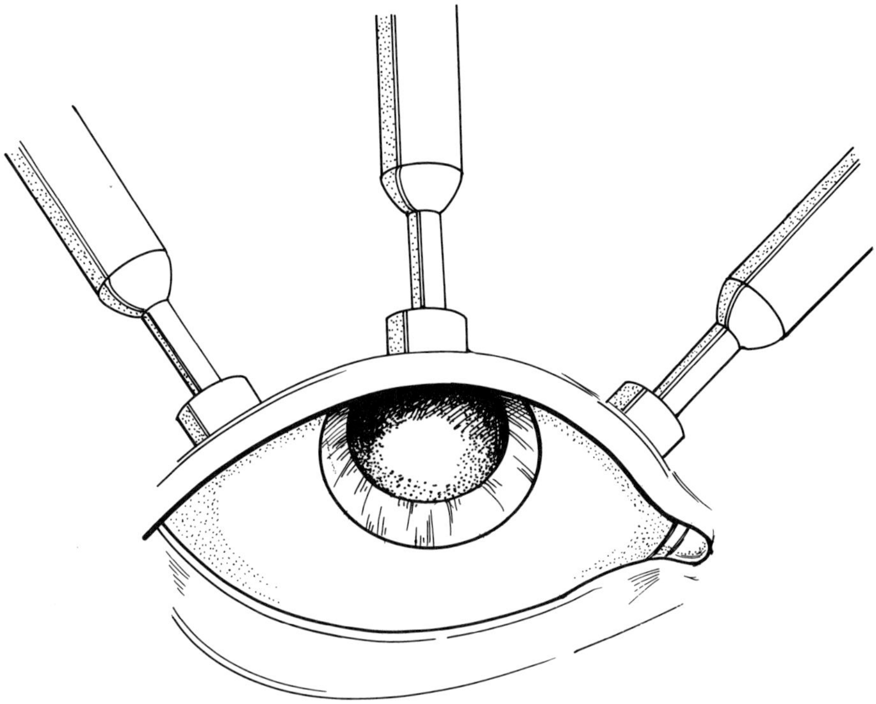

FIGURE 2–2

Diagram of scleral depressor placement on the eyelids for scleral depression.

The last part of the retinal examination is the examination of the macula and the optic nerve at the slit lamp. Use of the 90 diopter lens is helpful for stereoscopic details of the macula and the optic disc (Fig. 2–3). Use of the 60 diopter lens permits the evaluation of the vitreous interface with the internal limiting membrane of the retina. It is particularly useful to find the posterior vitreous detachment in patients who complain of a new onset of a floater. The 78 diopter lens is a combination of the 90 diopter and 60 diopter lens, but for viewing the vitreous, the best view is still obtained with the 60 diopter lens. All of these lenses at the slit lamp provide a binocular and stereoscopic view which is useful for examination of macular edema, localized serous retinal detachments, or hemorrhagic detachments of the retina in the macular area. The Hruby lens is excellent for the above as well.

The direct ophthalmoscope is still very useful to evaluate the optic disc and closeup view of the macula. This is an adjunct to the use of the slit-lamp biomicroscopic view of the macula using the 90 D, 78 D, or 60 D lenses (Fig. 2–4).

Lastly, after all the noncontact methods are used, the Goldmann contact lens is extremely useful to confirm the diagnosis of small retinal holes or investigate suspicious areas seen from the earlier indirect ophthalmoscopic examination. It is useful to examine the midperiphery to the equator as well as the ora serrata.

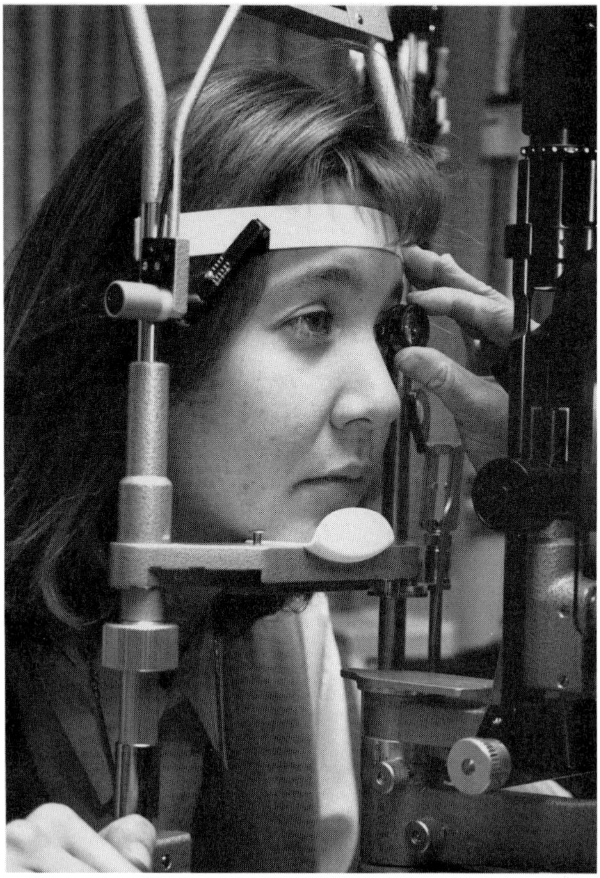

FIGURE 2-3

Patient being examined at the slit lamp with 90 D lens.

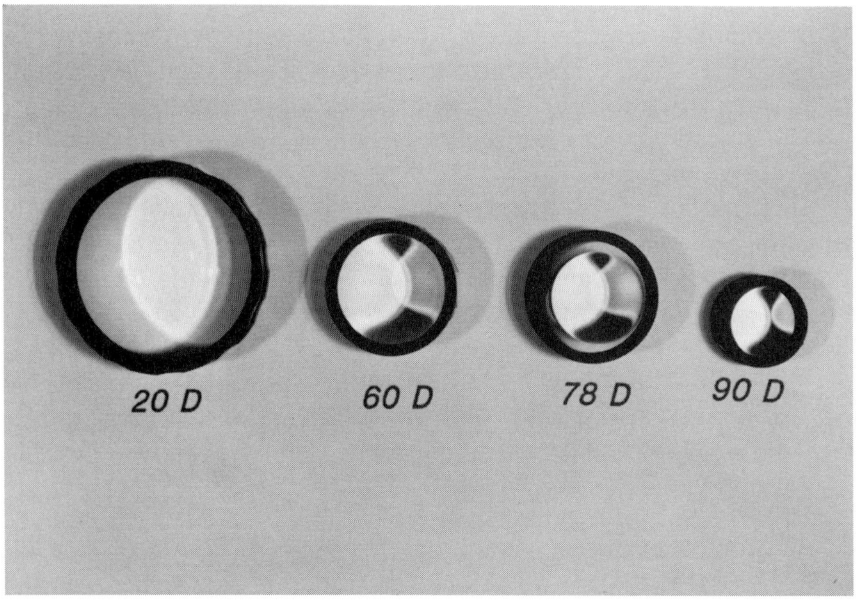

FIGURE 2-4

Ophthalmic lenses for examination of the retina.

DIAGNOSTIC TECHNIQUES

Photographs of the Retina

In a general ophthalmology practice or a retina subspecialty practice, it is important to document the exact location, size, shape, and color of the retinal lesion when trying to record it for the medical record. The photograph will be useful to show the patient and the family what the diagnosis is and to jar the examiner's own memory when the patient is examined again at a later date for a follow-up examination.

The best photographic documentation is 35 mm color slides, taken in stereo, with a fundus camera. These photographs of the macula will enable the clinician to view the retinal lesion for size and volume indices. For example, stereoscopic slides of diabetic macular edema can be seen with depth when viewed with a stereoscopic viewer. This information provides the clinician with information about eligibility for laser treatment. These slides also serve as a prelude to fluorescein angiography, to be discussed in the next section.

If unable to obtain color slides, documentation with a polaroid camera is useful. However, the lack of fine detail will not be especially helpful for treatment guidelines. A polaroid photographic record will always be useful in demonstrating to the patient the extent of the disease.

Fluorescein Angiography

Fluorescein angiography allows the visualization of the many layers of the retina and its circulation. It utilizes the principle that sodium fluorescein, a low-molecular-weight compound, fluoresces when excited by a blue light (465–490 nm) and will emit a yellow-greenish light (peak wave length of 520–530 nm).[1] Fundus cameras have built-in filters allowing for the fluorescence and emission of sodium fluorescein dye to be recorded on the black and white film.

Sodium fluorescein, 376 MW, freely diffuses out of the capillaries except those in the retina. Eighty percent of the sodium fluorescein dye is bound to plasma proteins. The remaining unbound fluorescein in the plasma layer lies between the blood vessel wall and the column of flowing erythrocytes. It is that column of dye that is detected in the angiogram.

Ten to 15 seconds after injection of fluorescein into the antecubital vein, the dye will reach the choroidal circulation via the short ciliary arteries. Choroidal flow is extremely rapid. Thus, rapid sequence photography in fluorescein angiography can visualize the patchy choroidal filling that occurs at the short ciliary arteries. The rapid perfusion of the choroid and the leakage of the dye from the choriocapillaries produces a background choroidal flush that has a mottled fluorescence because of the masking effect of the retinal pigment epithelium. The dye perfuses the retinal arteries then passes into the capillary bed, later collecting at the margins of the vein draining the area (arteriovenous phase).

As the dye diffuses out of the tissues, the fluorescein empties out of the retinal circulation and pools in the large choroidal vessels. Fluorescein is no longer seen on the rapid sequence photographs.

Fluorescein angiography is useful in evaluating diseases of the macula because it shows changes in blood flow, differential permeability of the retinal blood vessels, differential flow in the choroidal vasculature, and differential change in the normal barrier function of the retinal pigment epithelium to sodium fluorescein (Figs. 2–5 and 2–6).

Ultrasonography

Ophthalmic ultrasound uses wave frequencies of 8–10 MHz. These high frequencies allow for the fine resolution of the small structures in the eye. Clinical ultrasound utilizes the A-scan and B-scan. The A-scan provides a measurement of the time it takes for the acoustic wave to reach an interface and its return to the ultrasound probe.

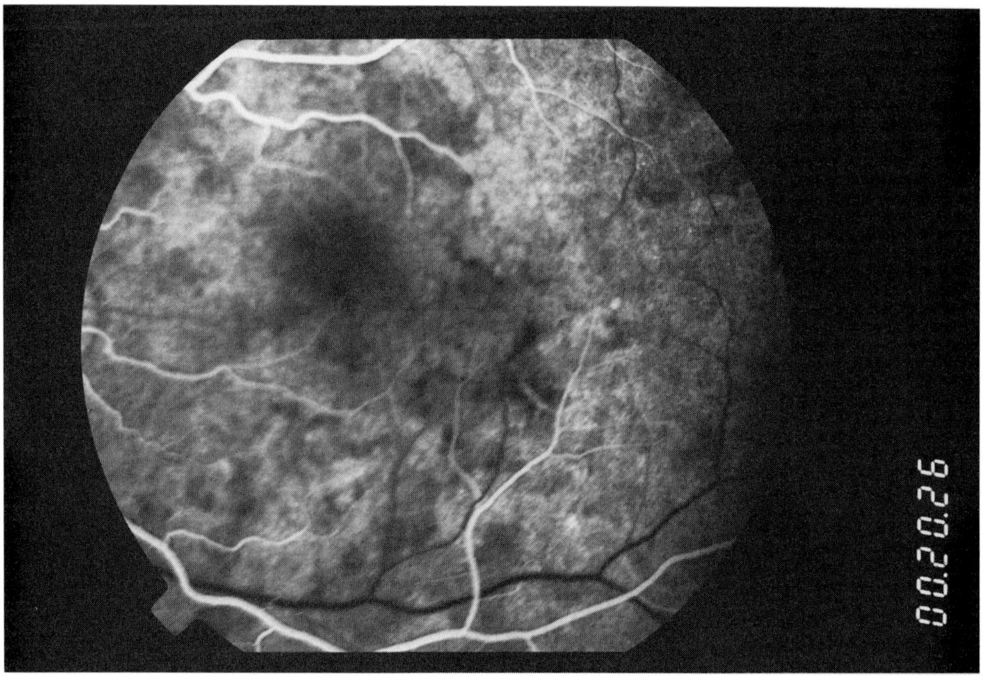

FIGURE 2–5

Early fluorescein transit, choroidal fluorescence.

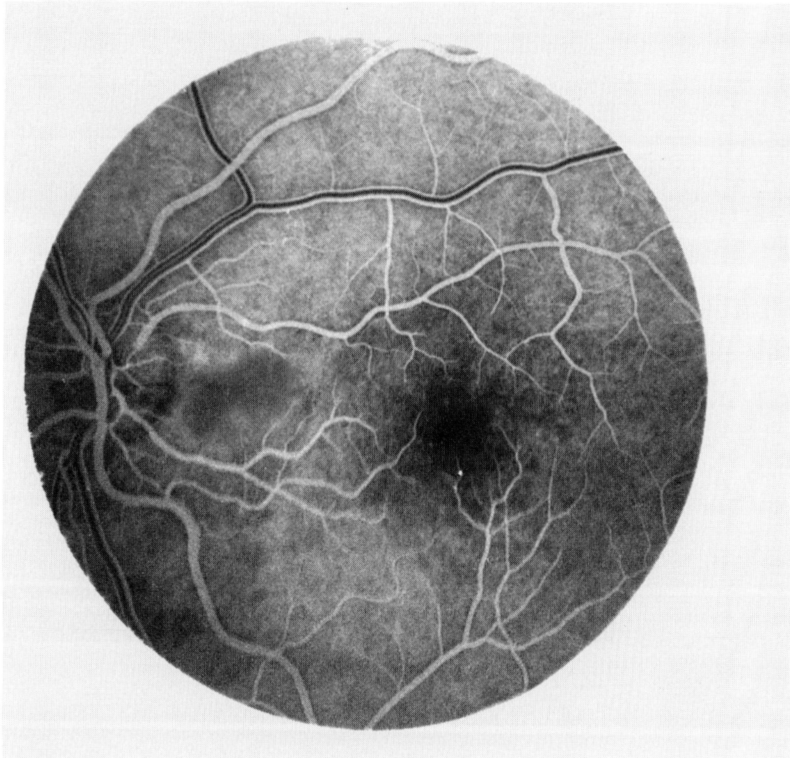

FIGURE 2–6

Arteriovenous phase of fluorescein transit.

The A-scan is used commonly in ophthalmology for the measurement of axial length, anterior chamber depth for cataract surgery. It plays a role in the measurement of tumors or other large lesions in the posterior pole.

The B-scan generates a two-dimensional view of the tissue interface under consideration. A section of tissue is "examined" by the transducer and the returning acoustic waves are represented as a series of echoes on the screen which then provide a "picture" of the tumor, hemorrhage, and retinal elevation seen in the eye.

Contact ultrasound units are widely available. There are two modes of examining the patient, through closed eyelids or direct contact on the limbus or cornea. Both techniques utilize the kinetic nature of the vitreous to view the posterior pole structures (Fig. 2–7).

Waterbath ultrasound units use the same principles as above but provide greater precision for the localization and size of tumors.

Electroretinography

The electroretinogram (ERG) is the record of the electrical response of the human retina to a flash of light. It is based on the principle

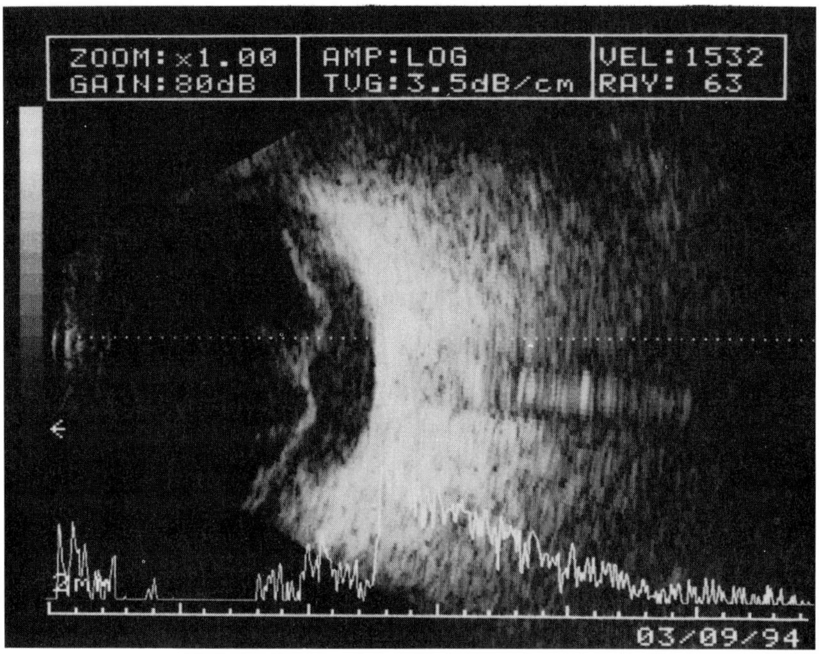

FIGURE 2-7

Ultrasound of a dense hyaloidal membrane and blood.

that the eye is like a battery and that a spontaneous electrical response can be elicited with the cornea acting as the positive electrode and the retina acting as the negative electrode.[2] As early as 1908, Einthoven, who is credited with developing the electrocardiogram, conceived of the ERG as having an initial negative segment, the a-wave, followed by a larger positive deflection, the b-wave.[3] However, it was not until the 1940's that clinical applications with a contact lens on the human eye was possible.[4] Recently, ERG textbooks for the clinician and modern computer-driven software programs have made ERG recordings a practical office examination technique.[5–7]

There are instances in daily clinical practice that the clinician is concerned about the visual potential of a patient with opaque media because of a dense cataract or an opaque cornea. In addition, the clinician is concerned about the patient with a vitreous hemorrhage from diabetic retinopathy, retinopathy from central retinal vein occlusion, and lastly, inherited retinal diseases. Ultimately the question of concern is, "Will the patient see?" or "Is the patient's retina functioning so that the cataract operation or corneal surgery will be successful?"

The ERG is measured using a contact lens electrode on the cornea serving as the active electrode, the indifferent electrode is placed on the forehead, and a ground electrode is placed on the ear. The eye is stimulated by using different intensities of light stimuli, in both the light-adapted (photopic) state and dark-adapted (scotopic) state. By processing the resultant action potential through preamplifiers and amplifiers, the response is recorded and displayed on an oscilloscope monitor or ink writer. Some units contain signal averaging electronic devices to collect and average the many small electrical responses and separate them from background noise (Figs. 2–8 and 2–9).

The ERG is described by two characteristics: the amplitudes of the waves and the response time (implicit time) with respect to the stimulus of light. Components of the ERG that are known and have been studied are (Fig. 2–10):

1. Early receptor potential (ERP)
2. a-wave
3. b-wave
4. c-wave
5. d-wave (off response)

The ERP is the first response that occurs 60 seconds after the stimulus of light. It is the first positive deflection followed by a slower negative deflection merging with the a-wave. Its origin is

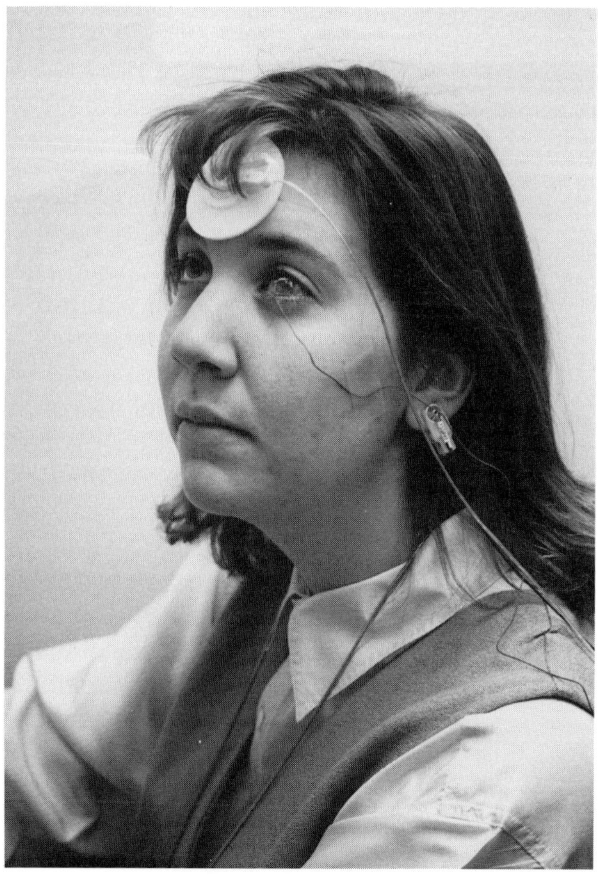

FIGURE 2–8

Patient with an electrode placed on the eye, ground electrode placed on the ear, and an indifferent electrode placed on the forehead.

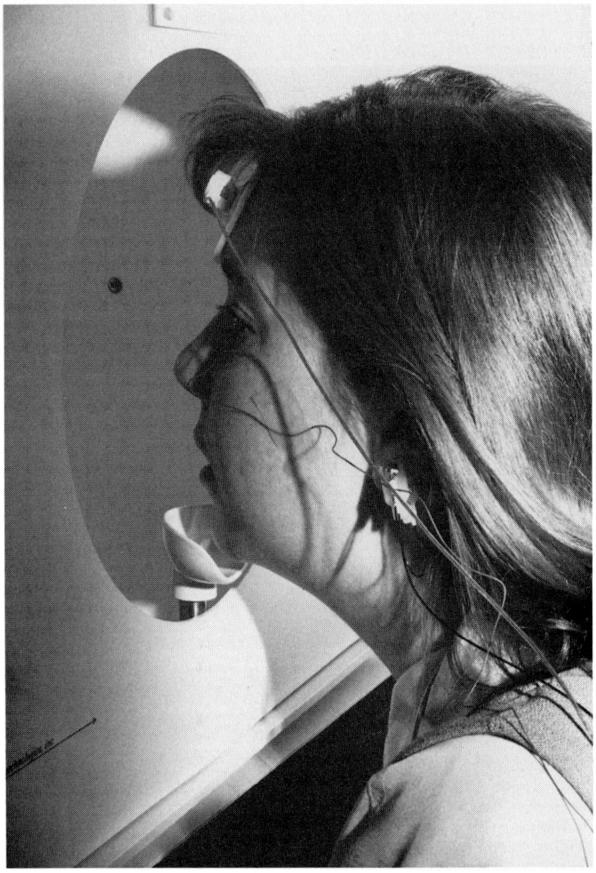

FIGURE 2–9

Patient's head and chin inside the Ganfgeld bowl for ERG testing.

thought to be the photoreceptor outer segments and may correspond to light absorption and chemical reactions of the photopigments. It is rarely used clinically.

After a light stimulus, the first clinically significant negative deflection of the recording is the a-wave. The a-wave is monophasic in the photopic state and biphasic (a_1 and a_2) in scotopic testing. It is more prominent in scotopic testing and may not be evident in the photopic state. The a-wave measures the response of the photoreceptors, rods, and cones. There are 130 million rods to 7 million cones. The ERG is a mass response testing all of these cells. Thus, if there are only isolated, small lesions, the ERG will be normal. If we are interested in the certain areas of the retina, we need to understand that the cone density of the foveola is very high, i.e., it contains 9000 cones, but the other 6.9 million cones are scattered outside the foveal region, and if normal, will contribute overwhelmingly to a normal ERG waveform. The cones respond to a deep red or bright light. Thus to test the cones, we must use the correct light stimulus and look to see where the cones are located, to understand what the waveform will mean. Rods, also part of the photoreceptors tested in the a-wave, are stimulated primarily with a dim blue light or dim light stimuli. The separation of the rod and cone response is useful in inherited retinal diseases (see Table 2–1). The vascular supply of the photoreceptors is the choroidal circulation, i.e., the ophthalmic artery. Thus, in ophthalmic artery occlusions, there is no a-wave. The a-wave is thought to originate in the photoreceptors of the retina.

The b-wave is the positive deflection following the a-wave. The b-wave reflects the response of the bipolar cell layer and the retinal circulation of the inner retina. At low intensities of light in the scotopic state, a monophasic, long-lasting positive deflection called the d-c potential is seen. As the light intensity increases, a rapid, large positive deflection occurs as the d-c potential decreases. It is this fast component is thought to originate in the Mueller cell layer. The ascending limb of the b-wave is called the oscillatory potential (Fig. 2–11). These five wavelets with their summed amplitudes and latencies are of renewed interest in the last 10 years in diabetic retinopathy studies.[8–12] They have been shown to be abnormal in diabetic patients with varying degrees of diabetic retinopathy.

The inner retinal layers up to and including the inner plexiform layer are served by the central retinal artery. With experimental ligation of the central retinal artery, one can see an absent b-wave.

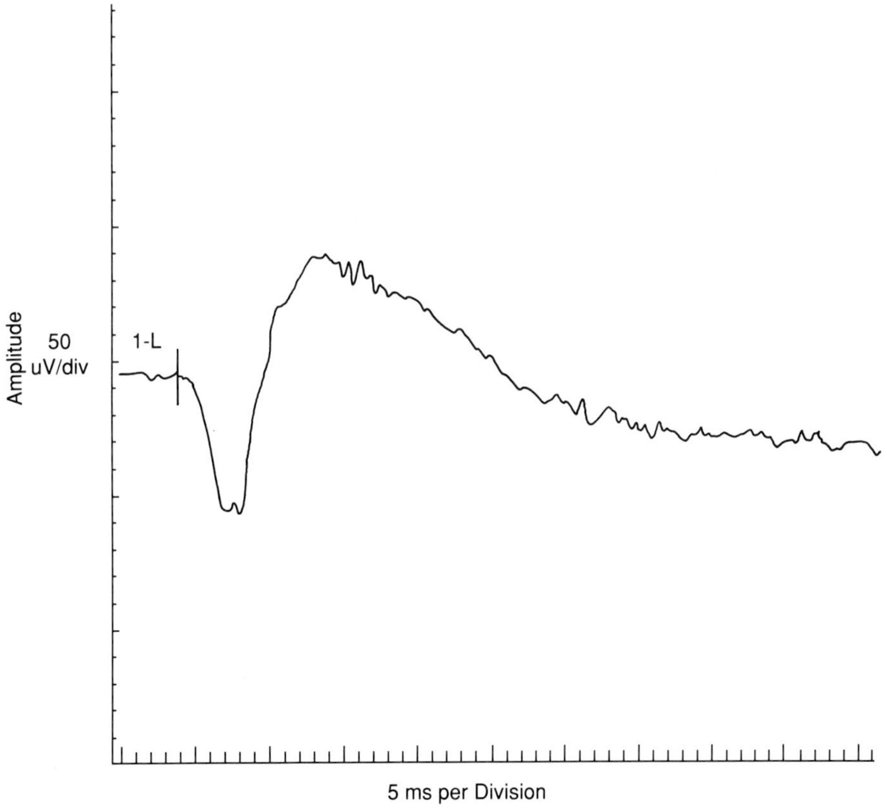

FIGURE 2–10

The large downward deflection is the a-wave; the upward deflection is the b-wave.

■ TABLE 2-1 Patient Preparation and Suggested ERG Protocol

Instrumentation

1. LKC
2. Nicolet
3. Sonometrics

Recording Environment

The room in which the ERG will be performed should be relatively lightproof when the room lights are turned off.

Patient Protocol

The patient's pupil is dilated, then the patient is brought into a room. With darkening of all lights for the period of dark adaptation from 30–45 minutes, the first part of the scotopic testing can be performed. The contact lens is inserted onto the cornea just prior to recording. The testing includes several intensities of light with variable intervals between the flashes. It is then followed by 1–2-minute period of light adaptation (the Ganzfeld bowl illumination can be turned on). The photopic testing can begin and end with the flicker fusion frequency.

Supplies

Burian Allen monopolar corneal contact electrode or Jet disposable electrodes (useful for patients with acquired immunodeficiency syndrome [AIDS]), Wratten red filter over a pen light or flashlight, electrocardiographic electrodes to serve as the indifferent electrode, earclip as a ground electrode, alcohol wipes, topical anesthetic drops, facial tissues, and irrigation solution for the cornea at the end of the procedure.

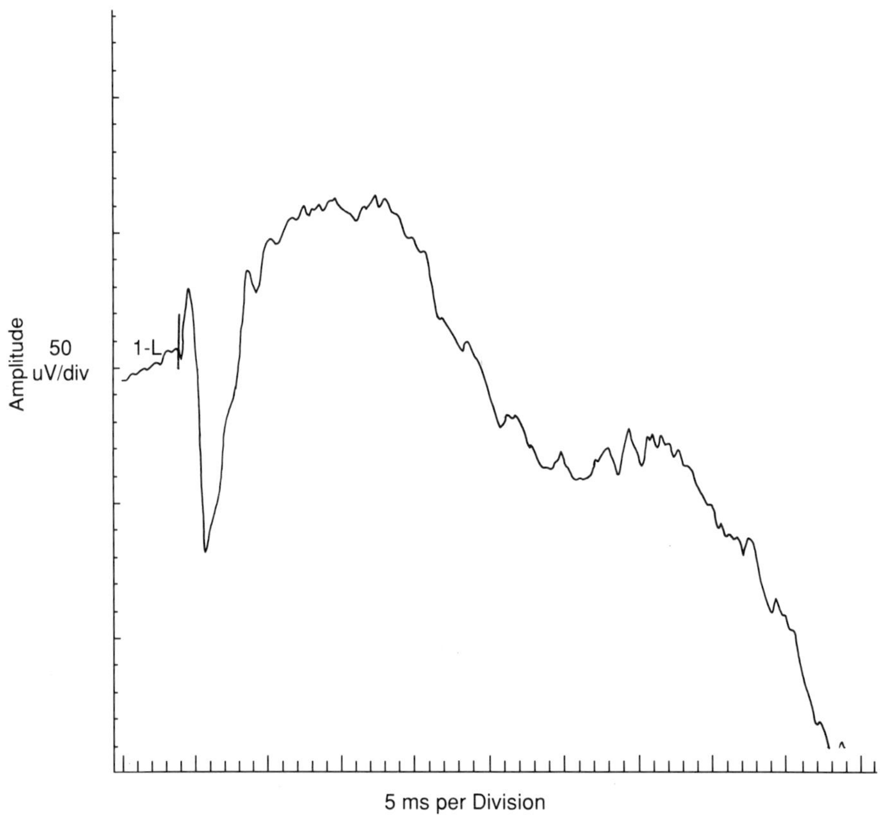

FIGURE 2-11

Note that the upward deflection has little wavelets leading to the maxima that is the b-wave. These wavelets are called the oscillatory potential.

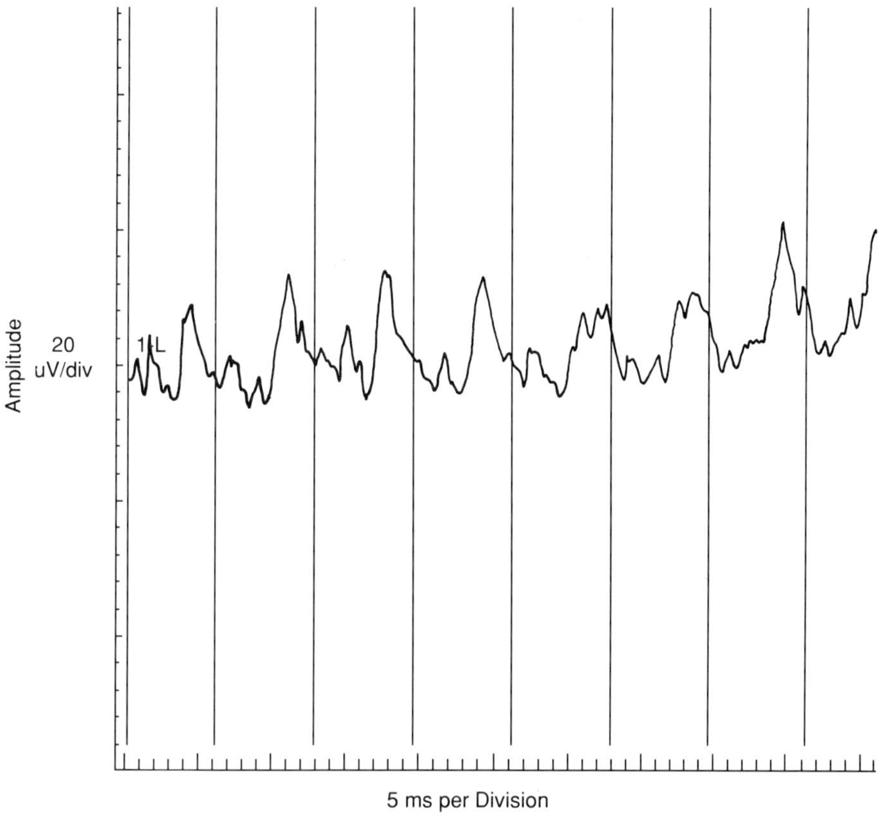

FIGURE 2–12

Flicker fusion frequency.

The c-wave is a small and inconsistent positive deflection following the b-wave. Its cellular origin is thought to be the pigment epithelium, however, this is not measured clinically.

The d-wave is either a positive or negative deflection occurring at the time when the light stimulus is turned off. Its postulated origin is the decay of the a-wave and slow d-c component of the b-wave. This is not measured clinically.

Flicker Fusion Frequency

At a light frequency of 30 per second, the ERG measures cone function only because rods cannot respond at that frequency. It is at this Flicker fusion frequency in humans, that each light flash no longer stimulates a corresponding single response (Fig. 2–12).

Clinical Electroretinography and Its Uses

In patients with opaque media, the clinician is interested in both components of the a- and b-wave because he is concerned with the function of the retina, the photoreceptors, as well as the inner retina where the vascular supply of the retina lies. For these patients, the ERG would serve to make a prognosis of vision.

In patients with vascular diseases as diabetic retinopathy, the ERG tests the vascular integrity of the inner retina, as reflected in the b-wave and its marked decrease in amplitude of the oscillatory potential. This is an especially important clinical parameter in those patients with severe proliferative diabetic retinopathy.

In patients with central retinal vein occlusion, the concern for the development of subsequent retinal ischemia and subsequent neovascular glaucoma is a common concern. The comparison of the b-wave to the a-wave, called the "b/a-wave ratio," is used to help clinicians follow the changes in these patients.[13] If the ratio is less than 1, we are concerned about the development of ischemia and the need for panretinal photocoagulation may be helpful in the prevention of neovascular glaucoma.

Clinical Interpretation of the ERG

NORMAL SCOTOPIC ERG (Fig. 2–13):

1. Large a-wave
2. Large b-wave
3. Longer implicit times than the photopic ERG

NORMAL PHOTOPIC ERG:

1. Small or no a-wave
2. Small b-wave
3. Shorter implicit times

Clinical ERG is a useful adjunct to the ophthalmic examination of the retina when there is a question about visual function. Although classically, the ERG has been used to test retinal function in inherited retinal and choroidal dystrophies, it is being used increasingly to test other entities where there is opaque media. Much of ophthalmology is concerned about the anatomy and physiology of visual function and ERG allows the clinician to learn more about the different cellular components of vision.

Electro-oculography

The electro-oculogram (EOG) records the voltage changes between the cornea to the back of the eye. As the patient looks back and forth at fixation lights, the electrodes at the inner and outer canthi record the voltage changes. This test is useful in measuring the metabolic activity of the retinal pigment epithelium. The EOG is recorded in two-minute intervals during 15 minutes of dark adaptation

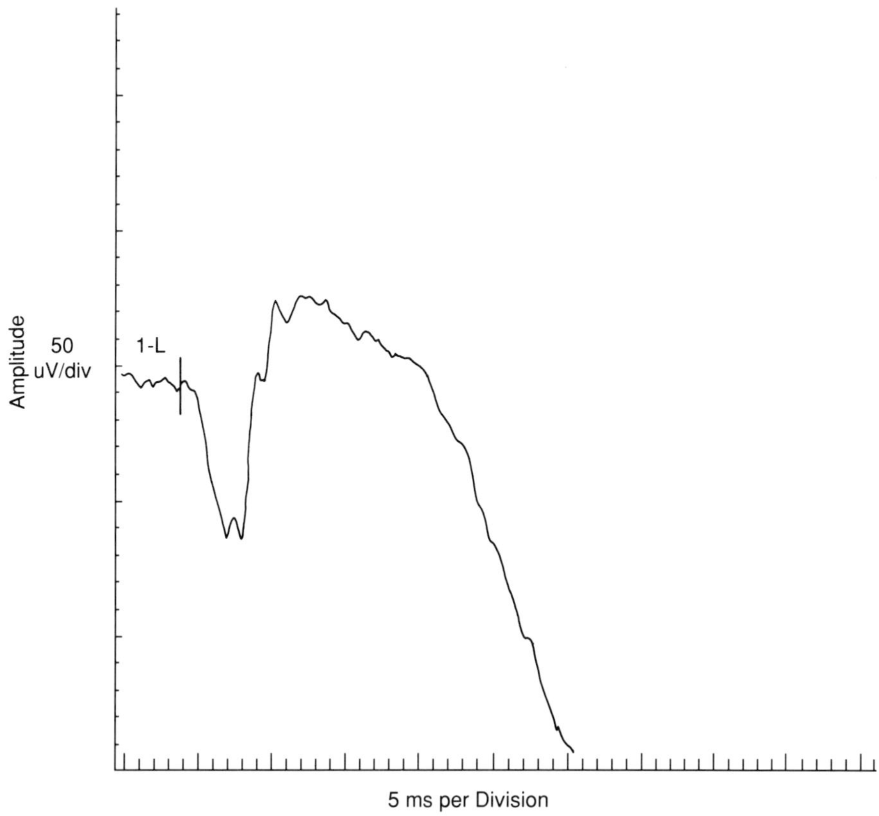

FIGURE 2–13

Normal scotopic ERG from a 32-year-old male.

followed by 15 minutes of light adaptation. The EOG in normal volunteers is 1.7 to 2 times larger during light than during dark adaptation. The Arden ratio is the light peak divided by the dark trough.

The EOG usually parallels the ERG findings. However, the main exception is Best's disease where the EOG is abnormal and the ERG may be normal.

Dark Adaptation

Dark adaptation is the evaluation of the ability of rod and cone mechanisms to recover sensitivity after exposure to light. This is done by changing threshold luminance of a test light in the upper retina, 15–20 degrees in the periphery.

Color Vision

Color vision is based on the neurophysiologic understanding of receptive fields.[14] A receptive field is a set of neural elements designed to detect differences in a stimulus. There are receptive fields set up to detect differences in brightness, patterns, motion, and color. The fields have excitatory and inhibitory regions. One region concentrically surrounds the other, e.g., a ganglion cell of the retina will increase its firing rate if the central (excitatory) portion of the photoreceptor field is stimulated and decrease its firing if the surround (inhibitory) portion of the field is stimulated. Such a receptive field is an "on-center off-surround" type. Receptive fields for color are similarly organized except that the excitatory and inhibitory portions of the field are opponent-color units. Thus, a red on-center, green off-surround cortical cell would increase its firing rate if reddish light fell near the field center on the retina and would decrease its firing rate if greenish light fell on the surrounding areas of the field. Color detection works by the detection of slight changes in wavelength being translated into a increase or decrease in spike firing rate.

By stimulus, we mean (1) wavelength (hue or color), (2) quanta of light per unit time from a unit area of radiating emitter (intensity, brightness, or luminance), and (3) saturation (purity or richness of color).[15]

Color pigments reside in each cones outer segment. Each cone pigment absorbs a broad range of wavelengths. A red-sensitive cone would absorb greatest amounts of red and lesser amounts from the other spectral regions. Ganglion cells discriminate between wavelength and intensity by requiring another factor, i.e., the presence of at least one other type of cone pigment, for instance, a green-sensitive one, the output of which feeds into the same ganglion cell. In this situation, the ganglion cell receives a signal derived from the two cones with each pigment absorbing quite different numbers of quanta based on their intrinsic sensitivities. Thus, a minimal requirement for color discrimination is the presence of at least two kinds of cone photopigment. Thus, normal color vision requires all three types of cone pigments: red-, green- and blue-sensitive cones to be functioning.

Ganglion cells outside the fovea receive rod input that increases the farther the stimulus is from the fovea. Rods contain the visual pigment rhodopsin (absorbs wavelengths at the blue-green region). Rods provide additional color information. In the dark-adapted state, the ganglion cell of the retina has both cone and rod input but the rods dominate in this state (scotopic). However, in the presence of a light background, the cones dominate the neural activity under the light (photopic) condition.

Individuals with a red-green deficiency related to the red-sensitive pigment loss were described originally, thus protanopia, the absence of vision of the first type. Another type of red-green deficiency is the loss of the green-sensitive pigment, and this is known as the second type, i.e., deuteranopia. Blue-yellow color blindness or the loss of the blue-sensitive or short wavelength cones is the third type, tritanopia.

The anomalous trichromats are color-deficient persons who require three primaries to match an unknown color but use them in anomalous amounts compared to the normal trichromat. They are "color weak" rather than "color blind." Thus, a protanomalous person needs more red in a red-green mixture to match a yellow.

Color vision testing is an adjunctive test which can be easily performed in the office. It serves to screen retinal diseases. Many inherited retinal diseases have associated color vision defects and have lesions in the cone system of the retina. For other patients who present with distortions of macular vision or other complaints, color vision testing may help highlight the acquired nature of the disease. For example, diabetic macular edema is known to have color vision abnormalities which can be followed and correlated with the amount of macular edema.[16]

Congenital and acquired hereditary congenital color vision defects are almost always "red-green" affecting 8 percent of the males, and 0.5 percent of females. Congenital color vision defects are bilateral and symmetric. These patients do not usually misname colors whereas patients with acquired defects report that the colors of familiar objects have changed. Acquired defects are usually called the "blue-yellow" variety and affect males and females equally. Congenital or hereditary color vision defects may not show any retinal lesions, however, in acquired color vision defects, there are frequently associated retinal lesions.

Guidelines for Color Vision Testing (Fig. 2–14)

1. All children at a very early age.
2. Patients on their first office visit.
3. All patients with decreased visual acuity.
4. All patients who report recent color disturbance or difference of color perception between the two eyes.
5. Those who have been diagnosed as color defective on an employment examination.
6. Patients taking chloroquine, plaquinil, or mellaril.

Testing of color vision can be accomplished by using Ishihara color plates (most commonly used clinically), Farnsworth D15 (retina specialists), and Farnsworth-Munsell D 100 (retinal electrophysiology labs).

Visual Field Testing

In certain macular diseases, it may be helpful to map out the central scotoma to demonstrate the areas of affected retina. This can be useful in patients with age-related macular degeneration who need laser therapy. The physician should try to map out the scotoma if the lesion is subfoveal to help guide the laser therapy and keep the laser treatment within the scotomatous areas.[17] The visual field test is useful in the follow up of patients with uveitis and diabetic macular edema as a parameter of the treatment.

Amsler Grid

Amsler Grid testing is useful in patients with macular disease (Fig. 2–15). It is also useful in patients with diabetic macular edema, age-related macular degeneration, and other macular lesions. It allows patients to test themselves and alert the physician if there are any changes in between follow-up examinations.

Macular Function Testing

Macular photostress testing tests the ability of the macula to recover from a bright flash of light.[18] It is easy to administer in the office.

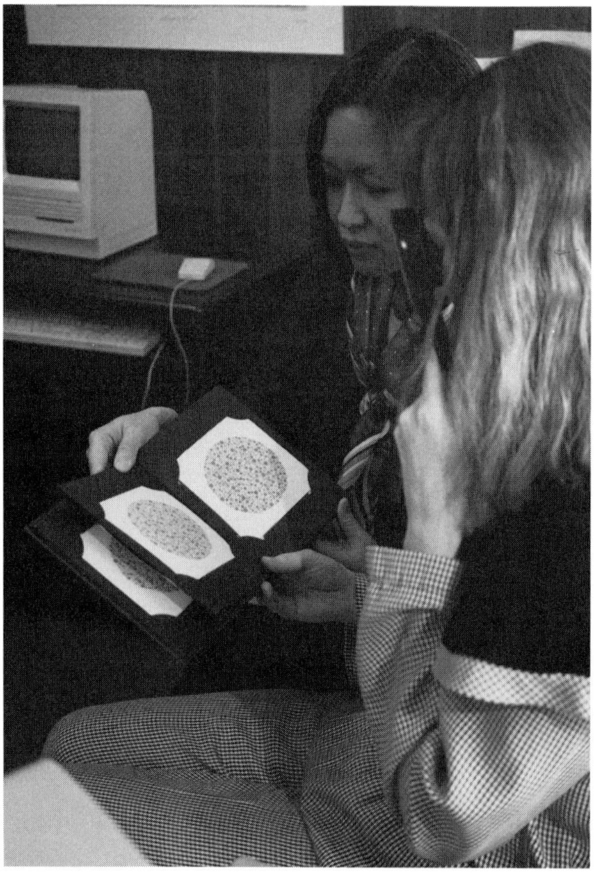

FIGURE 2–14

Patient being tested with Ishihara plates for color vision.

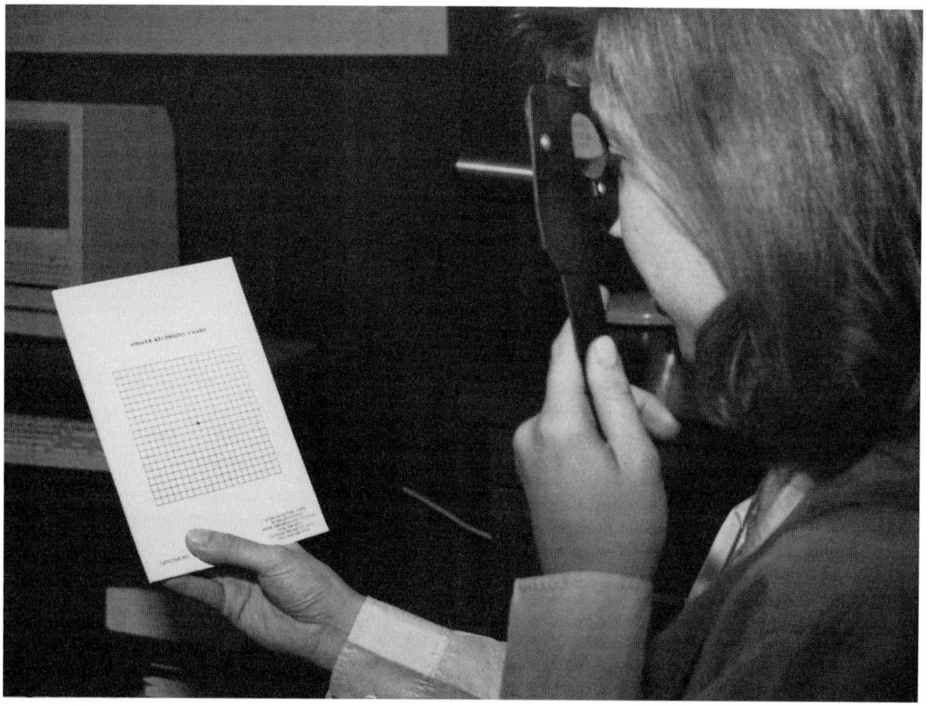

FIGURE 2-15

Patient being examined for macular defects with Amsler Grid.

This test utilizes the indirect ophthalmoscope, set at 6 volts and held 6 inches away from the patient, and the testing of the visual acuity before the macular photostress test and after the bright flash of light. After the flash of light, the examiner counts the number of seconds (recovery time) the patient needs to regain the ability to read the original line of Snellen visual acuity.

Contrast Sensitivity

Many of the automatic refractors test contrast sensitivity with glare testing. This allows the examiner to approximate the normal light conditions of outdoor sunlight. It allows the physician to appreciate the quality of vision that the patient experiences. This test is useful in assessment of functional visual acuity.

REFERENCES

1. Novotny HR, Alvis DL: A method of photographing fluorescence in circulating blood in the human retina. Circulation 1961; *24*:82–86

2. DuBois-Reymond E: Untersuchungen uber die tierische elektrizitat. p. 256. In Reumer G (ed): Vol. 2. Berlin, 1849

3. Einthoven W, Jolly W: The form and magnitude of the electrical response of the eye to stimulation at various intensities. QJ Exp Physiol 1908; *1*:373–416

4. Riggs LA: Continuous and reproducible records of the human retina. Proc Soc Exp Biol 1941; *48:*204–207

5. Carr RE, Siegel IM: Visual Electrodiagnostic Testing. Baltimore, Williams & Wilkins, 1982

6. Fishman GA: The Electroretinogram and Electro-oculogram in Retinal and Choroidal Disease. San Francisco, American Academy of Ophthalmology, 1975

7. Heckenlively JR, Arden GB: Principles and Practice of Clinical Electrophysiology of Vision. St. Louis, Mosby Year Book, 1991

8. Bresnick G, Korth K, Groo A, Palta M: Electroretinographic oscillatory potentials predict progression of diabetic retinopathy. Arch Ophthalmol 1984; *102:*1307–1311

9. Bresnick G, Palta M: Predicting progression to severe proliferative diabetic retinopathy. Arch Ophthalmol 1987; *106:*810–815

10. Bresnick G, Palta M: Oscillatory potential amplitudes. Arch Ophthalmol 1987; *105:* 929–933

11. Wu G, Jacobson L, Astor-Rueda R, et al: ERG changes in early diabetic retinopathy. Invest Ophthalmol Vis Sci 1990; *31:*126 (suppl.)

12. Holopigian K, Seiple M, Lorenzo M, et al: A comparison of phototopic and scotopic electroretinographic changes in early diabetic retinopathy. Invest Ophthalmol Vis Sci 1990; *31:*423 (suppl.)

13. Sabates R, Hirose T, McMeel JW: Electroretinography in the prognosis and classification of central retinal vein occlusion. Arch Ophthalmol 1983; *101:*232–235

14. Miller RF: The physiology and morphology of the vertebrate retina. p. 83. In Ryan SJ (ed): Retina. Vol 1. St Louis, CV Mosby, 1989

15. Pokorny J, Smith V: Color vision and night vision. p. 109. In Ryan SJ (ed): Retina. Vol 1. St Louis, CV Mosby, 1989

16. Jacobson L, Wu G, Weiter JJ: Ishihara plates as a screening test for diabetic macular edema. Ophthalmol 1990; *97:*151 (suppl.)

17. Coscas G, Soubrane G: Treatment for subfoveal choroidal new vessels in age-related macular degeneration. Arch Ophthalmol 1991; *109:*1258–1265

18. Wu G, Weiter JJ, Santos S, et al: The Macular photostress test in diabetic retinopathy and age-related macular degeneration. Arch Ophthalmol 1990; *108:*1556–1558

CHAPTER THREE

Congenital Anomalies

VASCULAR ANOMALIES

Congenital Telangiectasis or Coats Disease

Described by George Coats in 1908, Coats disease is an idiopathic condition associated with telangiectasia, irregular dilatation of retinal vessels with massive subretinal exudation or exudative retinal detachment.[1] It typically affects young males in a unilateral fashion. It is often a disease of childhood or adolescence but adults can be affected as well.

Anatomy and Physiology

Pathologic specimens have shown dilation of retinal veins, arteries, and capillaries with associated PAS-exudate in the outer retinal layers. Marked retinal vascular endothelial proliferation and hemorrhagic infarction of the retina may occur in some children with severe congenital telangiectasia.[2–4]

Clinical Presentation

Patients who present in childhood or in adolescence with telangiectasia usually have more widespread involvement and have poor vision in one eye. In patients with a milder form of the disease, it may present later in life and there may be fluctuations of vision corresponding to the amount of vascular leakage.

Diagnosis

Funduscopic examination showing massive exudation with varying degrees of retinal telangiectasia is key. Occasionally, the massive exudative detachment may seem like a mass and be confused with retinoblastoma in a child or a melanoma in an adult.

Fluorescein angiography will demonstrate the aneurysmal dilation of the capillary bed and the retinal arteries and veins. There may be capillary nonperfusion. The fluorescein dye also extravasates into the subretinal exudate. Retinal function remains intact in the area of telangiectasis, if retinal vascular permeability is not compromised.

Treatment

Laser photocoagulation and cryotherapy is used to ablate the telangiectatic vessels in order to preserve vision and prevent rubeotic glaucoma. Surgery may be necessary to drain the subretinal fluid and treat the telangiectatic vessels.

Coloboma of the Retina

Coloboma is usually seen in the region of the embryonic cleft, i.e., inferonasally and is often bilateral in 60 percent of the patients.[5] Histologically, the pigment epithelium seems to be primarily involved and is absent in the areas of the coloboma. The sensory retina is atrophic and gliotic. The choroid can be partially or completely absent. The accompanying sclera is thinned or even absent in the area of the coloboma (Fig. 3–1).

Treatment

There is no treatment.

Optic Nerve Pits and Optic Nerve Anomalies

An optic pit is a small, round convexity about ⅛ to ½ the diameter of the optic disc. Usually the optic pits are found in the inferotemporal quadrant of the optic disc.

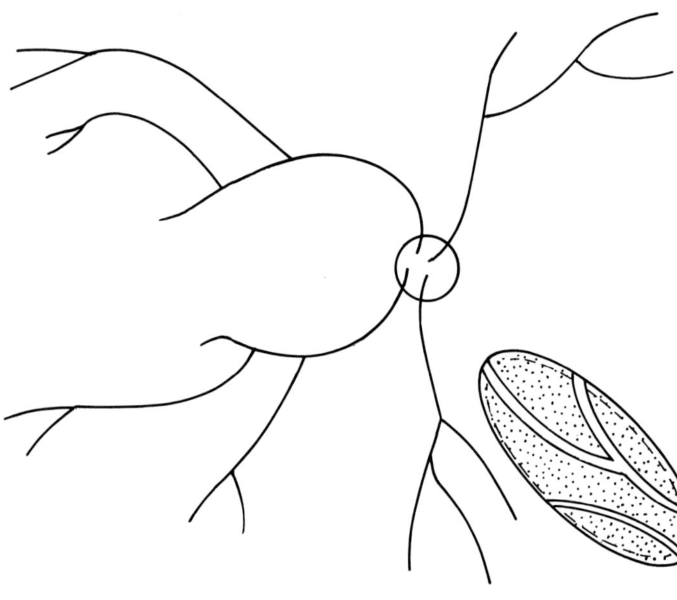

FIGURE 3–1

Coloboma of the retina, inferonasal position.

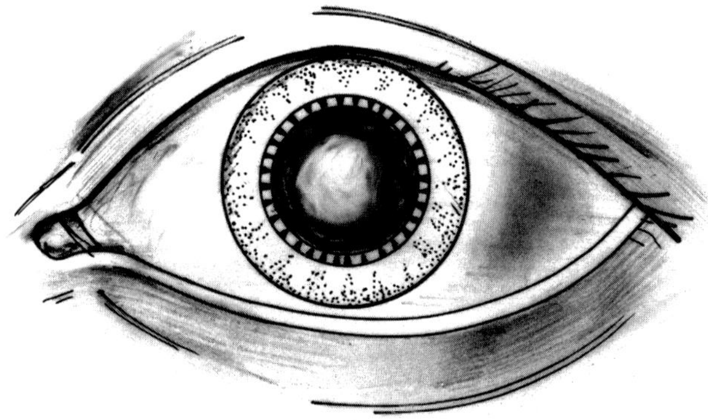

FIGURE 3-2

Persistent hyperplastic primary vitreous. Note elongated ciliary processes under the lens.

There can be associated macular changes and hemorrhages and pigmentary changes, cysts, and holes of the retina. There can be associated retinal detachments as well.

Subretinal fluid may be vitreous fluid that has leaked into the area through the pit or cerebrospinal fluid that has leaked around the pit and into the subretinal space.

Histology

The pit is an outpouching of neuroectodermal tissue surrounded by a connective tissue capsule. The pit passes posteriorly through a defect in the lamina cribosa and protrudes into the subarachnoid space.

Treatment

Surgery has been performed in those patients with optic pits with associated macular retinal detachments. Vitrectomy, air fluid exchange and gas tamponade, and laser photocoagulation have been tried with good results in some cases.[6,7] The type of treatment for this entity is evolving as these cases are rare and vitreoretinal surgical techniques are changing with new technology.

Persistent Hyperplastic Primary Vitreous

Persistent hyperplastic primary vitreous is a benign condition usually that is present at birth, affecting one eye. Remnants of the primitive hyaloid vascular system connects to the lens, causing a cataract and a posterior radial retinal fold with the micropthalmos (Fig. 3–2). The child usually presents with leukocoria unilaterally with a small eye, poor vision, and strabismus. This entity is in the differential diagnosis of leukocoria: retinopathy of prematurity, retinoblastoma, toxocariasis, Coats disease, and so forth.

Treatment

Surgical removal of the cataract and vitrectomy may be necessary. However, the anatomy of the eye is distorted with the ciliary processes being pulled forward, that the surgical landmarks are not as clear in other normal children with normal-sized eyes. Vision rehabilitation is a challenge in these small children.

REFERENCES

1. Coats G: Forms of retinal disease with massive exudation. Roy Lond Ophthalmol Hosp Rep 1908; *18:*440–525

2. Ehlers N, Jensen VA: Hereditary central retinal angiopathy. Acta Ophthalmol 1973; *51:*171–181

3. Farkas TG, Potts AM, Boone C: Some pathologic and biochemical aspects of Coats' disease. Am J Ophthalmol 1973; *75:*289–301

4. Tripathi R, Ashton N: Electron microscopical study of Coats' disease. Br J Ophthalmol 1971; *55:*289–301

5. Yanoff M, Fine BS: Ocular Pathology. Philadelphia, Harper & Row, 1982 p. 476

6. Schatz H, McDonald HR: Treatment of sensory retinal detachment associated with optic nerve pit or coloboma. Ophthalmol 1988; *95:*178–186

7. Cox MS, Witherspoon CD, Morris RE, Flynn HW: Evolving techniques in the treatment of macular detachment caused by optic nerve pits. Ophthalmol 1988; *95:*889–896

CHAPTER FOUR

Diabetic Retinopathy

EPIDEMIOLOGY

Diabetic retinopathy is the leading cause of blindness for the working-age American, between the ages of 20–64 years. It affects approximately 10–12 million Americans. An additional 8–10 million Americans may have diabetes, but do not know that they have the disease.[1] It accounts for 5,800 cases of legal blindness each year in America.[2]

The duration of diabetes is a factor in the development of diabetic retinopathy.[2–5] After 7 years of insulin-dependent diabetes mellitus (IDDM), approximately 50 percent of these patients have diabetic retinopathy.[3] After 20 years, duration of insulin-dependent diabetes, 90 percent of these patients have diabetic retinopathy.[5] In the first 5 years of insulin-dependent diabetes, diabetic retinopathy rarely develops.[2–5]

The natural history of noninsulin-dependent diabetes mellitus (NIDDM) is harder to describe since NIDDM may be present for many years before diagnosis. As a result, patients with NIDDM may present with severe diabetic retinopathy at time of diagnosis.[4]

ANATOMY AND PHYSIOLOGY

The anatomy of the lesions seen in diabetic retinopathy lies in the microvasculature of the retina. The retinal vessels lie in the inner retina, near the inner plexiform layer where hard exudates are seen. Microaneurysms seen in diabetic retinopathy seem to be superficial and are probably in the inner plexiform area. Macular edema lies in the cystic spaces of the outer plexiform layer (Fig. 4–1).

While the pathogenesis of diabetic retinopathy is not fully elucidated, we understand from pathological specimens that there is the loss of pericytes of the capillaries of the retina and associated basement membrane thickening.[6–7] The loss of pericytes is thought to cause microaneurysm formation and early leakage of blood and blood products. The leakage of blood products is a source of focal retinal edema and hard exudate rings seen in diabetic macular edema.

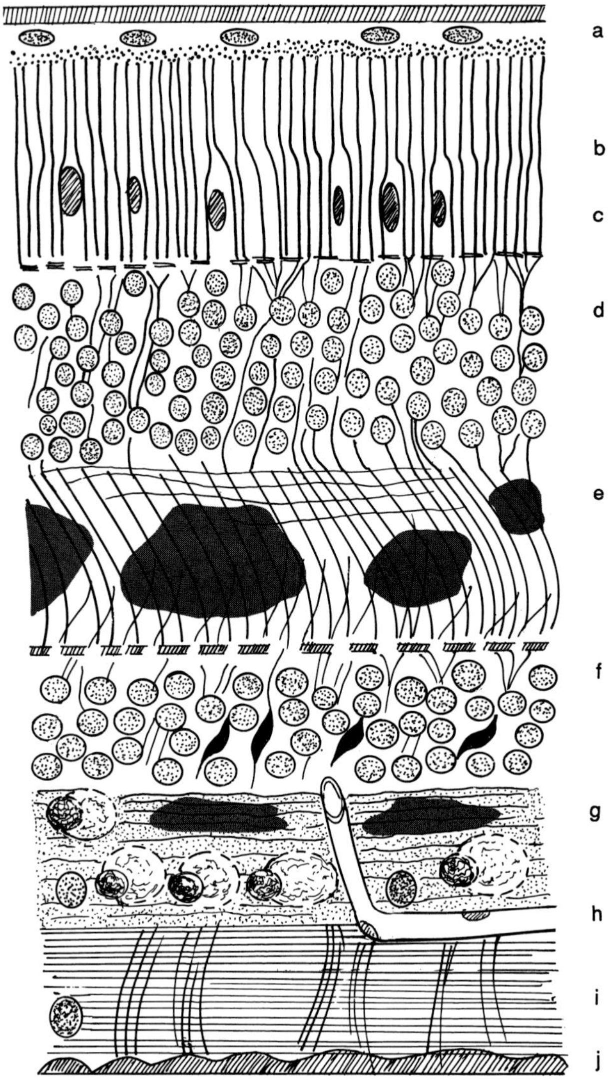

FIGURE 4-1

Diabetic retinopathy in relation to the layers of the retina. *a.* Retinal pigment epithelium; *b.* rods and cones; *c.* external limiting membranes; *d.* outer nuclear layer; *e.* outer plexiform layer: hard exudates are found here, and macular edema is found here; *f.* inner nuclear layer; *g.* inner plexiform layer: microaneurysms are located here; *h.* ganglion cell layer; *i.* nerve fiber layer; *j.* internal limiting membrane.

Retinal arteriolar obstruction results in ischemic nerve fiber layer infarcts, or better known as cotton wool spots or soft exudates. Large, dark blot hemorrhages are hemorrhagic infarcts. The arteriolar obstruction leads to venous stasis and the appearance of venous beading. White threadlike arterioles are signs of arteriolar obstruction. It is this stage that may play a role in ischemia and acts as a stimulus to neovascularization.[8]

The presence of new vessels marks the beginning of the most severe stage of diabetic retinopathy—proliferative diabetic retinopathy. Abnormal new vessels are made with abnormal vessel walls, prone to leakage of blood products and blood. The bleeding adjacent to the vitreous interface causes fibrovascular contracture and the formation of traction retinal detachments. Later on, there is vitreous hemorrhage combined with retinal detachment that leads to poor visual prognosis.

CLINICAL CLASSIFICATION

No Diabetic Retinopathy

In newly diagnosed adult-onset or insulin-dependent diabetics,[9,10] there are no fundus abnormalities seen with binocular indirect ophthalmoscope, slit-lamp biomicroscopy or Goldmann contact lens (Table 4–1).

Nonproliferative Diabetic Retinopathy

Nonproliferative diabetic retinopathy (NPDR) previously known as transitional diabetic retinopathy or preproliferative diabetic retinopathy (Fig. 4–2).[9]

Diabetic Macular Edema

It is thought that there are 75,000 new cases of macular edema per year (Table 4–2). There are 50,000 cases with treatable clinically significant macular edema per year, according to the Early Treatment Diabetic Retinopathy Study (Fig. 4–3).[13]

Fluorescein Angiography of Diabetic Macular Edema

In the arterial phase, there is hyperfluorescence of the microaneurysms which cause macular edema. It is in these fluorescein frames

■ **TABLE 4–1** Clinical Classification[9]

No Diabetic Retinopathy No microaneurysms and other characteristics absent. Follow up annually.
Mild NPDR A few scattered retinal hemorrhages and microaneurysms or venous loops in at least one field. See every 6–9 months with optimal control of serum glucose.
Moderate NPDR One or more of the following: Increased number of retinal hemorrhages and microaneurysms with or without intraretinal microvascular abnormalities or soft exudates. Follow up every 6 months.
Severe NPDR One or more of the following: Severe amount of retinal hemorrhages and microaneurysms, moderate number of intraretinal microvascular abnormalities in one or more fields and venous beading. Follow up every 4 months with possible scatter laser treatment when approaching "high-risk characteristics."[11,12]

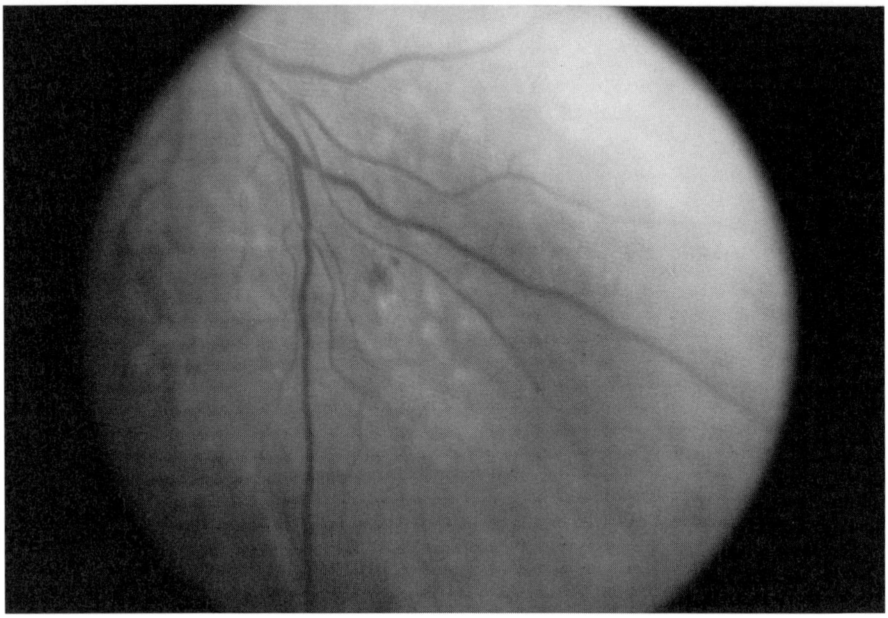

FIGURE 4-2

Microaneurysms.

that one identifies the microaneurysms which will be photocoagulated by laser. In the late phase fluorescein angiogram, there is late hyperfluorescence showing pools of leakage. In this last phase of transit, focal leakage and diffuse leakage are identified.

Proliferative Diabetic Retinopathy

Proliferative diabetic retinopathy is the most severe form of diabetic retinopathy in that it can lead to severe visual loss and loss of ambulatory vision in the past. Proliferative diabetic retinopathy (PDR) is defined as neovascularization of the retina, the iris, and the optic disc (Table 4–3). The criteria of "high-risk characteristics" has set the standard for emergency laser photocoagulation (Figs. 4–4 to 4–6).[10–12]

■ **TABLE 4-2** Macular Edema as Defined by the Early Treatment Diabetic Retinopathy Study[13]

1. Thickening of the retina at or within 500 μ of the center of the macula.
2. Hard exudates at or within 500 μ of the center of the macula, if associated with thickening of the adjacent retina.
3. A zone or zones of retinal thickening 1 disc diameter or larger in size, any portion of which is within 1 disc diameter of the center of the macula.[13]

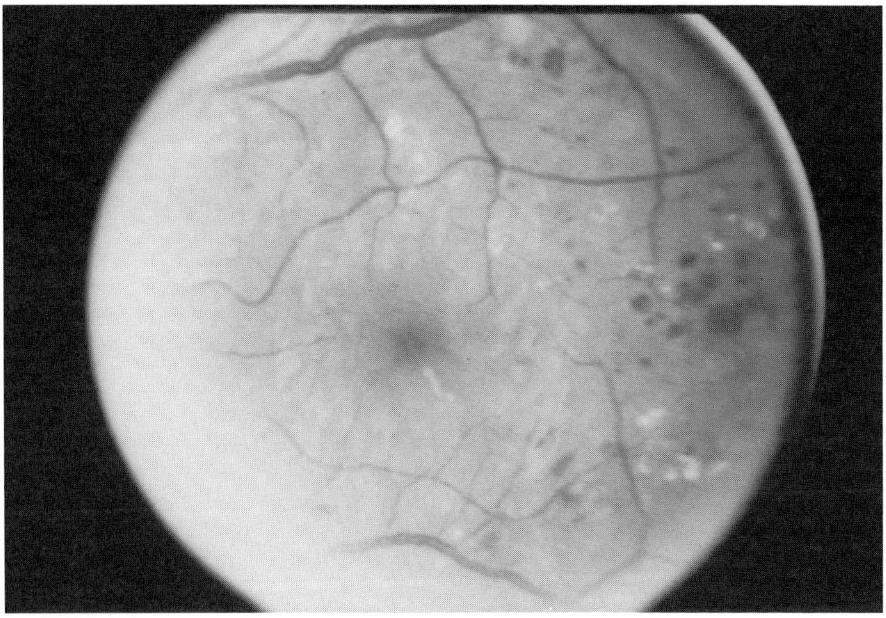

FIGURE 4–3

Clinically significant macular edema.

Pregnancy and Diabetes

The American Academy of Ophthalmology recommends that pregnant diabetic patients and gestational diabetic patients be seen during pregnancy.

The patient is examined in the first trimester, and if there is no diabetic retinopathy, the patient is seen again in the last trimester. However, if there are abnormal findings, the patient may need to be examined every trimester. If there is macular edema, the patient may need to see an ophthalmologist every month during the pregnancy (Figs. 4–7 to 4–11).[15]

At 6 weeks postpartum, the patient is seen again for follow up. At this time additional laser may be needed or there may be regression of the disease. However, in nursing mothers, there may be a prolonged phase of active diabetic retinopathy and follow up

■ **TABLE 4–3** Proliferative Diabetic Retinopathy

1. New vessels on the disc
2. New vessels elsewhere
3. Fibrous proliferation
4. Preretinal hemorrhage
5. Vitreous hemorrhage

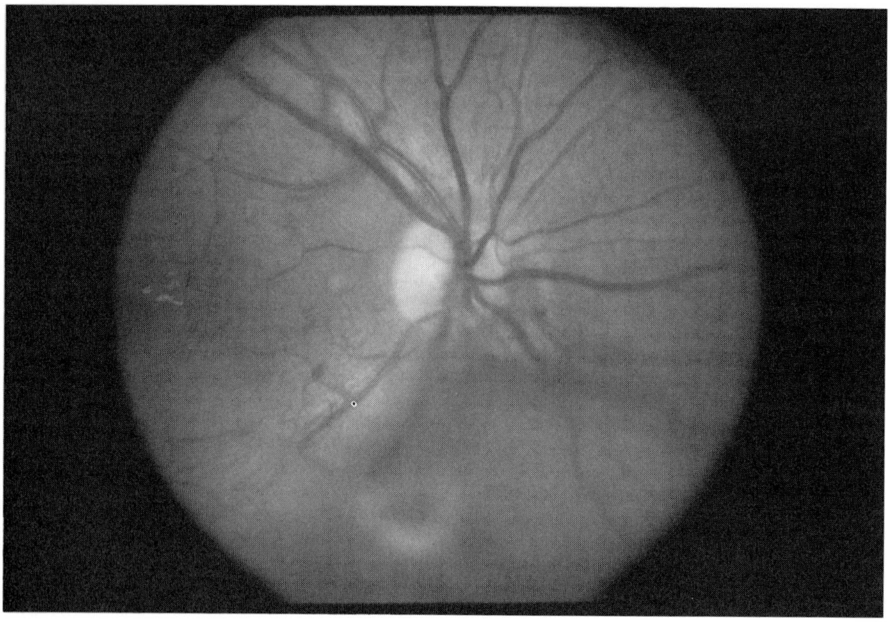

FIGURE 4-4

Proliferative diabetic retinopathy.

of every few months may be necessary. The progression of diabetic retinopathy during the postpartum period occurs as the patient's insulin requirements change. The patient's glycemic control may not be as stable as in other periods of her life.

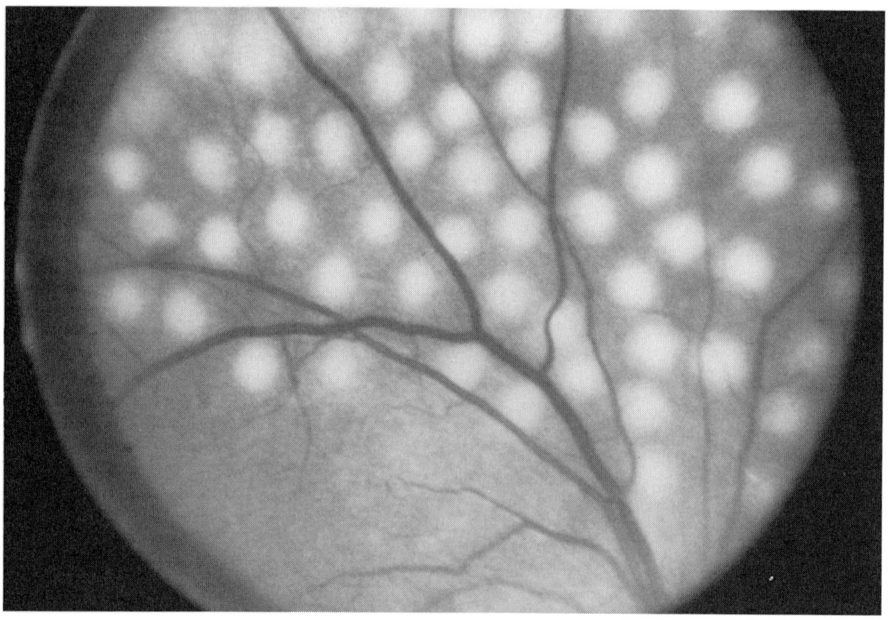

FIGURE 4-5

Photocoagulation on the retina.

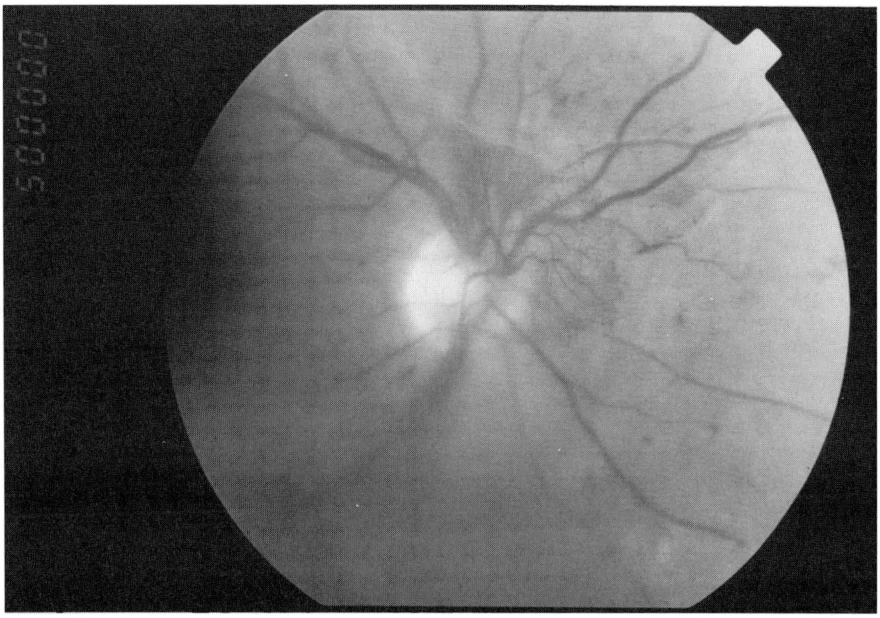

FIGURE 4–6

Vitreous hemorrhage and neovascularization of the disc.

Gestational Diabetes

Gestational diabetic patients are known to have vascular tortuosity but no other untoward effects.[16] However, it is important to follow these patients if they become increasingly more dependent on larger doses of insulin as they approach their third trimester. In addition, some of the gestational diabetic patients remain insulin-dependent during the postpartum course and will have mild to moderate NPDR depending on their glycemic control.

Ophthalmologists Interfacing with the Obstetrical Team

Diabetic patients prior to becoming pregnant, are recommended to visit the internist and obstetrician so that the patient may plan for excellent glycemic control prior to conception and during pregnancy. It is thought that euglycemia during pregnancy, i.e., achieving a HbA_{1c} as close to the normal range of 5.6–6.5 mg percent leads to a lower risk of fetal death and fetal malformations.[15,17–20]

The additional systemic complications of hypertension and proteinuria during a diabetic pregnancy can lead to massive diabetic macular edema and rapid acceleration of NPDR towards PDR in a matter of weeks.[21] Thus, close follow up is necessary if the patient has moderate NPDR.

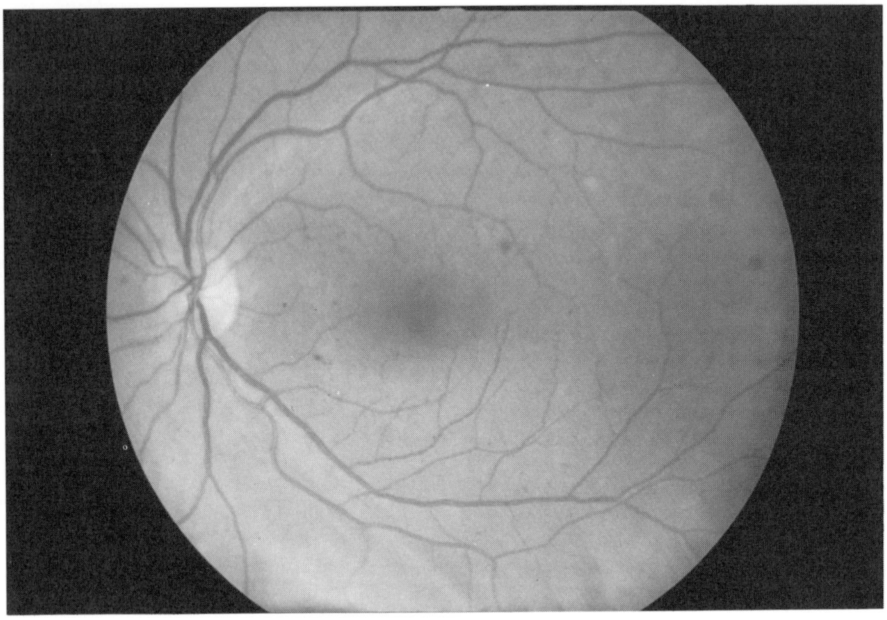

FIGURE 4–7

34-year-old pregnant female in the first trimester with a thirty-one-year history of diabetes mellitus. Vision OS: 20/20.

The ophthalmologist's role in the pregnant diabetic patient is to interact with the medical and obstetrical team. Often, the obstetrical team would like to know if elective caesarean section is necessary. Possible indications for caesarean section include (1)

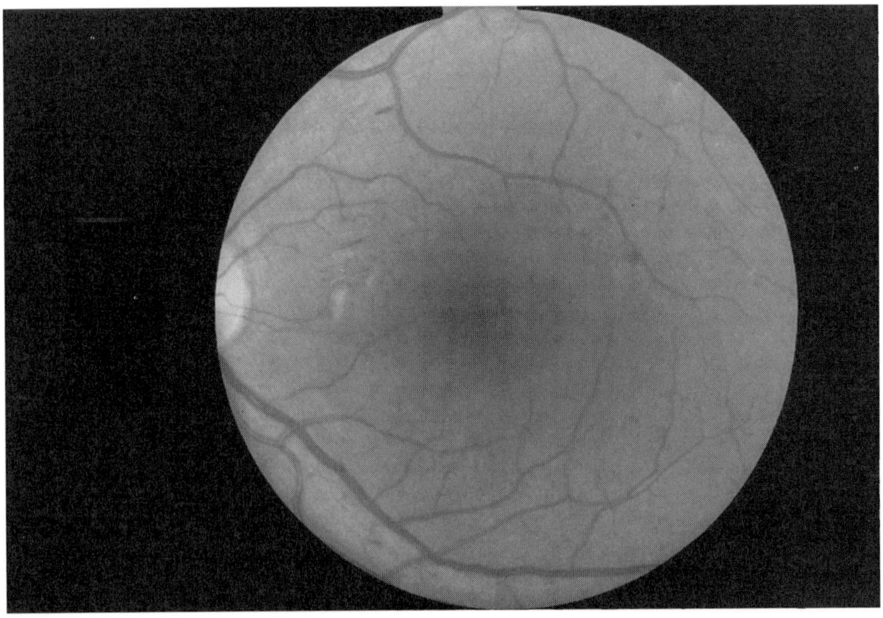

FIGURE 4–8

Same patient as in Figure 4–7 in the third trimester. Vision OS: 20/20.

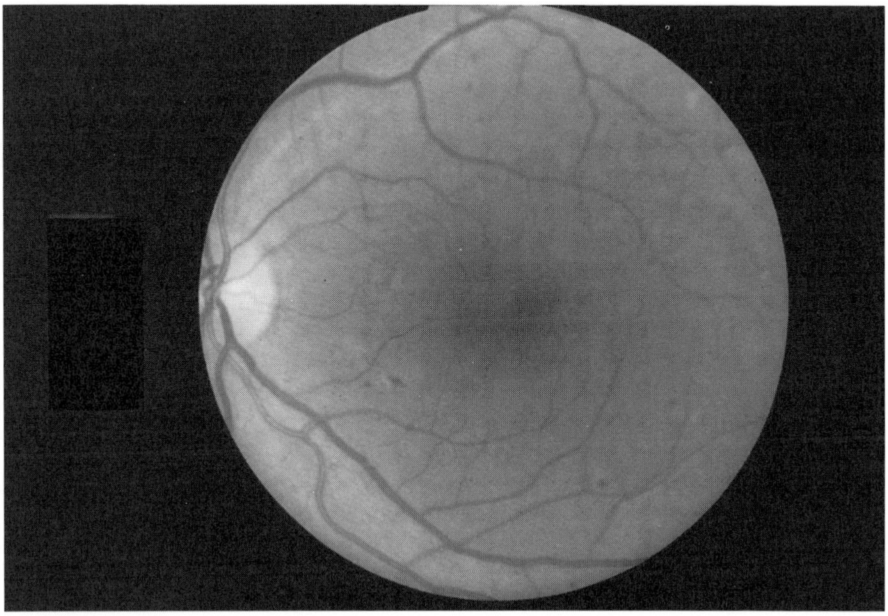

FIGURE 4–9

Same patient as in Figure 4–7, postpartum. Vision OS: 20/20.

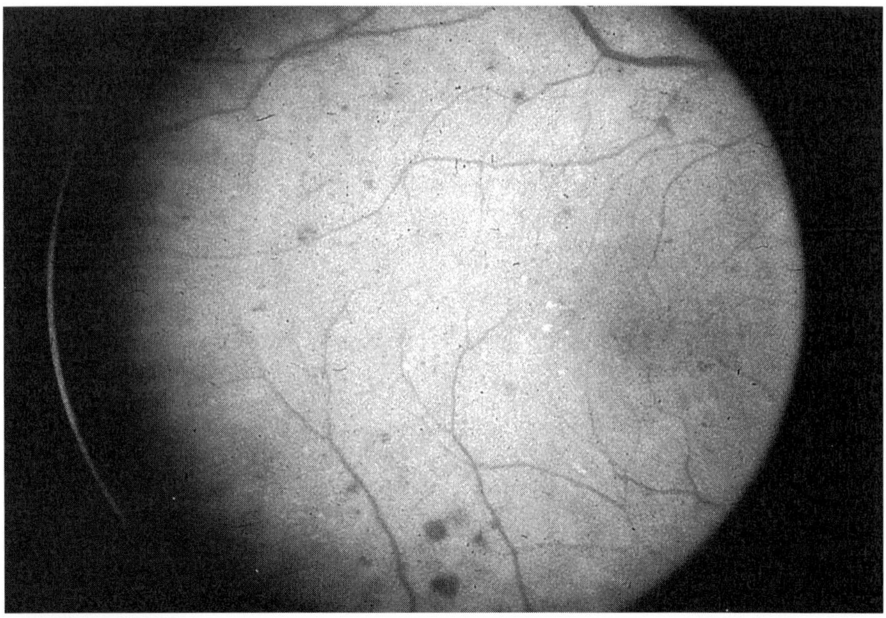

FIGURE 4–10

39-year-old female with a thirty-five-year history of diabetes mellitus and with newly developed hypertension during pregnancy. Patient is proteinuric and in the second trimester. Vision OD: 20/25.

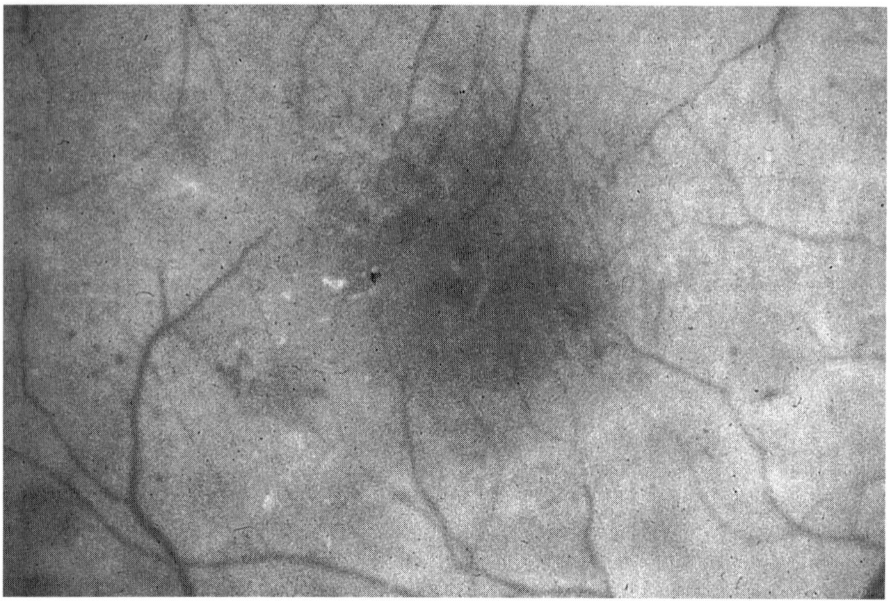

FIGURE 4-11

Same patient as in Figure 4-10 now in the third trimester. Vision OD: 20/40, with significant macular edema.

severe PDR, (2) only partially treated or documented progression of PDR despite laser photocoagulation, and (3) traction retinal detachment.

In this current age of excellent prenatal and perinatal care in the specialized medical centers, abortion is rarely recommended. The indications for abortion are (1) severe systemic complications of diabetes, e.g., renal failure, cardiac instability; (2) congenital pulmonary and cardiac malformations in the pregnant mother; and possibly (3) one-eyed patient with severe PDR at the start of her pregnancy with a history of poor glycemic control and other systemic diseases complicating the diabetes.

Fluorescein Angiography in the Pregnant or Nursing Patient

Fluorescein angiography has been found in the breast milk of nursing mothers. However, to date, there has been no adverse effects of fluorescein on the fetus or the infant. It is usually part of the informed consent for the pregnant and nursing mother that disclosure of the above is made.

In pregnant patients who do not wish fluorescein angiography, it is possible to perform laser photocoagulation without fluorescein angiography, taking care to avoid the central 500 μ of the foveal avascular zone or using a combined approach of grid macular laser and focal macular laser.[13,14]

Diagnosis

The diagnosis is made by careful examination of the retina with binocular indirect ophthalmoscopy to see the posterior pole, equatorial region and midperiphery. The Hruby, 90 diopter, or Goldmann lenses are used to view the macula carefully.

The purpose of the retina examination is to look for:

1. Swelling, thickening of the retina, retinal edema, or macular cysts
2. Microaneurysms, their number, size, and type (Fig. 4–12)
3. Intraretinal microvascular abnormalities (Fig. 4–13)
4. Venous loops (Fig. 4–14) and venous beading (Fig. 4–15)
5. Areas of featureless retina, i.e., loss of fine capillaries seen at the posterior pole in a patient with macular edema
6. Retinal neovascularization
7. Cotton wool spots
8. Arteriolar abnormalities
9. Types of hemorrhages, intraretinal and preretinal, and size and shape of the hemorrhages

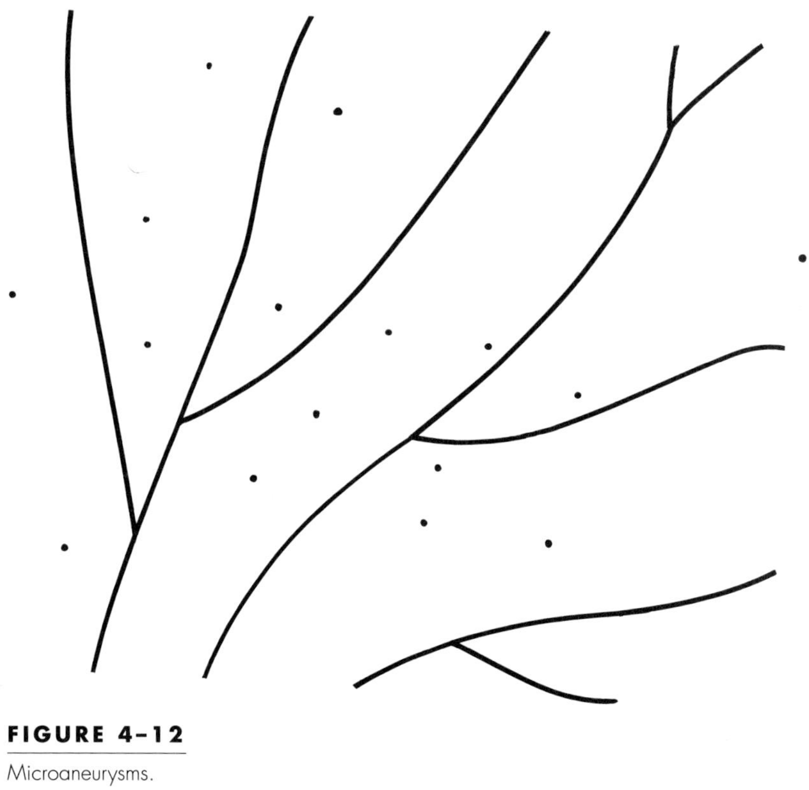

FIGURE 4–12

Microaneurysms.

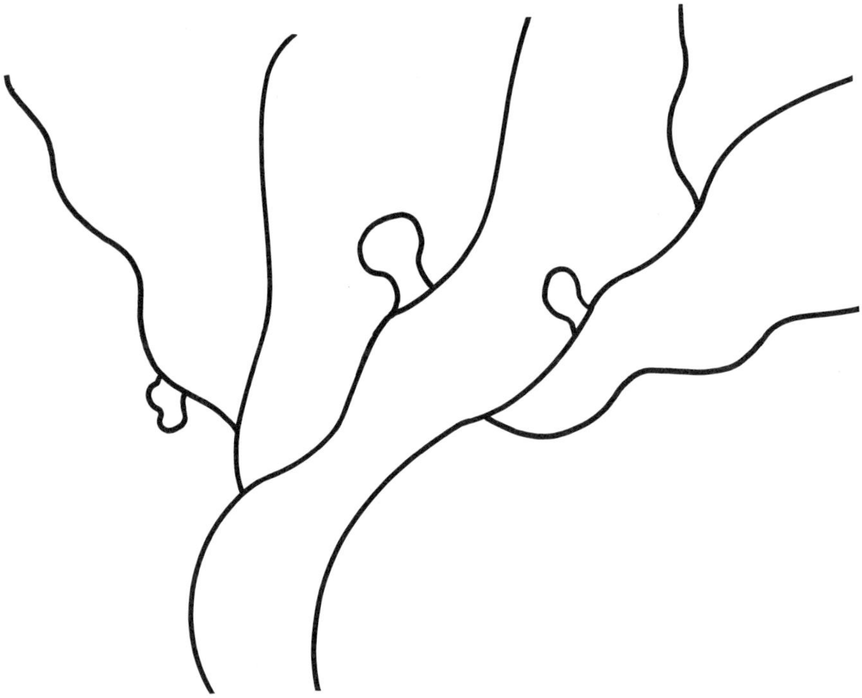

FIGURE 4-13

Intraretinal microvascular abnormalities.

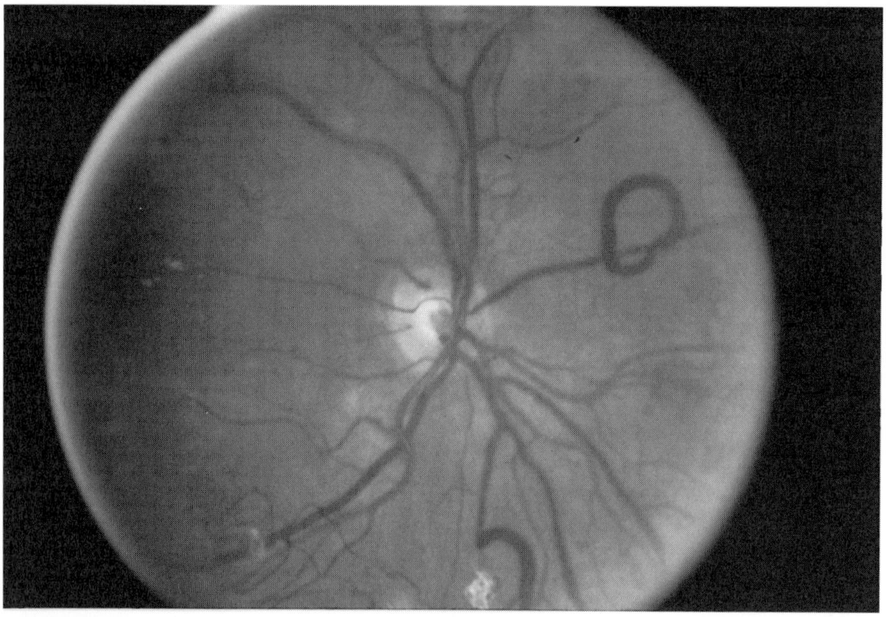

FIGURE 4-14

Venous loops.

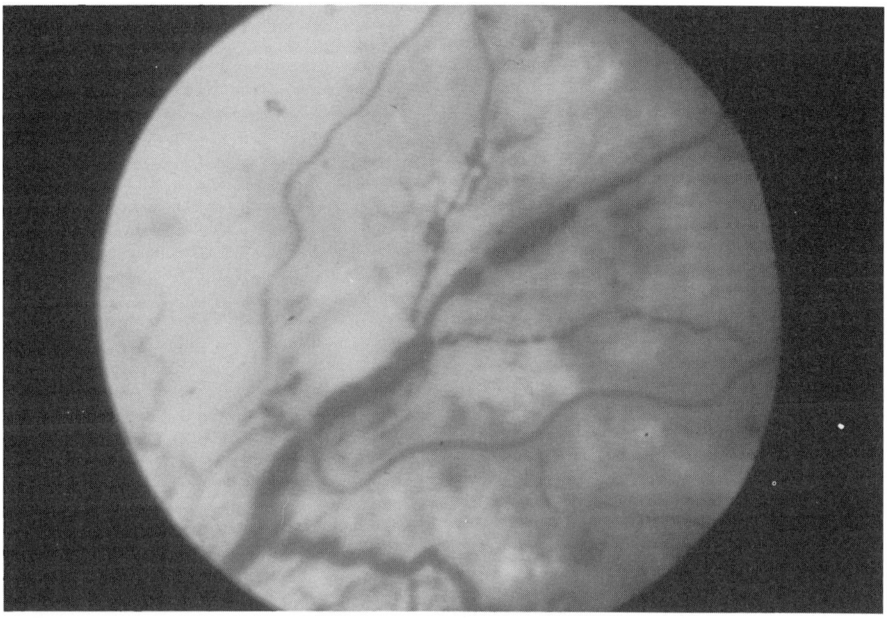

FIGURE 4–15
Venous beading.

Treatment

NONPROLIFERATIVE DIABETIC RETINOPATHY

Follow up with internal medicine physicians and diabetologists is recommended for good consistent glycemic control. In cases of very severe NPDR, one can consider treatment with laser photocoagulation, especially in patients with poor history of compliance or clinic attendance (Figs. 4–16 to 4–20).

MACULAR EDEMA

Once the diagnosis of macular edema is made by slit-lamp biomicroscopy, fluorescein angiogram is used to identify the lesions to be treated by focal macular laser photocoagulation.[13]

PROLIFERATIVE DIABETIC RETINOPATHY

Laser panretinal photocoagulation is recommended for eyes reaching high-risk characteristics. Urgent consideration is made for those eyes not meeting high-risk characteristics but have rubeosis of the iris or have neovascular glaucoma.[12]

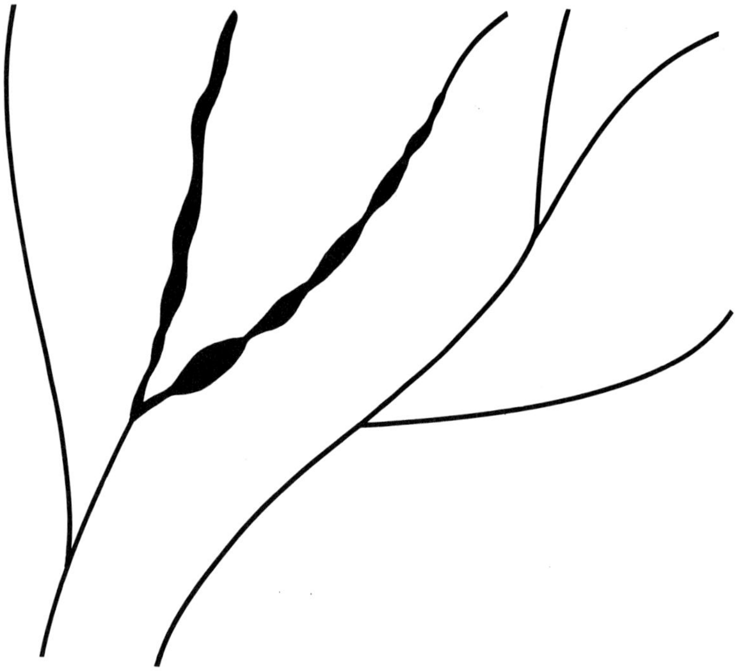

FIGURE 4–16

Venous beading.

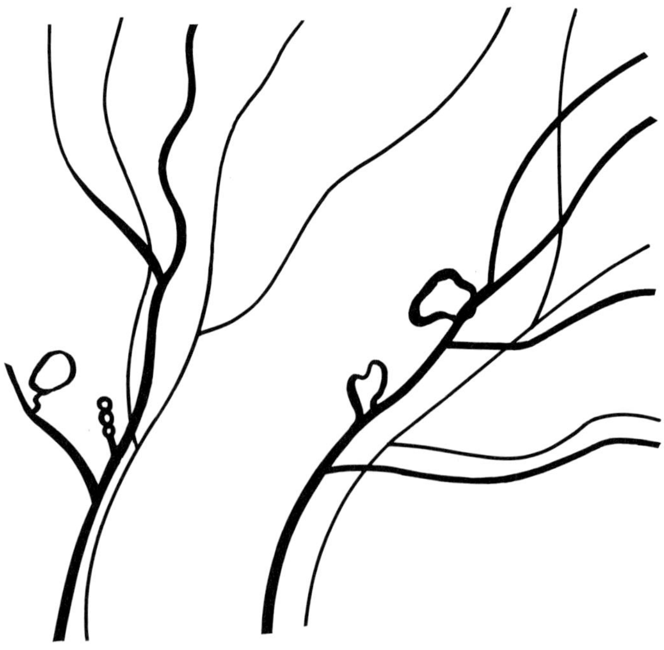

FIGURE 4–17

Venous loops.

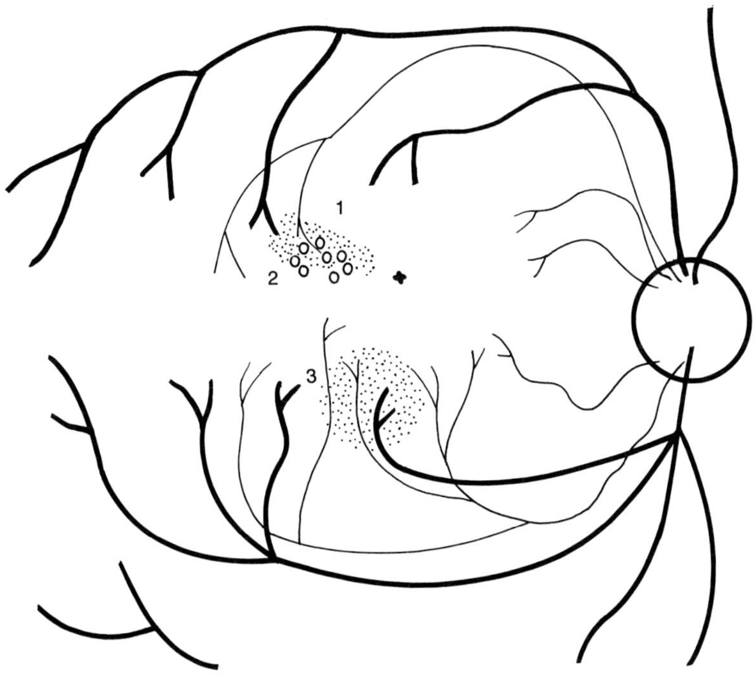

FIGURE 4–18

1. Thickening of the retina at or within 500 μ of the center of the macula. *2.* Hard exudates at or within 500 μ of the center of the macula. *3.* A zone of thickening 1 disc diameter in size, a portion of which is within 1 disc diameter of the center of the macula.

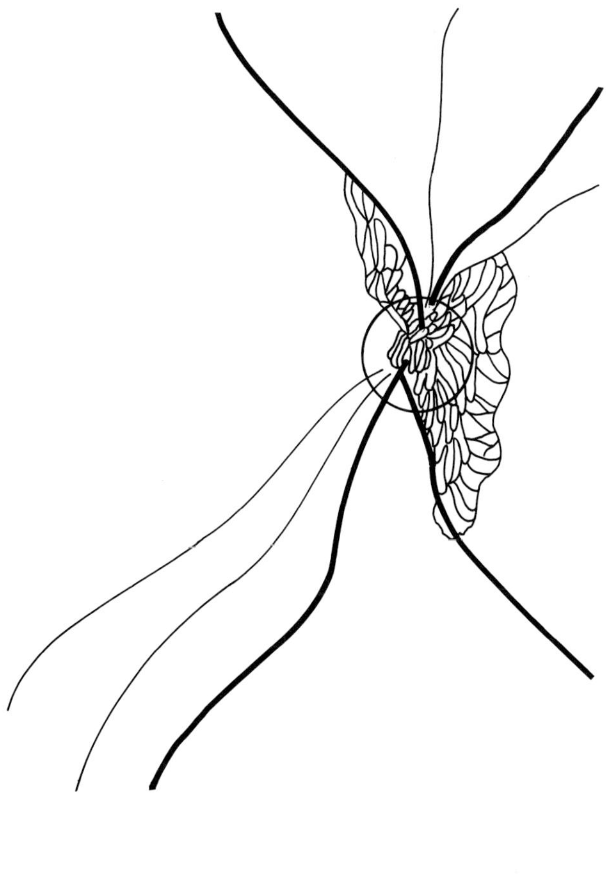

FIGURE 4–19

Neovascularization of the optic disc. Note the feathery nature of the new vessels at the optic disc.

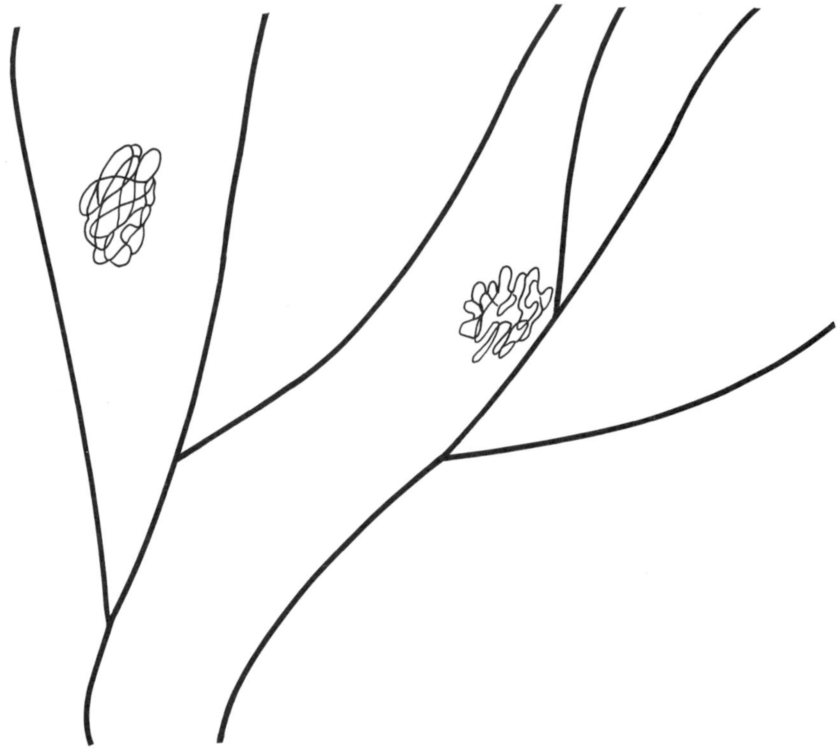

FIGURE 4-20

Neovascularization elsewhere. Note the location between large vessels. Feathery nature makes this entity hard to see.

VITREOUS HEMORRHAGE

As PDR progresses to neovascularization of the retina and the optic disc, the natural history of diabetic retinopathy leads to vitreous hemorrhage. As the neovascular fronds leak and cause leakage of blood next to the hyaloidal surface, fibrous scarring and additional vitreous traction on the same neovascular fronds occur. This process starts the cycle of additional bleeding leading to more traction and more bleeding. The cycle leads to the formation of a traction retinal detachment either in the extramacular area or around the arcades surrounding the macular area. At this last phase, vitrectomy surgery is performed as an emergency process in order to preserve the macula.

■ **TABLE 4-4** High-risk Characteristics and Indications for Laser Photocoagulation[12]

New vessels on the disc with vitreous hemorrhage
New vessels elsewhere with new vessels on the disc
New vessels on the disc with greater than ⅓ disc diameter of new vessels on the disc
New vessels elsewhere with vitreous hemorrhage

Diagnosis

Ultrasound evaluation is useful in these eyes when no clear view of the retina is available. The ultrasound delineates the extent of the retinal detachment. Using low attenuation of sound waves, one can measure the size and locate the extent of small traction retinal detachments.[22–25]

Surgery

The Diabetic Retinopathy Vitrectomy Study (DRVS) found that visual outcome of vitreous surgery for nonclearing vitreous hemorrhage established that younger patients with Type I, insulin-dependent diabetes benefitted from early surgical intervention whereas older patients with Type II, noninsulin dependent diabetes, showed no benefit from early surgery. Indications for surgery include nonclearing vitreous hemorrhage, visual acuity at the 5/200 level or worse for one month in Type I diabetics, hemorrhage with similar vision of 6 months duration in Type II diabetics. However, in diabetic patients with vitreous hemorrhage and extramacular traction retinal detachment but with good vision, benefit was also seen with vitreous surgery.

In cases of vitreous hemorrhage and cataracts, surgical techniques have progressed to the combined procedures of extracapsular surgery or phacoemulsification with intraocular lens implant when vitrectomy has been successful.[26–27]

REFERENCES

1. Aiello LM: Treatment of diabetic macular edema-timing, strategies, laser. Diagnosis and management of the ocular complications of diabetes mellitus. Tufts University School of Medicine–New England Eye Center, MA Saturday, June 26, 1993

2. Klein R, Klein BEK, Moss SE: Visual impairment in diabetes. Ophthalmol 1984; *91:*1–9

3. Klein R, Klein BEK, Moss SE et al: The Wisconsin Epidemiologic Study of Diabetic retinopathy. II. Prevalence and risk of diabetic retinopathy when age at diagnosis is less than 30 years. Arch Ophthalmol 1984; *102:*520–526

4. Klein R, Klein BEK, Moss SE et al: The Wisconsin Epidemiologic Study of Diabetic retinopathy. III. Prevalence and risk of diabetic retinopathy when age at diagnosis is 30 years or more years. Arch Ophthalmol 1984; *102:*527–532

5. Palmberg P, Smith M, Waltman S et al: The natural history of retinopathy in insulin–dependent juvenile onset diabetes. Ophthalmol 1981; *88:*613–618

6. Frank RN: On the pathogenesis of diabetic retinopathy. Ophthalmol 1984; *91:*626–634

7. Cogan DG, Toussaint D, Kuwabara T: Retinal vascular patterns. IV. Diabetic retinopathy. Arch Ophthalmol 1961; *66:*366–378

8. King GL, Johnson S, Wu G: Possible growth modulators involved in the pathogenesis of diabetic proliferative retinopathy. p. 303. In Westermark B, Betsholtz C, Hokfelt B (eds): Growth Factors in Health and Disease. New York, Elsevier, 1990

9. Early Treatment Diabetic Retinopathy Study Research Group. Fundus photographic risk factors for progression of diabetic retinopathy. ETDRS Report Number 12. Ophthalmol 1991; *98:*823–833

10. Diabetic Retinopathy Study Report Number 1. Preliminary report on effects of photocoagulation therapy. Am J Ophthalmol 1976; *81:*1–14

11. Diabetic Retinopathy Study Report Number 2. Photocoagulation of proliferative diabetic retinopathy. Ophthalmol 1978; *85:*82

12. Diabetic Retinopathy Study Report Number 3. Four risk factors for severe visual loss in diabetic retinopathy. Arch Ophthalmol 1979; *97:*654–655

13. Early Treatment Diabetic Retinopathy Study Report Number 1. Photocoagulation for diabetic macular edema. Arch Ophthalmol 1985; *103:*1796–1806

14. Early Treatment Diabetic Retinopathy Study Report Number 9. Early photocoagulation for diabetic retinopathy. Ophthalmol 1991; *98:*766–785

15. Sinclair SH, Nesler C, Foxman B et al: Macular edema and pregnancy in insulin–dependent diabetes. Am J Ophthalmol 1984; *97:*154–157

16. Boone MI, Farber ME, Jovanovic-Peterson L, Peterson CM: Increased vascular tortuosity in gestational diabetes mellitus. Ophthalmol 1989; *96:*251–254

17. Hanson U, Persson B, Thunell S: Relationship between haemoglobin A_{1C} in early type 1 (insulin–dependent) diabetic pregnancy and the occurrence of spontaneous abortion and fetal malformation in Sweden. Diabetologica 1990; *33:*100–104

18. Lucas MJ, Leveno KJ, Williams ML et al: Early pregnancy glycosylated hemoglobin, severity of diabetes and fetal malformations. Am J Obstet Gynecol 1989; *161:*426–431

19. Dicker D, Feldberg D, Samuel N et al: Spontaneous abortion in patients with insulin–dependent diabetes mellitus: the effect of preconceptual diabetic control. Am J Obstet Gynecol 1988; *158:*1161–1164

20. Gestation and Diabetes in France Study Group. Multicenter survey of diabetic pregnancy in France. Diabetes Care 1991; *14:*994–1000

21. Mills JL, Simpson JL, Driscoll SG et al: National Institute of Child Health and Human Development-Diabetes in Early Pregnancy Study. Incidence of spontaneous abortion among normal women and insulin-dependent diabetic women whose pregnancies were identified within 21 days of conception. N Engl J Med 1988; *319:*1617–1623

22. Diabetic Retinopathy Vitrectomy Study Report Number 2. Early vitrectomy for severe vitreous hemorrhage in diabetic retinopathy. Two–year results of a randomized trial. Arch Ophthalmol 1985; *103:*1644–1652

23. Diabetic Retinopathy Vitrectomy Study Report Number 3. Early vitrectomy for severe proliferative diabetic retinopathy in eyes with useful vision. Results of a randomized trial. Ophthalmol 1988; *95:*1307–1320

24. Diabetic Retinopathy Vitrectomy Study Report Number 4. Early vitrectomy for severe proliferative diabetic retinopathy in eyes with useful vision. Clinical application of results of a randomized trial. Ophthalmol 1988; *95:*1331–1334

25. Diabetic Retinopathy Vitrectomy Study Report Number 5. Early vitrectomy for severe vitreous hemorrhage in diabetic retinopathy. Four year results of a randomized trial. Arch Ophthalmol 1990; *108:* 958–964

26. Kokame GT, Flynn HW Jr, Blankenship GW: Posterior chamber lens implantation during diabetic pars plana vitrectomy. Ophthalmol 1989; *96:*603–610

27. Blankenship GW, Flynn HW Jr, Kokame GT: Posterior chamber lens insertion during diabetic pars plana lensectomy and vitrectomy for complications of proliferative diabetic retinopathy. Ophthalmol 1989; *96:*603–610

CHAPTER FIVE

Other Proliferative Vitreoretinopathies

SICKLE CELL RETINOPATHY

Epidemiology

In the United States, severe ocular complications occur with homozygous hemoglobin sickle cell disease. Sickle-cell hemoglobin C disease (HbSC) and sickle cell beta-thalessemia are less often responsible.[1]

In the United States, the prevalence of the sickle cell trait in African-Americans is 8–10 percent and the number of homozygous persons approaches 1 in 400 births.[1]

Anatomy and Physiology

The sickle cell hemoglobinopathies are due to the inheritance of a gene for a structurally abnormal betaglobin chain subunit of adult hemoglobin, the beta-s chain of HbS (alpha-2 beta-s). The structural abnormality of the beta-s globin chain consists of a single amino acid substitution or replacement of valine instead of the normal glutamic acid at position number 6 of the beta-polypeptide chain.

HbS can be found in the heterozygous state (HbSS, sickle cell anemia, or sickle cell disease) in association with other structural hemoglobin variants (HBSC and SD disease) and in association with beta-thalassemia or sickle beta-thalassemia syndromes. The structural abnormality of HbC, a nonsickling hemoglobin, also consists of a single amino acid substitution at residue 6 of the betaglobin chain L in beta-c chain where lysine replaces glutamic acid.[2]

Clinical Course

The retinopathy of this disease is caused by the abnormal shape of the red cells that are less deformable than normal, especially in hypoxic conditions. Ischemic manifestations are due to the in-

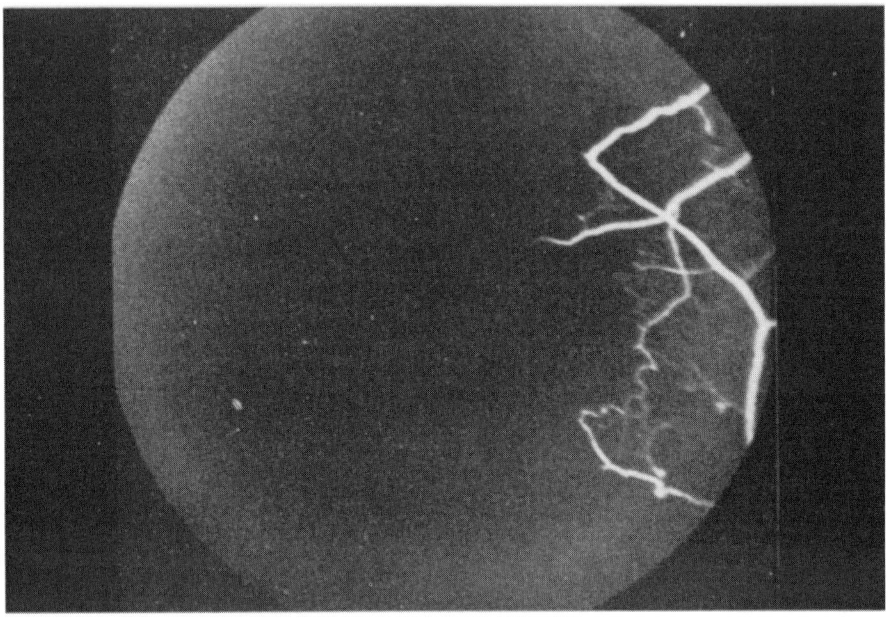

FIGURE 5-1

Fluorescein angiogram of the periphery showing loss of capillaries.

creased viscosity that these cells produce. Most significantly, they block the capillaries, venules, and often even the arterioles, leading to widespread vascular occlusion most marked in the retinal periphery (Fig. 5–1).[1] The retinal arterioles are narrowed and are seen to terminate abruptly while the veins are dilated and tortuous. The retinal surface is pale and ischemic and the ischemic area gradually fades into the more normally perfused retina. The most peripheral retina is frequently infarcted and the most posterior retina becomes ischemic.[3] Thus, proliferative retinopathy develops. The proliferative retinopathy is heralded by the development of large "shunt" vessels with the surrounding capillaries completely occluded. The new vessels have a characteristic fanshaped appearance and always grow toward and into the avascular peripheral retina. The development of the proliferative lesions can lead to vitreous hemorrhages and traction retinal detachments like those found in diabetes (Fig. 5–2).[3]

Clinical Findings in the Retina

1. Arterioventricular communications or shunts
2. Seafans (Figs. 5–3 and 5–4)
3. Focal Intraretinal Hemorrhage
4. Subretinal hemorrhage (salmon-patch hemorrhage): Seen at the junction of perfused and nonperfused retina

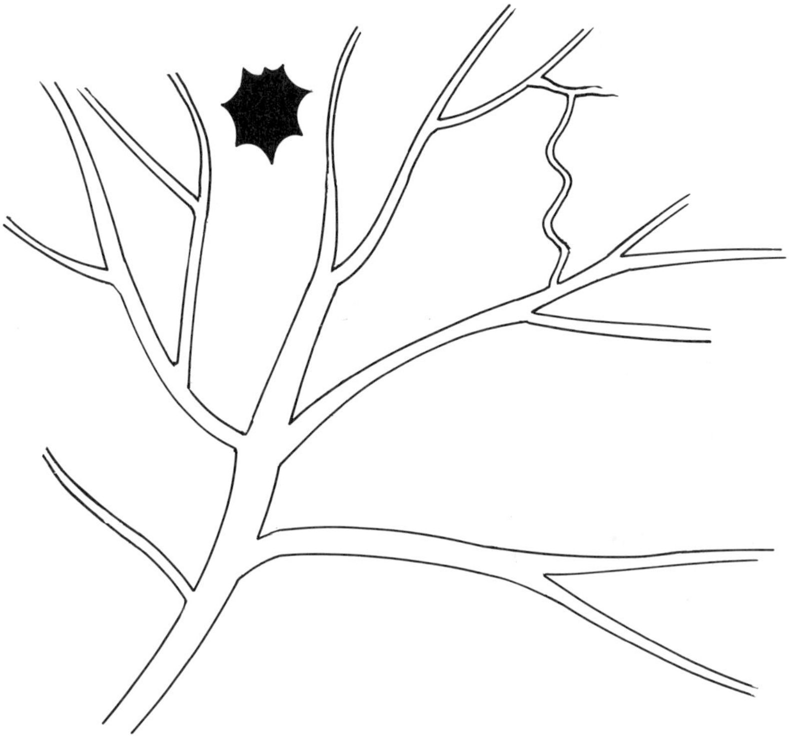

FIGURE 5–2

Black sunburst.

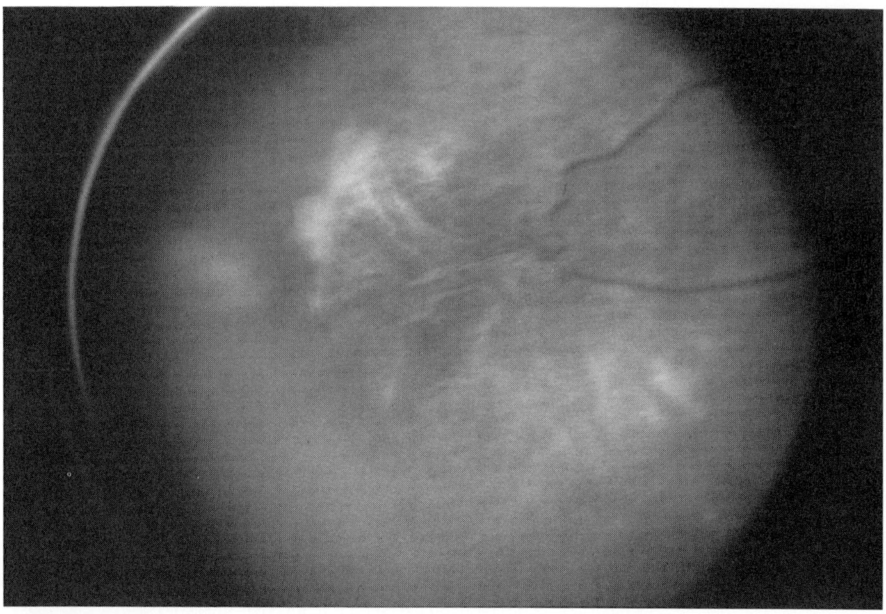

FIGURE 5–3

Seafan.

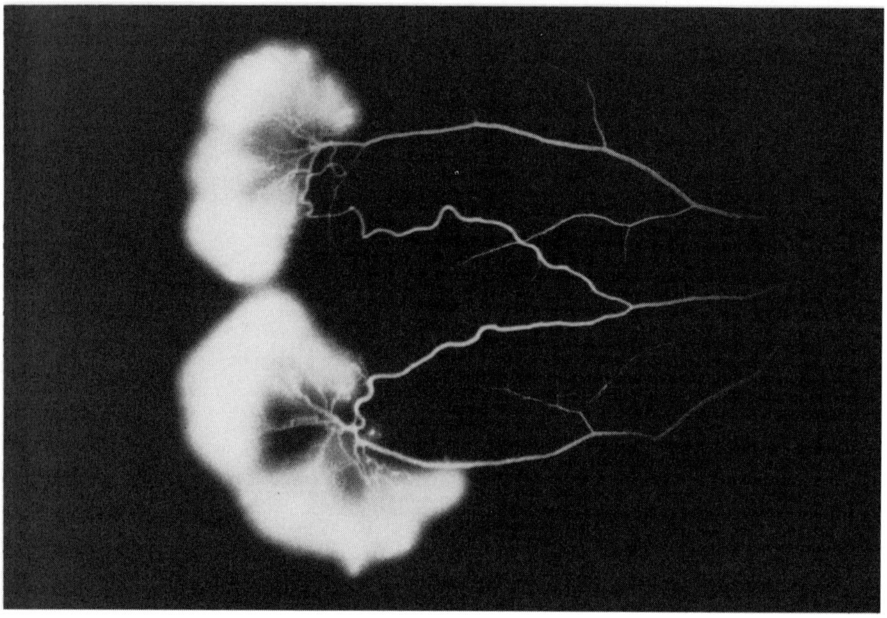

FIGURE 5-4

Fluorescein angiogram of seafan.

5. Iridescent patch of hemosiderin or late retinal pigment epithelium atrophy
6. Black sunburst: Black patch of hyperplastic retinal pigment epithelium
7. Hyperpigmented scar

Treatment

Because the disease process leads to a process of autoinfarc-tion of the retina, much of the disease is self-limited. However, in cases where vitreous hemorrhage has occurred, the surgeon can consider vitrectomy. However, if there is only a small area of vitreous hemorrhage and one can identify the area of neovascularization that is bleeding, the surgeon can perform focal laser photocoagulation or cryotherapy to the site.[4] Rarely in cases of retinal holes or rhegmatogenous retinal detachment or traction retinal detachment, vitrectomy with scleral buckling may be necessary.[5] Retinal holes can occur at sights at the base of the seafans.

Anterior segment necrosis or ischemia is a rare yet feared complication of scleral buckling surgery in these patients. Hydration of the patient and use of oxygen are recommended.

Segmental laser scatter photocoagulation to the involved ischemic quadrant can cause regression of the retinal neovascular areas.[4,6,7]

Diagnosis

Sickle cell preparation
Hemoglobin electrophoresis
Complete blood count with differential

Fluorescein Angiography

The foveal capillary net may be disturbed with small areas of capillary nonperfusion in asymptomatic patients. In addition, the fluorescein angiogram will mirror the clinical findings such as seafan formation and retinal neovascularization.

Visual Prognosis

Serious visual loss from sickle cell retinopathy, i.e., retinal neovascularization, vitreous hemorrhage and retinal detachment are more characteristic of sickle cell-hemoglobin C disease and sickle-cell thalassemia disease rather than sickle cell disease. Rarely proliferative sickle retinopathy has been described in patients with milder hemoglobinopathies, i.e., AS and AC disease.

RETINOPATHY OF PREMATURITY

Epidemiology

Retinopathy of prematurity (ROP) is the proliferation of abnormal retinal vessels that occurs in low-birthweight, premature newborns. Originally named retrolental fibroplasia in 1942, it described a white mass of retinal proliferation behind the lens.[8] During this time, the incidence of ROP was 25–30 percent of all premature infants who were diagnosed with this entity.

In 1952, Patz and coworkers found that there was an association between high concentrations of oxygen and ROP. There was a dramatic decrease in the incidence of the disease in the 1960's and 1970's as the use of oxygen was decreased to 5 percent in the newborn nurseries.[9]

However, in the last 20 years, the technological advances of neonatology have increased the survival rate of very low-birthweight and premature infants. Consequently, there has been a resurgence of ROP to the level of 25 percent of all premature infants. In infants weighing less than 900 g, the incidence of ROP is 89 percent as reported by Flynn and coworkers.[10] Most cases of ROP are of the less severe nature and the majority regresses. The most severe levels of disease, stage III or worse, remain at the level of 5–10 percent.[10]

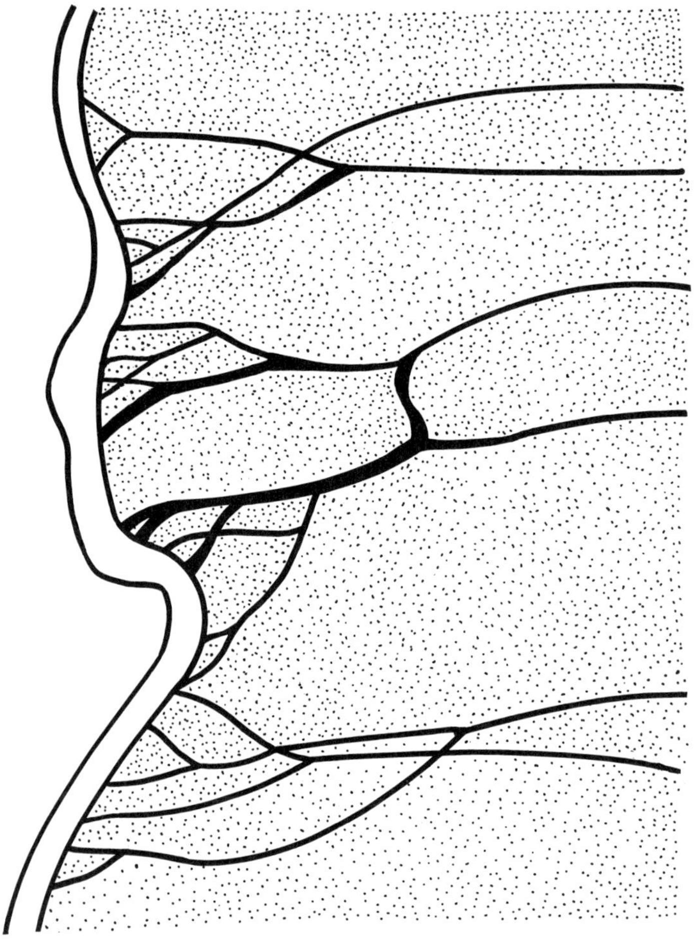

FIGURE 5–5
Stage I: Demarcation line.

Clinical Course and Pathophysiology

Stage I[11]

In the normal premature eye, the division between vascular and avascular retina is not clinically apparent. Fine branches of retinal vessels extend toward but do not reach the ora serrata. The earliest manifestation of acute ROP, Stage I, is the formation of a demarcation line between vascular (rearguard) and avascular (vanguard) retina. This demarcation line is white, flat, and thin. This early stage of ROP is transient in many cases (Fig. 5–5).

Stage II

As ROP progresses, the demarcation line develops into the ridge (also known as shunt or mesenchymal shunt), a thickened and three-dimensional demarcation line. Spontaneous regression with minimal residual scarring occurs in more than 80 percent of patients with mild acute ROP (Fig. 5–6).[10]

Stage III

As the fibrovascular ridge develops, there are large neovascular vessels which are engorged. These vessels are becoming raised and elevated (Fig. 5–7).

Stage IV

As a natural progression, the large vessels mentioned in Stage III bleed and cause contracture of the retina and subtotal retinal detachment occurs (Fig. 5–8).

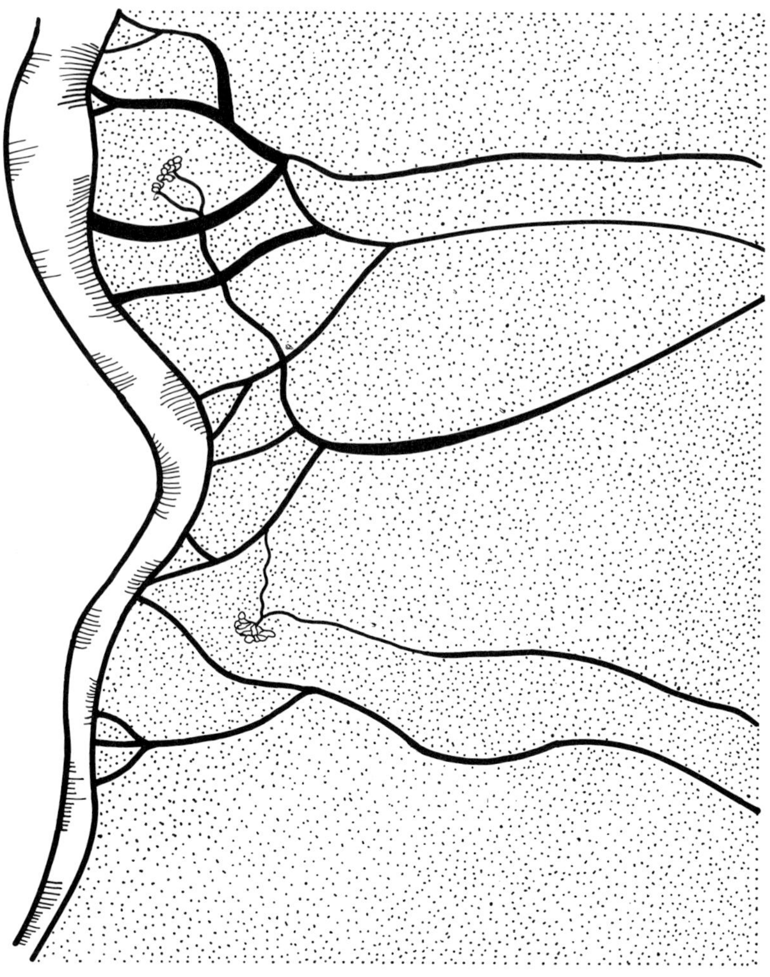

FIGURE 5–6
Stage II: Elevated ridge.

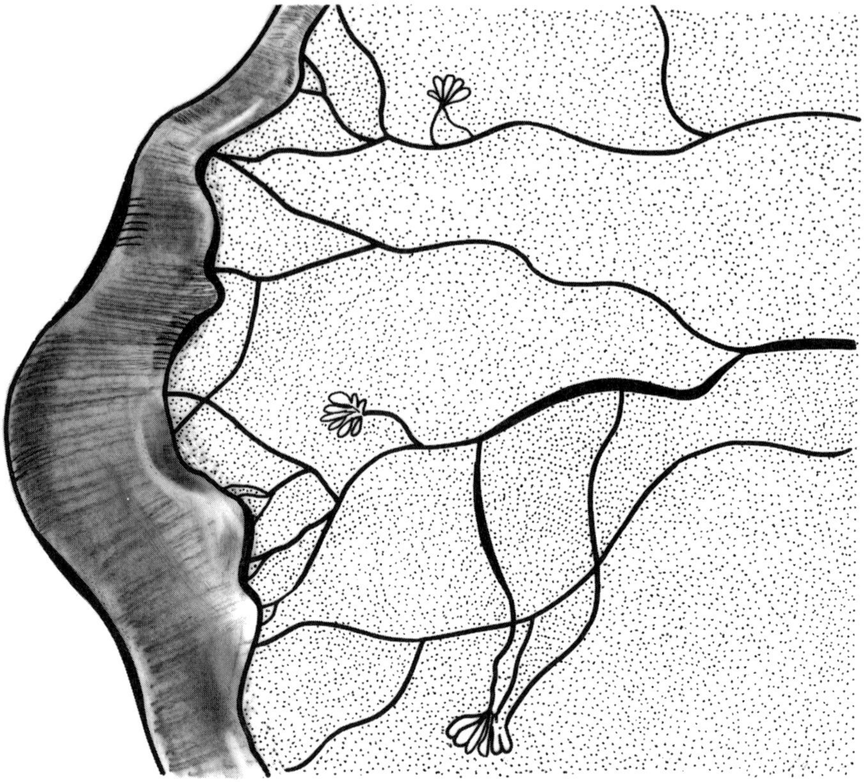

FIGURE 5-7

Stage III: Moderately elevated fibroproliferation.

Stage V

As the subtotal retinal detachment progresses, the retinal detachment becomes complete. The configuration of the retina is either an open funnel retinal detachment or a closed funnel retinal detachment, not unlike proliferative vitreoretinopathy cases. In some cases, the funnel configuration is combined, e.g., open funnel at the posterior pole but narrows as the retina approaches anteriorly towards the lens (Figs. 5–9 and 5–10).

Theories of Pathogenesis

High Oxygen Concentration

It was felt that elevated oxygen levels cause vasoconstriction of the retinal vessels and subsequent closure. The endothelial cells adjacent to the closed capillaries proliferate and consequently new vessel growth occurs. However, ROP can occur with minimal oxygen supplementation and pathologic specimens do not demonstrate this in retinas of newborn infants who have received supplemental oxygen.[12,13]

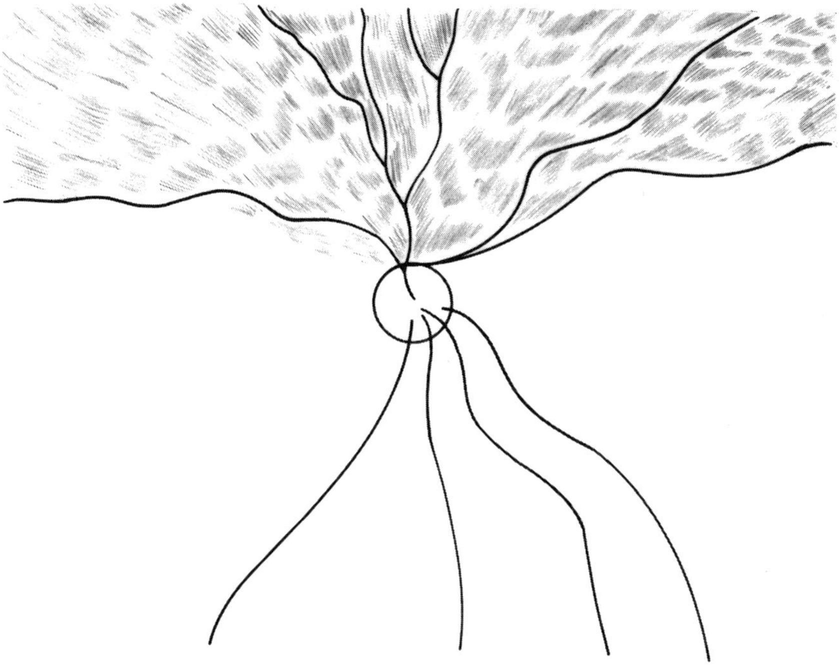

FIGURE 5–8

Stage IV: Retinal detachments, superiorly is detached retina.

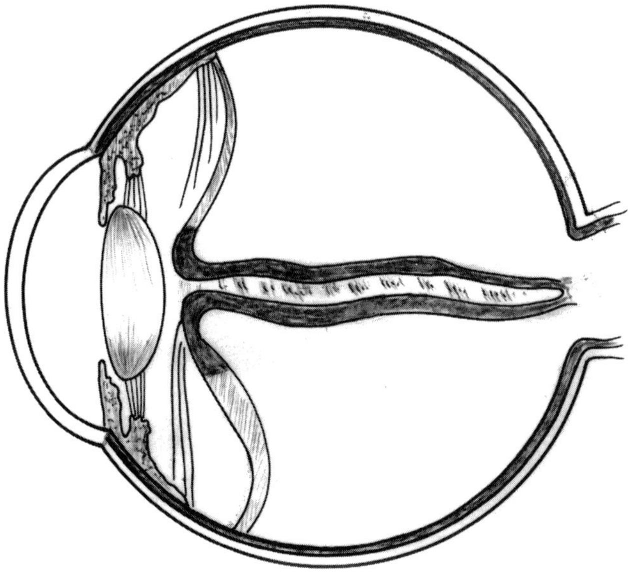

FIGURE 5–9

Stage V: Total retinal detachment.

Spindle Cell Model

With prematurity, there are immature spindle cells that are exposed to an environment rich with oxygen-free radicals at birth. These immature infants are unable to scavenge the free radicals. Thus, the free radicals cause injury to the spindle cells. Consequently, the

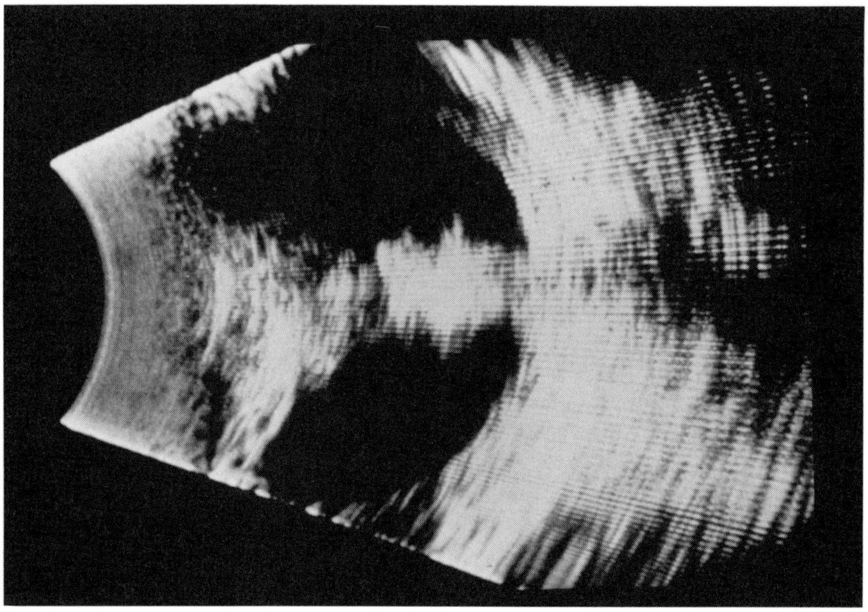

FIGURE 5-10

Total retinal detachment by ultrasound.

injured spindle cells that now have lost the ability to canalize into normal capillaries are also releasing angiogenic factors. This theory is compatible with immaturity and does not require increased oxygen supplementation.[14,15]

Animal Models

Various animal models, such as kittens, puppies, rabbits, baboons, and rats, have been used. However, in each of these animal models, retinal embryogenesis is not like that of the human preterm infant.[16–18]

International Classification of ROP

The International classification of ROP was started in 1984 to make studies of the natural history and treatment more comparable (Fig. 5–11).[11] The classification considers the scarring sequelae independently from the acute disease process. This classification is based on three clinical parameters: the stage of vascular proliferation, the location of the disease, and the extent of involvement.

The stage of vascular proliferation refers to the degree of vascular proliferation. A plus designation is added if vascular

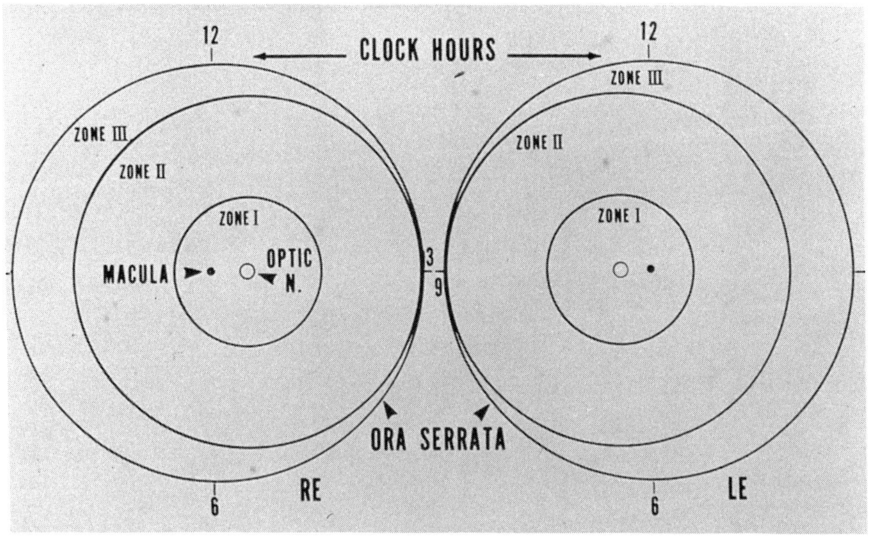

FIGURE 5-11

International classification of ROP. (From Archives of Ophthalmology 1984; 102:1130-1134, copyright 1984, American Medical Association, with permission.)

dilation and tortuosity involve the vessels in the posterior pole or the iris vessels.

■ **TABLE 5-1.**

Stage 1	Demarcation line	
Stage 2	Ridge	
Stage 3	Ridge with extraretinal fibrovascular proliferation	
Stage 4	Subtotal retinal detachment	
Stage 4a	Extrafoveal	
Stage 4b	Including fovea	
Stage 5	Total retinal detachment	
Funnel:	Anterior	Posterior
	Open	Open
	Narrow	Narrow
	Open	Narrow
	Narrow	Open

Location and extent are described by zones.

Zone 1: A circle surrounding the optic disc that extends to twice the distance from the optic disc to the fovea. This approximates the most posterior 60 degrees of the fundus.

Zone 2: Concentric and anterior to zone 1 and extends nasally to the ora serrata but does not reach the temporal ora.

Zone 3: Remaining temporal crescent of anterior retina.

The extent of disease is measured in clock hours.

Risk Factors:

1. Prematurity as determined by gestational age.
2. Birth weight: Infants smaller than 1000 g are at highest risk for the development of ROP. Infants larger than 1500 g rarely develop the disease.
3. Oxygen supplementation: O_2 saturation (percentage of oxygen delivered) and duration of oxygen therapy are associated with the severity of ROP. However, it is important to note that ROP can occur in the absence of oxygen delivery.
4. Sepsis
5. Intraventricular hemorrhage
6. Acidosis

Treatment

Cryotherapy has now been recommended for Stage III threshold disease.[19,20] It has been shown in a randomized clinical trial that 46 percent of untreated eyes versus 26 percent of treated eyes had an unfavorable outcome, such as retinal folds or retinal detachment.[20]

Cryotherapy is applied to the anterior edge of avascular retina. The indications for cryotherapy are shown below.

Laser treatment with the indirect laser ophthalmoscope has also been found to be just as effective.[21] Stage V ROP, surgery carries a 38–40 percent success rate. However, there has been some discussion as to whether the vision attained by these infants after surgery is indeed useful vision or worth spending the enormous healthcare dollars to achieve ambulatory vision.[22]

Fluorescein Angiography

Fluorescein angiography is occasionally done when examination under anesthesia is performed.

■ **TABLE 5–2.**

Stage	Zone	Extent	DIS
ST 3+	1	Any	Prethreshold
ST 2+ or 3	2	Any	Prethreshold
3+	1 or 2	5 Contiguous	Threshold
3+	1 or 2	8 Cumulative	Threshold

■ **TABLE 5-3.** Late Complications of Mild–Moderate ROP

Glaucoma
Strabismus
Cataract
Peripheral-retinal breaks
Microcornea
Band keratopathy–corneal deposits
Optic atrophy
Systemic complications
  Seizures
  Neurologic complications
Regressed ROP and complications
Poor VA
Myopia
Strabismus
Amblyopia
Abnormal macular development

Diagnosis

Examination with 20 D lens or 30 D lens is useful to see the retina. Scleral depression is necessary to see the ora serrata. Screening is usually performed in infants whose birthweight is less than 1500 g or having received more than 50 days of supplemental oxygen. Examinations are usually done on infants who are 4–6 weeks of age. In some infants who are born very premature, one should look for iris vascular tortuosity, which is an indication of plus disease and also, one must consider looking for "rush" disease, in which the ROP develops very rapidly within days.

If disease is seen in the infants, biweekly or weekly examinations are advisable to monitor progression of the disease and treatment would be necessary.

Differential Diagnosis

Stages I and II resemble changes in persistent hyperplastic primary vitreous.[21] The stages III, IV and V in ROP resemble those changes seen in Coats disease caused by congenital telangiectasis, angiomatosis retinae and familial exudative vitreoretinopathy, and incontinentia pigmenti.[23–31]

EALES DISEASE

In Eales disease there is a posterior pole retinal neovascularization associated with areas of peripheral retinal occlusion that are of unknown etiology.[25] The disease occurs in young men between the ages of 20 and 30 years who present at an ophthalmologist's office because of floaters from a vitreous hemorrhage or decreased vision due to cystoid macular edema. Although there is a higher than normal incidence of reactivity to tuberculin protein, there is no evidence to suggest active tuberculosis in these patients. There is no evidence of vitreous or retinal inflammation (Fig. 5–12).

Fluorescein Angiography

Areas of peripheral nonperfusion and proliferative retinopathy occur along the junction of perfused and nonperfused retina.

Treatment

Scatter photocoagulation is useful in those nonperfused retinal areas in patients with recurrent vitreous hemorrhage. In cases of recurrent vitreous hemorrhage, vitrectomy may be necessary to avoid retinal detachment. Lastly macular edema may occur and laser photocoagulation may be useful to those patients who develop circinate maculopathy.

RADIATION RETINOPATHY

Progressive retinovascular changes with associated macular edema, capillary nonperfusion, and retinal and disc neovascular-

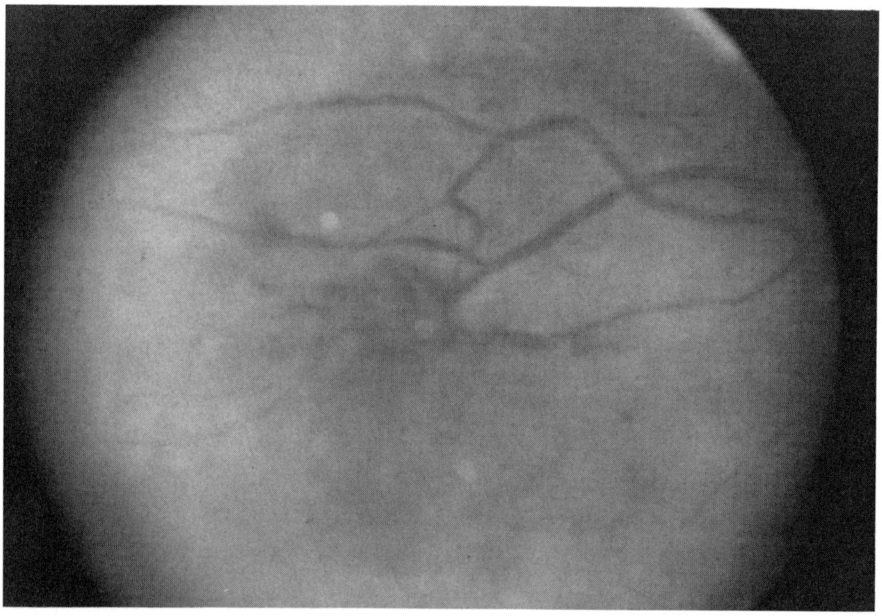

FIGURE 5-12

Eales disease.

ization occur in those eyes which have been exposed to radiation. Radiation retinopathy may be identical to the changes seen in patients with diabetic retinopathy, venous occlusive disease, or branch retinal artery occlusions. Radiation damage can occur with as little as 1500 rad of external beam irradiation. Diagnosis or radiation retinopathy can be confirmed by a careful history and review of the patient's medical records.

Treatment

Focal and grid laser photocoagulation have been attempted to treat the macular exudates.[26,27] Scatter laser photocoagulation has been used in cases with disc and retinal neovascularization to prevent the development of neovascular glaucoma.

FAMILIAL EXUDATIVE VITREORETINOPATHY

Familial exudative vitreoretinopathy is an autosomal dominant-inherited disorder that resembles ROP but occurs in patients with no history of prematurity or neonatal oxygen supplementation.[29,30]

Its earliest and mildest forms show:

1. Areas of peripheral retinal whitening without scleral depression ("white without pressure")
2. Peripheral cystoid degeneration
3. Vitreous band formation
4. Vitreous traction
5. Minimal or no retinal vascular changes are present in the temporal periphery
6. Retinal neovascularization
7. Fibrous proliferation
8. Exudation and localized retinal detachment in the area between the equator and ora serrata with traction and dragging of the major retinal vessels and macula in a temporal direction (Fig. 5–13).

Fluorescein Angiography

Areas of capillary nonperfusion anterior to the equator, dilated retinal vessels, retinal neovascularization, and dye leakage into fibrovascular masses can occur.

Treatment

Surgery is sometimes necessary in severe traction retinal detachment and rhegmatogenous retinal detachment.

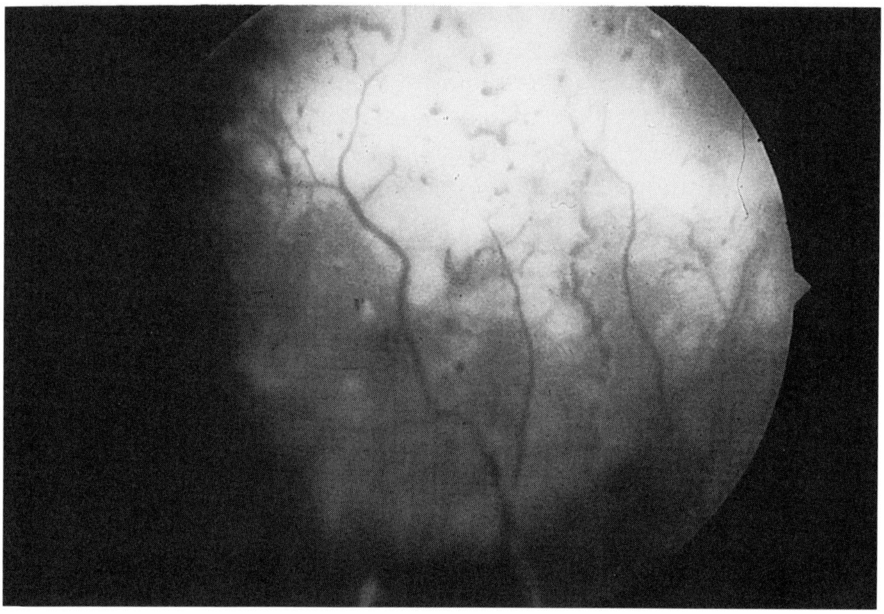

FIGURE 5-13

Familial exudative vitreoretinopathy.

NORRIE'S DISEASE

Norrie's disease is a recessive X-linked congenital retinal dysplasia that mimicks the clinical appearance of advanced ROP.[31] Infants with Norrie's disease manifest leukocoria earlier than ROP infants. Norrie's disease is associated with deafness and mental retardation.

INCONTINENTIA PIGMENTI

Incontinentia pigmenti is an X-linked dominantly-(lethal in males) inherited ectodermal dysplasia also known as Bloch-Sulzberger syndrome, that involves the eye (35 percent of the cases), hair, teeth, and the central nervous system (30 percent of the cases). Most cases are seen in female infants.[32]

The skin of the extremities and trunk is involved soon after birth with bullous, erythematous lesions that may progress to the verrucous stage and may further progress to the flat pigmented whorls and splotches, as well as a linear fashion around the rib cage area. The pigmentation may fade and disappear in later years. Alopecia and dental hypoplasia are frequent.

Central nervous system disorders include seizures, spastic paralysis, and mental retardation.

Ocular anomalies are: strabismus, cataract, myopia, nystagmus, blue sclera, corneal opacities, pigmentary changes in the fundus, retinal vascular anomalies, optic atrophy, retinal dysplasia, pseudoglioma, and phthisis bulbi.

Abnormalities of the periheral retinal vasculature near the temporal equator include vascular dilation, arteriovenous anastomosis, preretinal fibrous proliferation, vascular proliferation, exudation, and absence of the retinal vessels peripheral to these changes.

Fluorescein Angiography

Vascular proliferation and shunts can be seen.

Treatment

Laser photocoagulation has been attempted and may cause a regression of the vascular proliferation.

REFERENCES

1. Nagpal KC, Goldberg MF, Rabb MF: Ocular manifestations of sickle hemoglobinopathies. Surv Ophthalmol 1977; *21:* 391–411

2. Bunn H, Forget BG: Sickle cell disease. p. 685. In Nathan DG, Oski FA (eds.): Hematology of Infancy and Childhood. 2nd ed. Philadelphia, WB Saunders, 1981

3. Goldberg MF: Classification and pathogenesis of proliferation sickle retinopathy. Am J Ophthalmol 1971; *71:* 649–665

4. Goldberg MF, Acacio I: Argon laser photocoagulation of proliferative sickle retinopathy. Arch Ophthalmol 1973; *90:* 35–38

5. Jampol LM, Green JL Jr., Goldberg MF, Peyman GA: An update on vitrectomy surgery and retinal detachment repair in sickle cell disease. Arch Ophthalmol 1982; *100:* 591–593

6. Hanscom TA: Indirect treatment of peripheral retinal neovascularization. Am J Ophthalmol 1982; *93:* 88–91

7. Rednam KRV, Jampol LM, Goldberg MF: Scatter retinal photocoagulation for proliferative sickle cell retinopathy. Am J Ophthalmol 1982; *93:* 594–599

8. Terry TL: Extreme prematurity and fibroblastic overgrowth of persistent vascular sheath behind each crystalline lens I. Prelim Report. Am J Ophthalmol 1942; *25:* 203–204

9. Patz A, Hoeck LE, De La Cruz E: Studies on the effect of high oxygen administration in retrolental fibroplasia I. Nursery Observations. Am J Ophthalmol 1952; *35:* 1248–1253

10. Flynn JT, Bancalari E, Bachynski BN et al: Retinopathy of prematurity. Diagnosis, severity, and natural history. Ophthalmology 1987; *94:* 620–629

11. The Committee for the Classification of Retinopathy of Prematurity. An International Classification of Retinopathy of Prematurity. Arch Ophthalmol 1984; *102:* 1130–1134

12. Patz A, Eastham A, Higginbotham DH, Kleh T: Oxygen studies in retrolental fibroplasia in experimental animals. Am J Ophthalmol 1953; *36:* 1511–1522

13. Lanman JT, Guy LP, Dancis J: Retrolental fibroplasia and oxygen therapy. JAMA 1954; *155:* 223–226

14. Kretzer FL, Mehta RS, Johnson AT et al: Vitamin E protects against retinopathy of prematurity through action on spindle cells. Nature 1984; *309:* 793–795

15. Kretzer FL, Hittner HM: Spindle cells and retinopathy of prematurity: interpretation and predictions. Birth Defects 1988; *24:* 147–168

16. Gole GA: Animal models of retinopathy of prematurity. p. 53. In Silverman WA, Flynn JT (eds.): Retinopathy of Prematurity. Boston, Blackwell, 1985

17. Kretzer FL, Mehta RS, Goad D, Hittner HM: Animal models in research on retinopathy of prematurity. p. 79. In McPherson AR, Hittner HM, Kretzer FL (eds.): Retinopathy of Prematurity—Current Concepts and Controversies. Toronto, BC Decker, 1986

18. Penn JS, Thum LA: The rat as an animal model for retinopathy of prematurity. Prog Clin Biol Res 1989; *314:* 623–642

19. Cryotherapy for Retinopathy of Prematurity Cooperative Group. Multicenter trial of cryotherapy for ROP. Preliminary results. Arch Ophthalmol 1988; *106:* 471–479

20. Cryotherapy for Retinopathy of Prematurity Cooperative Group. Multicenter trial of cryotherapy for ROP. 3-1/2 year outcome–structure and function. Arch Ophthalmol 1993; *111:* 339–344

21. McNamara JA, Tasman W, Brown GC, Federman JL: Laser photocoagulation for stage 3+ Retinopathy of Prematurity. Ophthalmol 1991; *98:* 576–580

22. Quinn GE, Dobson V, Barr CC et al: Visual acuity in infants after vitrectomy for severe retinopathy of prematurity. Ophthalmol 1991; *98:* 5–13

23. Pruett RC, Schepens CL: Posterior hyperplastic primary vitreous. Am J Ophthalmol 1970; *69:* 535–543

24. Ridley ME, Shields JA, Brown GC, Tasman W: Coats' disease: evaluation of management. Ophthalmology 1982; *89:* 1381–1387

25. Renie WA, Murphy RP, Anderson KC et al: The evaluation of patients with Eales' disease. Retina 1983; *3:* 243–248

26. Gass JDM: A fluorescein angiographic study of macular dysfunction secondary to retinal vascular disease. VI. X-irradiation, carotid artery occlusion, collagen vascular disease, and vitritis. Arch Ophthalmol 1968; *80:* 606–617

27. Chaudhuri PR, Austin DJ, Rosenthal AR: Treatment of radiation retinopathy. Br J Ophthalmol 1981; *65:* 623–625

28. Thompson GM, Migdal CS, Whittle RJM: Radiation retinopathy following treatment of posterior nasal space carcinoma. Br J Ophthalmol 1983; *67:* 609–614

29. Criswick VG, Schepens CL: Familial exudative vitreoretinopathy. Am J Ophthalmol 1969; *68:* 578–594

30. Slusher MM, Hutton WE: Familial exudative vitreoretinopathy. Am J Ophthalmol 1979; *87:* 152–157

31. Hansen AC: Norrie's disease. Am J Ophthalmol 1968; *66:* 328–332

32. Watzke RC, Stevens TS, Carney RG Jr.: Retinal vascular changes of incontinentia pigmenti. Arch Ophthalmol 1976; *94:* 743–746

CHAPTER SIX

Retinal Vascular Diseases

ARTERIAL SYSTEM

Branch Retinal Artery Occlusion

Pathophysiology

Branch artery occlusion has associated systemic disease involvement. Most commonly, for branch retinal artery occlusion, the etiology has involved embolic phenomena,[1,2] intraluminal thrombosis,[3] hemorrhage with atherosclerotic plaque,[4] spasm,[5–7] vasculitis,[2,8] dissecting aneurysm,[9] hypertensive arteriolar necrosis,[10] and circulatory collapse.[11] Eighty percent of eyes affected with branch retinal occlusion improve to 20/40 or better although residual visual field defects remain (Fig. 6–1).

Associated Diseases:

Arterial hypertension
Diabetes mellitus
Carotid atherosclerosis and cardiac valvular disease
Collagen vascular disorders
Trauma
Coagulopathies
Local ocular abnormalities

Clinical Course

The patient experiences an acute loss of vision in part of the visual field. The patient complains of a spot on the visual field at near, i.e., when reading a book. Sometimes, the patient just notices a "grayness" of vision. The prognosis for return of good vision (20/40 or better) is excellent.

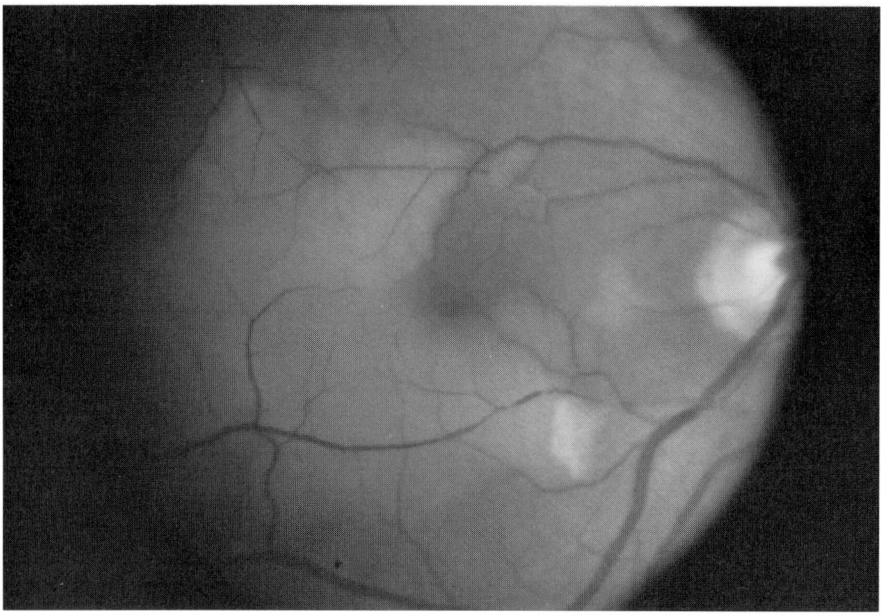

FIGURE 6–1
Branch retinal artery occlusion, OD.

Diagnosis

On indirect ophthalmoscopy, the retina shows narrowed retinal arteries and dilated retinal veins. Retinal hemorrhages can be seen in the affected quadrant of the retinal artery. Cotton wool spots can be present. Spontaneous retinal arterial pulsations and retina arterial emboli can also be seen. Usually the temporal vessels are involved.[12] Neovascularization of the iris and retina are rare, but rubeosis iridis and retinae are more common in patients with diabetes mellitus. Some patients with a branch retinal artery occlusion go on to develop another branch retinal artery occlusion at a different site or a central retinal artery occlusion.

Fluorescein Angiography

Delayed choroidal filling of the eyes, increased retinal arteriovenous transit time, late staining of the larger retinal vessels, especially the arteries, macular edema, microaneurysms, and areas of retinal capillary nonperfusion can be seen.

Treatment

There is no treatment for this entity. But, it is important to treat the underlying systemic disease, e.g., hypertension and diabetes or carotid artery disease.

Central Retinal Artery Occlusion

The pathophysiology of central retinal artery occlusion is the same as that in branch retinal artery occlusion. In central retinal artery occlusion, patients usually have an underlying systemic disorder: hypertension (66 percent),[1] cardiac valvular disease (25 percent),[1] carotid atherosclerotic disease (45 percent)[13] and diabetes (25 percent).[1]

Clinical Course

The patients present with abrupt, painless visual loss. The patient notices a profound loss of visual acuity and a darkening of vision that occurs suddenly without warning. Patients usually do not seek immediate medical attention, and subsequently, their vision remains at count finger or light perception level.

Diagnosis

The visual acuity is usually count finger or hand motion.[1] The patients have narrowed retinal arteries, superficial retinal whitening in the posterior pole, and a cherry-red spot in the foveola. However, in acute central retinal artery occlusion, the cherry red spot may not be present. An afferent pupillary defect is present. During acute central retinal artery occlusion, there may be only darkening and attenuation of the arterial vessels and an afferent pupillary defect. Beyond the macular area, the retinal whitening is less pronounced. The retinal whitening resolves within 4–6 weeks and a pale optic disc is then seen (Fig. 6–2).

In cases of central retinal artery occlusion, look for emboli. There are three types of emboli:

1. Platelet thrombin emboli that are dull, grayish white, oval bodies which can move into more distal vessels. Single or multiple, they are most often seen at a bifurcation.
2. Cholesterol emboli are found in groups. They are yellowish white or yellow bodies in the temporal peripheral arterial tree. They may or may not be associated with obstruction. When cholesterol emboli are seen near the optic nerve head, one has to consider their role in obstructive central retinal artery occlusion.
3. Calcific emboli are usually single, solid, white, nonrefractile bodies. Calcific emboli are thought to be derived from the aortic or mitral valve. These are usually near the optic nerve head. Periarterial sheathing caused by emboli may be more prominent than the emboli.

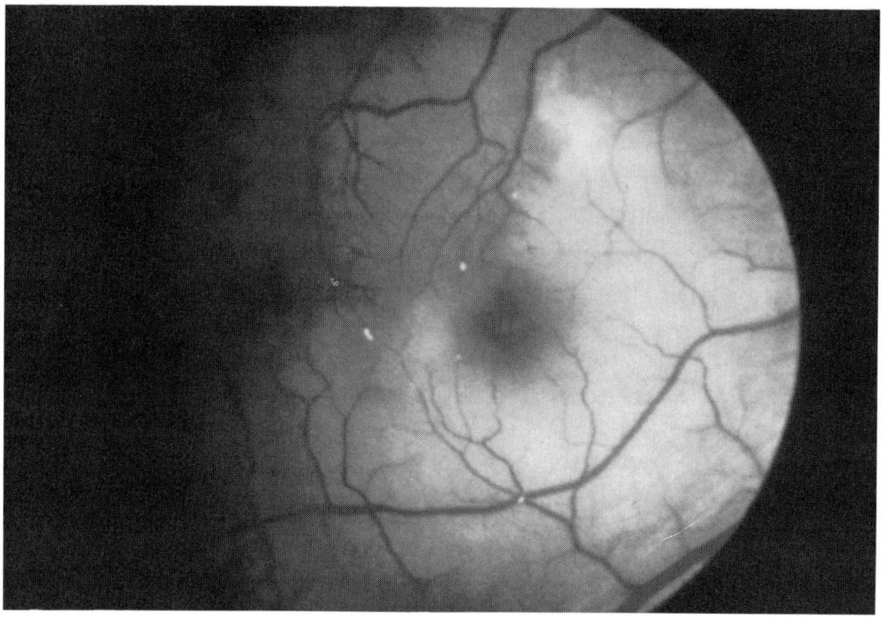

FIGURE 6–2

Central retinal artery occlusion, OD.

Fluorescein Angiography

Delayed arterial filling, increased retinal circulation time in the area of the affected arterial tree, is seen.

In complete occlusion of the central retinal artery, no fluorescein dye enters the eye by the artery, but fluorescein dye fills the optic nerve capillaries via the ciliary artery circulation passing through collateral channels and also fills the proximal branches of both the central retinal vein and artery. In some instances, the fluorescein flows around the embolus and in others, it goes around the embolus via collateralization. In other cases, there may be alternating nonfluorescent zones with fluorescent zones caused by aggregated packets of erythrocytes, and hyperfluorescent zones caused by stagnant plasma.

Treatment

There is no effective treatment for improving vision in patients with central retinal artery occlusion. Treatment is aimed at sudden decrease in intraocular pressure, such that the perfusion pressure behind the obstruction will push away an obstructing embolus by a sudden change in the pressure gradient. Anterior chamber paracentesis has been advocated when the central retinal artery occlusion is less than 24 hours. Although irreversible damage has been shown to occur after 90–100 minutes of complete central retinal artery occlusion in the subhuman primate model,[14] such total obstruction is not seen clinically in humans. Intravenous acetazolamide may be also used to induce a rapid decrease in intraocular pressure. Inhalation of 95 percent oxygen (O_2) and 5 percent carbon dioxide (CO_2) is used: CO_2 inhalation to dilate the retinal vessels and 100 percent oxygen to produce a normal PO_2 at the retinal surface via diffusion from the choroid in the setting of a central retinal artery occlusion.[15]

Giant cell arteritis can be a cause of central retinal artery occlusion and an erythrocyte sedimentation rate should be obtained in all patients. Aggressive corticosteroid therapy should be undertaken since the second eye can be involved within hours of the central retinal artery occlusion.

Cilioretinal Artery Obstruction

Cilioretinal arteries enter on the temporal aspect of the optic disc, separately from the retinal arterial system. The flow of blood in the cilioretinal arteries is concomitant with the choroidal circulation. Cilioretinal artery fluorescein flow occurs 1–2 seconds before the retinal arterial fluorescence.

Clinical Course

Isolated cilioretinal artery obstruction has a good visual prognosis. The majority achieve 20/40 vision or better.[16]

Cilioretinal artery obstruction can occur with central retinal vein occlusion. Again, the visual prognosis in patients with cilioretinal artery obstruction is excellent and no treatment is indicated. Two–thirds of the eyes will achieve 20/40 or better visual acuity.[16]

Cilioretinal artery with ischemic optic neuropathy carries the worst prognosis of vision: 20/400 to NLP. This variant comprises about 5 percent of all cilioretinal artery obstructions. Look out for giant cell arteritis in this case.

Ophthalmic Artery Obstruction

Clinical Course

Sudden visual loss is the hallmark of ophthalmic artery obstruction. The visual acuity is usually no light perception. Marked ocular ischemia and rubeosis iridis is not noted in this entity except rarely. The intraocular pressure is lower in the affected side as well as in the case of central retinal artery occlusion.

Diagnosis

Funduscopic examination shows intense retinal opacification resulting from inner and outer retinal ischemia that may extend beyond the posterior pole.

After a period of weeks, the retinal opacification resolves and leaves retinal pigment epithelial disturbances as a result of choroidal vascular compromise. Optic pallor follows as a late sequela.

Fluorescein Angiography

There is delay in choroidal and arterial circulation times.

Electroretinography

The electroretinogram is classic in differentiating ophthalmic artery occlusion from central retinal artery occlusion: there is the absence of the a-wave and b-wave. With central retinal artery occlusion, there is only a reduced b-wave.

Arterial Embolism

Emboli

1. Platelet thrombin emboli: Dull, grayish white, single or multiple, and are most often lodged at a bifurcation.
2. Cholesterol emboli: Multiple and yellowish white or iridescent globules seen in the peripheral arterial tree in the temporal retinal periphery.
3. Calcific emboli: Single, solid, white, nonrefractile ovoid or angulated emboli, may be derived from the aortic or mitral valve, usually near the optic nerve head.

Embolic arterial disease can occur with the intravenous use of illicit drugs and from facial injections of medication, usually steroids that are inadvertently injected into the arterial system.

Talc Retinopathy

Injected talc particles gain access to the ocular circulation through congenital shunts or by the chronic use of crushed talc-containing tablets in the presence of pulmonary obstructive disease severe enough to cause the development of pulmonary shunts. The particles lodge in the choriocapillaris and in the small vessels of the retina. They can be seen as crystalline intravascular emboli and patients can have good vision. Only if the emboli lodge in the perimacular arterial circulation is there significant loss of vision.[17–19]

VENOUS SYSTEM (SEE CHAPTER 13)

Branch retinal vein occlusion (Fig. 6–3)
Central retinal vein occlusion (Fig. 6–4)
Hyperviscosity syndromes

The blood itself may be hyperviscous and more prone to clotting and vaso-occlusive disorders can result. Increased blood viscosity is associated with various pathological conditions in which vascular thrombosis or occlusion is a feature.[20]

MACROANEURYSM

Macroaneurysms are oval or round dilations of retinal arterioles, occurring in the posterior pole. The superotemporal artery is the most common site of involvement. Most are unilateral.

Clinical Course

Patients are affected in the sixth and seventh decade of life and associated vascular problems are hypertension and arteriosclerotic and cardiovascular problems. There is decreased vision due to

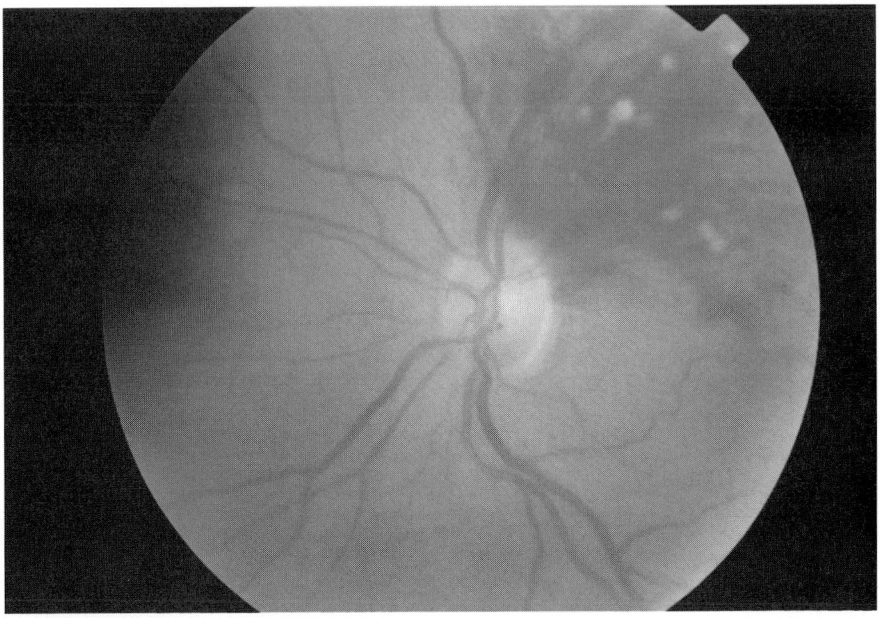

FIGURE 6–3
Branch retinal vein occlusion, OS.

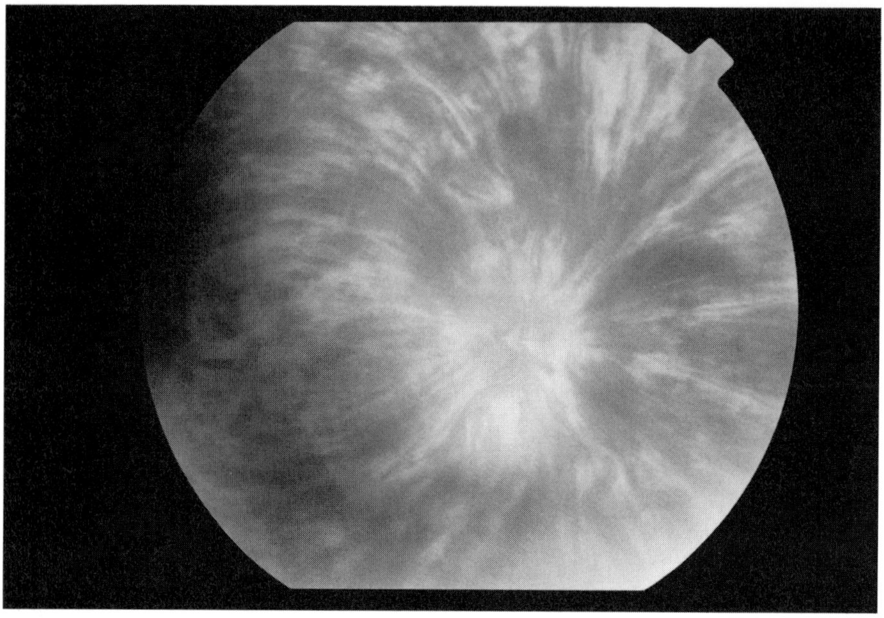

FIGURE 6–4
Central retinal vein occlusion, OD.

retinal edema, exudate, or hemorrhage. Vitreous hemorrhage can occur as well as subretinal hemorrhage.

Diagnosis

Indirect ophthalmoscopy and slit-lamp biomicroscopy will show these macroaneurysms in the superotemporal quadrant of the posterior pole. There can be associated retinal edema, exudate, or hemorrhage.

The visual prognosis can be excellent especially in the situation of spontaneous regression of the macroaneurysm. There can be associated poor visual prognosis because of complications such as vitreous hemorrhage or massive exudation in the macular area.

Fluorescein Angiography

The macroaneurysm fills in the early arterial phase of the angiogram. There can be staining of the vessel wall or marked fluorescein leakage. Leakage of surrounding dilated capillaries may be seen as well.

Treatment

There is no clear indication for treatment by laser photocoagulation unless lipid exudation affects the fovea. Then, direct laser photocoagulation of the offending macroaneurysm can be performed. With laser photocoagulation, the potential of occluding the distal portion of the arteriole and a subsequent macular scotoma, must be considered.

RETINAL TELANGIECTASIA

Coats Disease

Coats disease is an idiopathic condition in which telangiectatic and aneurysmal retinal vessels are associated with massive subretinal exudation, originally described by George Coats in 1908 (Figs. 6–5 and 6–6).[21]

Coats outlines three types:

1. Massive subretinal exudate, choroidal mononuclear infiltrate, and no demonstrable vascular abnormalities.
2. Subretinal exudate, multiple retinal vascular abnormalities with intraretinal hemorrhage, and no choroidal inflammatory infiltrate.
3. Subretinal exudate and frank arteriovenous malformations (angiomatosis retinae).

This condition can occur in two age groups: children before the age of 10 and in adults. The adult form has been frequently associated with hypercholesterolemia.[22,23]

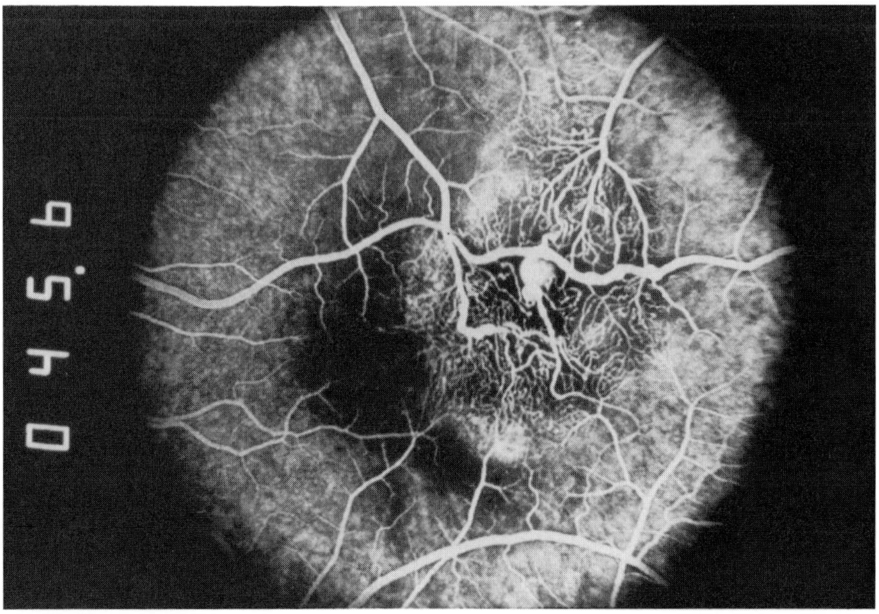

FIGURE 6–5

Fluorescein angiogram of a patient with Coats disease.

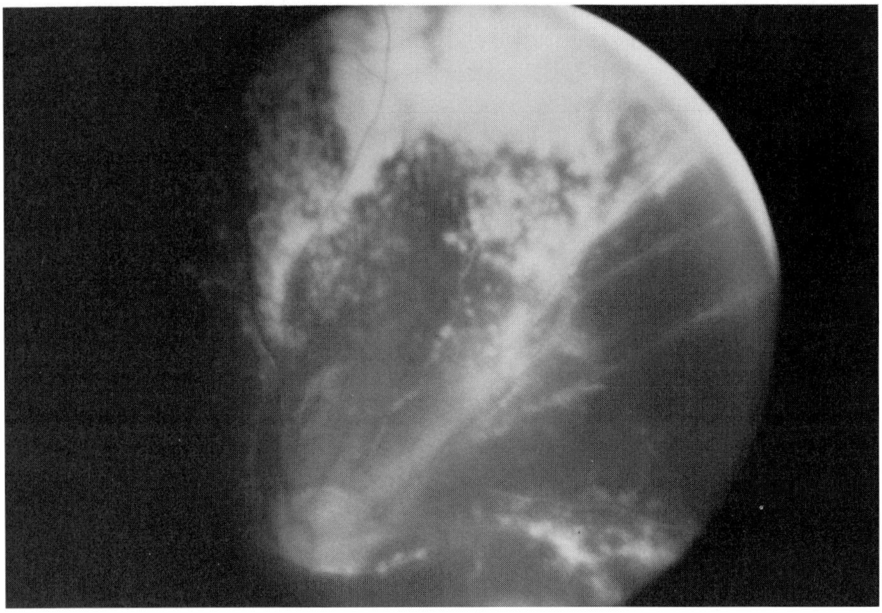

FIGURE 6–6
One-year-old infant with Coats disease.

Pathologic examination shows loss of both vascular endothelium and pericytes with subsequent mural disorganization and loss of the blood retinal barrier.[24]

Clinical Course

Children have been known to present with this condition in the first 6 months of life and there is speculation that the disease can occur at birth. Strabismus or a white reflex is often noted by the parents and the child is brought in to see an ophthalmologist. In adults, there is loss of vision from the exudation.

Fluorescein Angiography

Telangiectasia, aneurysms, beading of vessel walls, and various vascular communicating channels are seen. These vessels show persistent leakage.

Diagnosis

Massive subretinal exudation with abnormal retinal vasculature should bring to mind this entity especially in young children and adolescents.

For children, Coats disease is in the differential diagnosis of retinoblastoma, retinopathy of prematurity and retinal detachment,

Toxocara canis, persistent hyperplastic primary vitreous, and congenital cataract.

Coats disease, at any age, may be confused with Eales disease, vasculitis, collagen vascular disease, tumors, branch retinal vein occlusion, or idiopathic juxtafoveal telangiectasis.

Treatment

Laser photocoagulation to the anomalous retinal vessels responsible for the massive exudation has been tried. Cryotherapy and drainage of the subretinal fluid followed with diathermy or cryotherapy has been tried as well. However, the complications of treatment can be vitreous hemorrhage, inflammation, and retinal fibrosis.

Idiopathic Parafoveal Telangiectasia[25]

Congenital Parafoveal Telangiectasis:

Group 1A Unilateral congenital parafoveal telangiectasis

Male predominance

Mean age of onset is 40 years

Temporal half of macula, 1–2 disc diameters, clustered at the horizontal raphe, macular edema and exudate is the cause of visual loss in these patients.

Visual acuity = 20/25-20/40

Spontaneous resolution has occurred

Acquired Parafoveal Telangiectasis:

Group 1B Unilateral idiopathic parafoveal telangiectasis (Fig. 6–7)

Male predominance

Capillary telangiectasia 1 clockhour at edge of FAZ. This may or may not be accompanied by hard exudates.

Visual acuity = 20/25

Acquired Parafoveal Telangiectasis:

Group 2 bilateral acquired parafoveal telangiectasis

Male to female ratio equal

5th–6th decade

Temporal or entire perifoveal network, minimal macular edema and exudation, biomicroscopy reveals minimal to mild dilation of retinal capillaries with slight retinal edema.

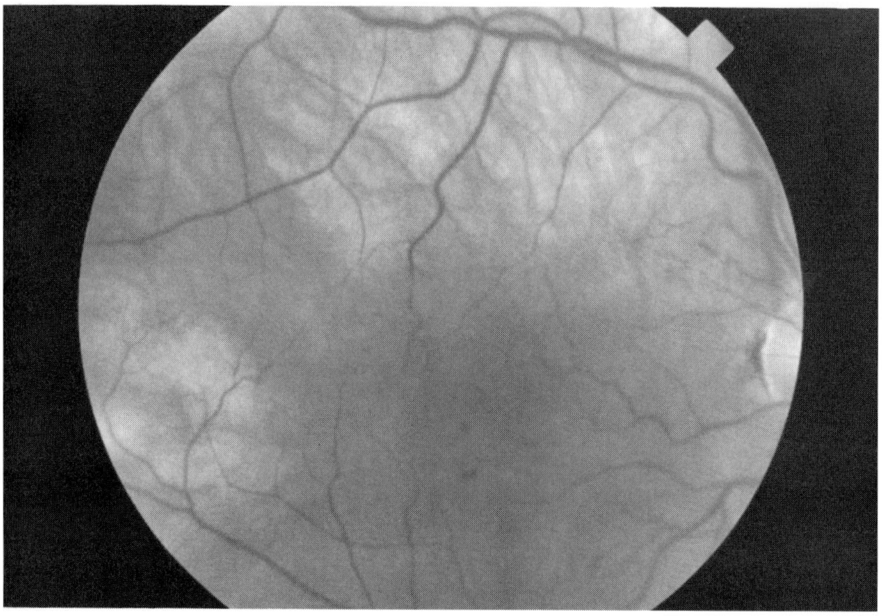

FIGURE 6–7

Idiopathic parafoveal telangiectasia in a 50-year-old male, OD.

SPECIFIC AND UNUSUAL FEATURES

1. See superficial glistening white dots
2. Right-angled retinal venules
3. Chronically, see retinal pigment epithelial hyperplasia along the right-angled venules
4. Yellow ⅓ disc diameter lesion in center of foveal avascular zone (not to be confused with Best's disease or adult vitelliform)
5. Subretinal neovascularization

FLUORESCEIN ANGIOGRAPHY

Dilated ectatic perifoveal capillaries and the above-mentioned retinal features are seen.

Idiopathic and Perifoveal Telangiectasis:

Group 3 Bilateral, idiopathic, perifoveal telangiectasis, and capillary occlusion

Age 50 years

Unclear about male or female preponderance

Bilateral progressive obliteration of perifoveal network, optic disc pallor.

Associated with diabetes and may be seen as a prediabetic state.[26]

FLUORESCEIN ANGIOGRAPHY

Dilated ectatic perifoveal capillaries and the above-mentioned retinal features.

TREATMENT

Because this is a rare entity and vision usually is 20/40 or better, laser photocoagulation has not been widely used nor recommended.

REFERENCES

1. Brown GC, Magargal LE: Central retinal artery obstruction and visual acuity. Ophthalmology 1982; *89:* 14–19

2. Appen RE, Wray SH, Cogan DG: Central retinal artery occlusion. Am J Ophthalmol 1975; *79:* 374–381

3. Perraut LE, Zimmerman LE: The occurrence of glaucoma following occlusion of the central retinal artery. A clinicopathologic report of six cases with a review of the literature. Arch Ophthalmol 1959; *61:* 845–865

4. Dahrling BE: The histopathology of early central retinal artery occlusion. Arch Ophthalol 1965; *73:* 506–510

5. Carroll D: Retinal migraine. Headache 1970; *10:* 9–13

6. Graveson GS: Retinal arterial occlusion in migraine. Br Med J 1949; *2:* 838–840

7. Silberberg DH, Laties AM: Occlusive migraine. Trans Pa Acad Ophthalmol Otolaryngol 1974; *27:* 34–38

8. Karjalainen K: Occlusion of the central retinal artery and branch retinal arterioles. Acta Ophthalmol (suppl.)(Copenh) 1971; *109:* 5–96

9. Wolter JR, Hansen KD: Intimo-intimal intussusception of the central retinal artery. Am J Ophthalmol 1981; *92:* 486–491

10. Leishman R: The eye in general vascular disease. Br J Ophthalol 1957; *41:* 641–701

11. Gold D: Retinal arterial occlusion. Trans Am Acad Ophthalol Otolaryngol 1977; *83:* 392–408

12. Brown GC, Shields JA: Cilioretinal arteries and retinal arterial occlusion. Arch Ophthalmol 1979; *97:* 84–92

13. Shah HG, Brown GC, Goldberg RE: Digital subtraction carotid angiography and retinal arterial obstruction. Ophthalmol 1985; *92:* 68–72

14. Hayreh SS, Kolder HE, Weingeist TA: Central retinal artery occlusion and retinal tolerance time. Ophthalmol 1980; *87:* 75–78

15. Landers MB: Retinal oxygenation via the choroidal circulation. Trans Am Ophthalmol Soc 1978; *76:* 528–556

16. Brown GC, Moffat K, Cruess A, et al: Cilioretinal artery obstruction. Retina 1983; *3:* 182–187

17. Atlee WE Jr: Talc and cornstarch emboli in eyes of drug abusers. JAMA 1972; *219:* 49–51

18. Bluth LI, Hanscom TA: Retinal detachment and vitreous hemorrhage due to talc emboli. JAMA 1981; *246:* 980–981

19. Jampol LM, Setogawa T, Rednam KRV, Tso MOM: Talc retinopathy in primates: a model of ischemic retinopathy I. Clinical studies. Arch Ophthalmol 1981; *99:* 1273–1280

20. Ring CP, Pearson TC, Sanders MD, Wetherley-Mein G: Viscosity and retinal vein thrombosis. Am J Ophthalmol 1976; *60:* 397–410

21. Coats G: Forms of retinal disease with massive exudation. Roy Lond Ophthalmol Hosps Rep 1980; *18:* 440–525

22. Egerer I, Tasman W, Tomer TL: Coats' disease. Arch Ophthalmol 1974; *92:* 109–112

23. Yeung JWS, Harris GS: Coats' disease: a study of cholesterol transport in the eye. Can J Ophthalmol 1976; *11:* 61–68

24. Tripathi R, Ashton N: Electron microscopical study of Coats' disease. Br J Ophthalmol 1971; *55:* 289–301

25. Gass JD, Oyakawa RT: Idiopathic juxtafoveolar retinal telangiectasis. Arch Ophthalmol 1982; *100:* 769–780

26. Green WR, Quigley HA, de la Cruz Z, Cohen B: Parafoveal retinal telangiectasis: light and electron microscopic studies. Trans Ophthalmol Soc UK 1980; *100:* 162–170

CHAPTER SEVEN

Age-related Macular Degeneration and Other Acquired Disorders

AGE-RELATED MACULAR DEGENERATION

Epidemiology

Age-related macular degeneration (ARMD) is the leading cause of blindness in Americans 55 years or older. It is one of the leading reasons patients attend ophthalmology and low-vision clinics. In the 1977 Framingham report, it was estimated that 6.4 percent of patients between the ages of 65–74 and 19.7 percent of patients aged 75 or older had evidence of ARMD in one or both eyes.[1] Other studies have shown that almost 30 percent of people 75 years or older have some manifestation of ARMD.

Anatomy and Physiology

The anatomic foci of abnormal physiology occurs at the retinal pigment epithelium (RPE).[2] It is the layer that is sandwiched between the photoreceptors and the choroidal blood supply that nourishes these outer layers of the retina.

Each RPE cell is in contact with 25 rods. Each rod sheds 100 discs each day. In a lifetime, 70 million discs may be phagocytosed by one RPE cell. In one hypothesis, as these RPE cells degenerate with age, undigested residual bodies are lipofuscin and these are seen as drusen or a constellation of drusen which then leads to other fundus abnormalities in ARMD (Fig. 7–1).[3–5]

Bruch's membrane is sandwiched between the RPE cell layer on one side and the choriocapillaris on the other. Bruch's membrane has elastin and collagenous layers that allow for the free movement

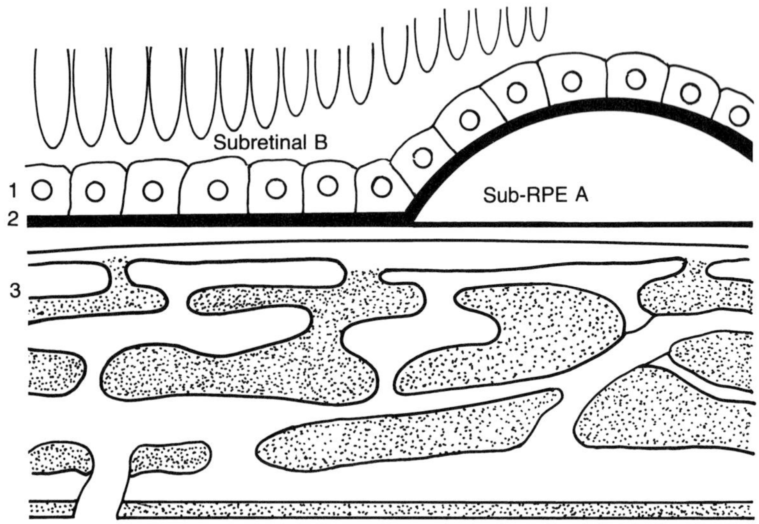

FIGURE 7–1

1. Retinal pigment epithelium; *2*. Bruch's membrane; *3*. Choriocapillaris; *a*. Serous retinal pigment epithelium detachment; *b*. Serous detachment of the retina.

of nutrients into the retina and waste products back toward the choriocapillaris. In the aging process, there is a loss of the elastin layer and thus there is a breakdown of Bruch's membrane. This leads to the decreased permeability of the waste products and thus an accumulation of waste products, such as lipofuscin, in the RPE cell and Bruch's membrane interface.

Such a disruption of Bruch's membrane allows for the extrusion of the waste products of metabolism and forms localized pockets of separation between Bruch's membrane and the RPE; these pockets are referred to as soft drusen. This same loss of integrity of Bruch's membrane causes cell death or cell atrophy of the neighboring RPE layer. With the cell death of localized areas of the RPE, there is loss of the pump mechanism of the RPE, and subsequently, there is the formation of small serous RPE detachments.

In addition, the breakdown of Bruch's membrane allows the ingrowth of the choriocapillaris to form new membranes under the retina, hence the term, subretinal neovascular membranes.

The repair process leads to macrophage and choriocapillaris pericyte activity to remove cellular debris. Replacement with fibrous scar tissue occurs later which leads to the formation of a "disciform scar" in many endstages of eyes with ARMD.

There are two types of ARMD: dry or inactive and exudative. Ten to 20 percent of all ARMD is the exudative type, however, and is the major cause of blindness (Figs. 7–1 and 7–2).[1]

Dry Age-related Macular Degeneration

It is thought that greater than 50 percent of the population have dry age-related macular degeneration after the age of 70.

Drusen, from the German word *druse,* are a crust of crystals lining a rock cavity. They are yellowish deposits lying deep in the retina.

Hard drusen are small, round, and discrete bodies. On fluorescein angiogram, these hard drusen fluoresce brightly in the early phase and fade soon after background choroidal fluorescence (Fig. 7–2).[6,7]

Soft drusen resemble a RPE detachment and are more at risk for developing subretinal neovascularization. Soft drusen pathologically represent focal accumulations of a continuous layer of debris, their margins are indistinct and can become confluent. In addition, soft drusen may pool fluid that the pigment epithelium is unable to pump out, hence the definition of localized RPE detachments (Fig. 7–3).

Mixed drusen are flatter than they are soft, more atrophic with mild late staining on fluorescein angiography (Fig. 7–4).

Nodular drusen or basal laminar drusen can be seen in the younger ARMD patient. One can consider them to be like the

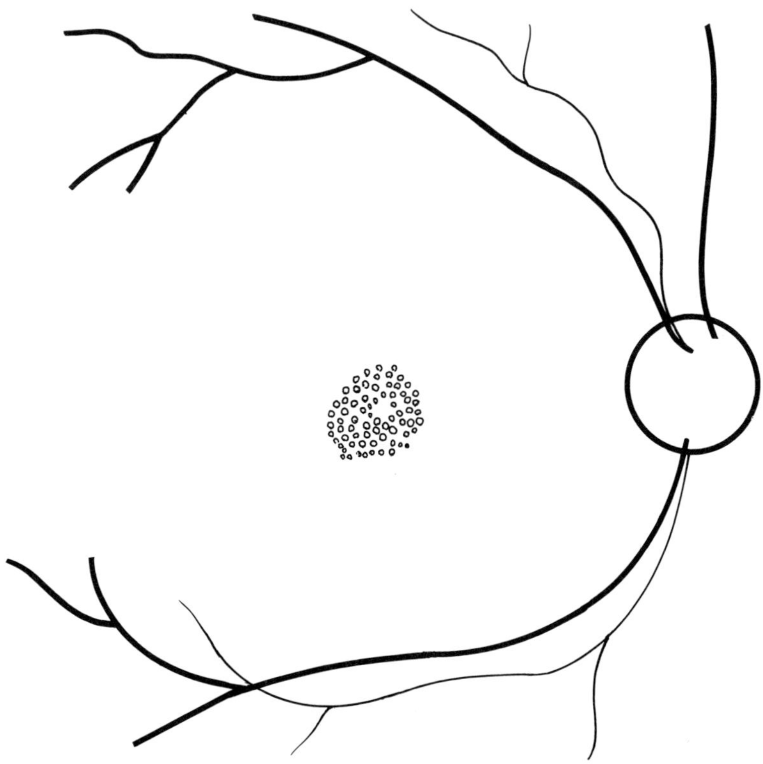

FIGURE 7–2
Hard drusen.

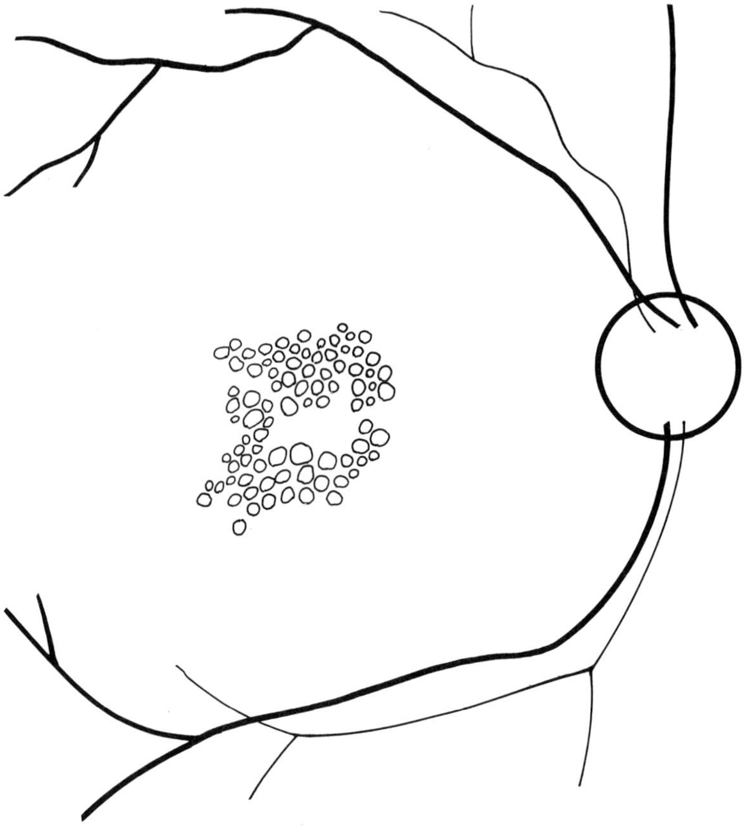

FIGURE 7–3
Soft drusen.

corneal guttata but the RPE equivalent. They fade on fluorescein angiography.[8]

Calcific drusen are refractile small deposits and are seen in clusters. Over time, their characteristics may change.

Exudative Age-related Macular Degeneration

Serous RPE detachment is more translucent than soft drusen and there may be an associated history of previous RPE cell compromise, i.e., central serous choroidopathy when the patient was younger. There also can be diffuse bilateral, but asymmetrical changes.[9]

Choroidal Neovascular Membrane

A well-defined choroidal neovascular membrane has a classic lacy pattern seen on fluorescein angiography at the choroidal phase of the angiogram.[9,10] It is treatable with laser photocoagulation if greater than 200 μ from the foveal avascular zone center. This type of well-defined membrane is only 25 percent of all choroidal neovascular membranes.

In poorly defined/occult neovascular membranes, the pattern of fluorescein leakage does not identify a site of origin and the fluorescein shows diffuse leakage. The majority of choroidal neovascular membranes are of this type:

1. Exudate or hemorrhage at the edge of lesion
2. Uneven elevation of RPE detachment
3. Areas of irregularly elevated RPE and pigment
4. Associated sensory retinal detachment
5. Choroidal folds
6. "Notch" sign
7. Irregular or slow filling on fluorescein angiography
8. RPE tear

"Self-limited" subretinal neovascular membranes occur in the elderly, older than age 80 years, with minimal leakage on the fluorescein angiogram and can resolve spontaneously over time.

In hemorrhage RPE detachment, definite neovascularization is present.

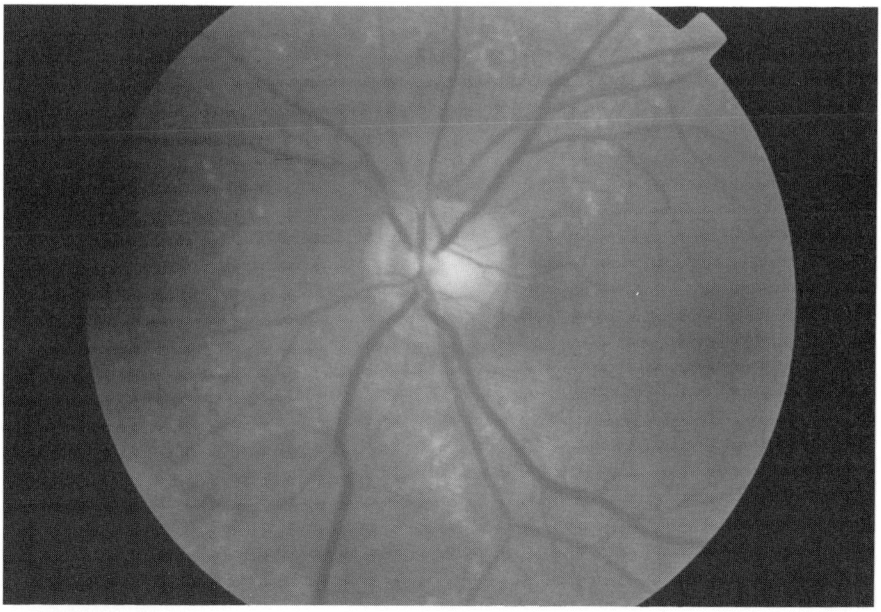

FIGURE 7–4

Mixed drusen.

Vitreous hemorrhage clears in 75 percent of patients, but the prognosis for vision is guarded.

Risk Factors

The cause of ARMD is unclear. However, some risk factors proposed include aging and light toxicity. The longer one lives past the age of 75, the greater the likelihood of developing ARMD. It is unclear whether it is the long-term cumulative exposure to light and ultraviolet radiation that causes the sequence of events leading to an accumulation of the byproducts of metabolism, e.g., lipofuscin, and hence the clinical presentation of ARMD.

Treatment

Vitamins

Vitamins A, C, E, and beta carotene have been postulated to prevent the oxidative damage from superoxide radicals in animal models; however, the clinical trials are still in progress and have not shown any efficacy. Zinc has been suggested because it is a cofactor for many of the metalloenzymes in human cell membrane interactions. However, there is no proven efficacy. In addition, there are side effects involving gastritis, copper deficiency, anemia, and cardiovascular disease.

Sunglasses

Ultraviolet-filter sunglasses should block less than 510 nm wavelengths, but all commercially available glasses block less than 400 nm wavelengths. Again, there is no proven efficacy.

Laser Photocoagulation

1. Well-defined choroidal neovascular membranes: The Macular Photocoagulation Study (MPS)[11] shows that in well-defined choroidal neovascular membranes that are 200 µ from the foveal center, laser reduces severe visual loss and postpones visual loss by 18 months or longer.
2. Serous RPE detachment: Light-grid pattern of photocoagulation may be useful.
3. Subfoveal neovascular membranes: The latest results of a controlled clinical trial reported in 1991[12] indicate that laser helps the long-term prognosis of vision over 2 years of follow up; however, after laser, there is an immediate reduction of vision.

Mainstay of Care

1. Home use of the Amsler Grid.
2. Frequent visits to the ophthalmologist.
3. Fluorescein angiography for any suspicious symptoms or clinical findings.

Low Vision Aids

1. Magnifiers, illuminators
2. Closed-circuit television
3. Talking books, large print books, talking watches
4. Telescope lenses
5. Signature guides

OTHER ACQUIRED MACULAR DISEASES

Presumed Ocular Histoplasmosis Syndrome

Anatomy and Physiology

The site of pathologic change is in the choroid and in one autopsy examination,[13] choroidal granulomas have been found to correlate with areas of macular drusenlike changes. In the presumed ocular histoplasmosis syndrome, the etiologic organism is thought to be the fungus, *Histoplasma capsulatum*, a dimorphic soil mold found in central and eastern United States. However, this organism is not found commonly in the eyes of patients with this disorder.

It is thought that focal choroiditis damages the choriocapillaris, RPE, and Bruch's membrane complex, produces an exudative detachment of the retina, may leave a focal area of atrophic RPE cells, or causes a hemorrhagic retinal detachment from neovascularization, similar to the process in ARMD. The process may leave an atrophic chorioretinal scar. Later, with recurrent episodes of inflammation, there may be a recurrence of the above active processes and finally a disciform scar may form.

Clinical Course

SYMPTOMS

Sudden blurring of vision, metamorphopsia, and a positive scotoma in one eye can occur.

On physical examination, there is a localized serous or hemorrhagic detachment of the retina involving the macula. Frequently, there is dark gray, round, or oval ring of pigment present in the serous retinal detachment. In the other eye, there may be peripapillary scars, old circumscribed, round, "punched out" lesions or scars scattered in the retina.

On fluorescein angiography, there is the leakage that one sees with subretinal neovascularization or, in the case of atrophic scars, late staining is seen.

Treatment

Similar treatment is advocated as in ARMD. Greater success can be attained in these patients with laser when the lesion is outside the foveal avascular zone. In others, however, the lesion may extend under the fovea and there is still controversy surrounding the efficacy of laser in these lesions. The ongoing clinical trial will answer this question in the 1990's. Prophylactic laser photocoagulation of scars near the macula has not been found to be useful.

Treatment with corticosteroids has not been found to be helpful in the treatment of macular lesions. Antifungal therapy does not change the macular lesions, either. As with ARMD, home use of the Amsler Grid and frequent examinations by the ophthalmologist is the mainstay of therapy.

Myopic Degeneration

Epidemiology

Myopia is the sixth leading cause of blindness in the United States.[15] Simple or congenital myopia is refractive error that tends to be stationary and nonprogressive. There are no associated retinal findings. However, degenerative myopia means greater than 6 diopters of myopia associated with elongation of the axial length and progressive choroidal degeneration of the posterior pole (Figs. 7–3 to 7–5).

Anatomy and Physiology

Visible breaks in Bruch's membrane can occur along with concomitant decrease in vision. The breaks in Bruch's membrane are associated with the same pathophysiologic mechanisms seen in ARMD.

It is believed that progressive elongation of the eye occurs and there are subsequent distention of the posterior pole and a resultant thinning of the retina and choroid.[16,17]

Clinical Course

Ruptures in Bruch's membranes are also called "lacquer cracks" in this entity. Macular hemorrhages may be seen along the break in

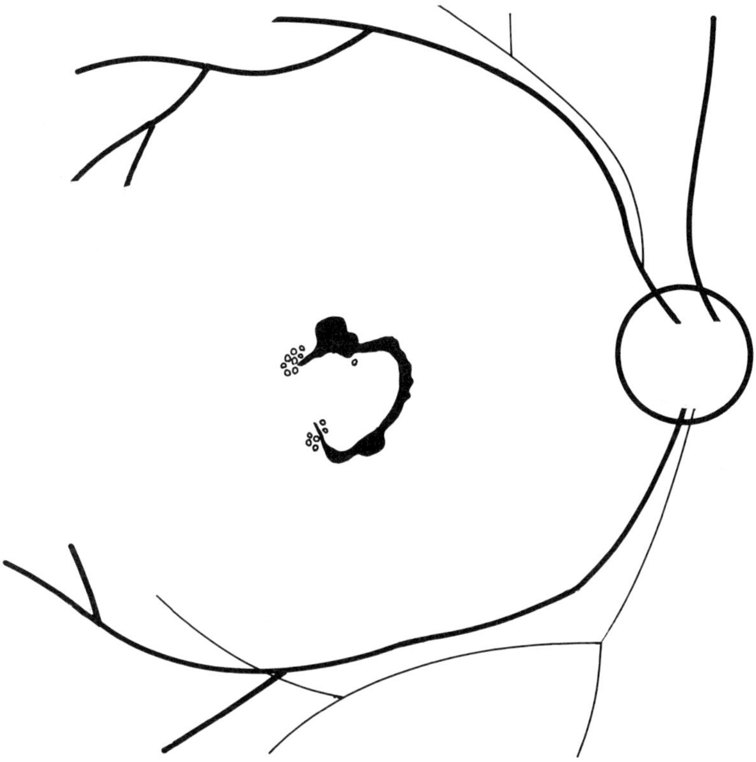

FIGURE 7–5

Choroidal neovascular membrane.

Bruch's membrane. Choroidal neovascularization can also be seen (Figs. 7–6 and 7–7).

Treatment

These neovascular membranes often affect the foveal area and laser photocoagulation is not feasible. However in some myopic membranes which are not under the foveal avascular zone, laser photocoagulation may be helpful, as in cases of ARMD.

Surgical techniques using autologous sclera to support the posterior staphyloma have been tried with limited success.

Angioid Streaks

Epidemiology

Angioid Streaks is a condition associated with pseudoxanthoma elasticum, osteitis deformans (Paget's disease), sickle cell anemia, senile elastosis of the skin, and Ehlers-Danlos syndrome.

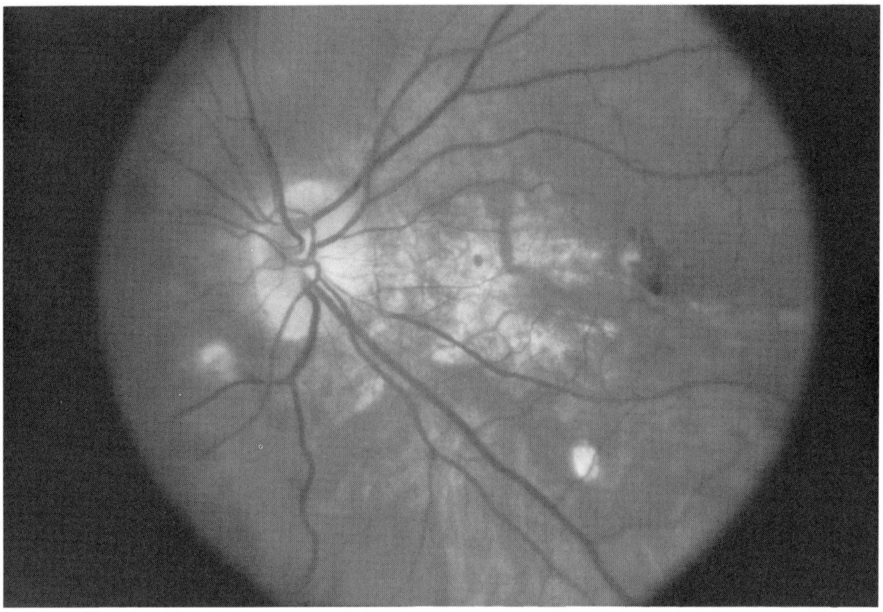

FIGURE 7-6

Myopic patient with decreased vision, 20/50, OD.

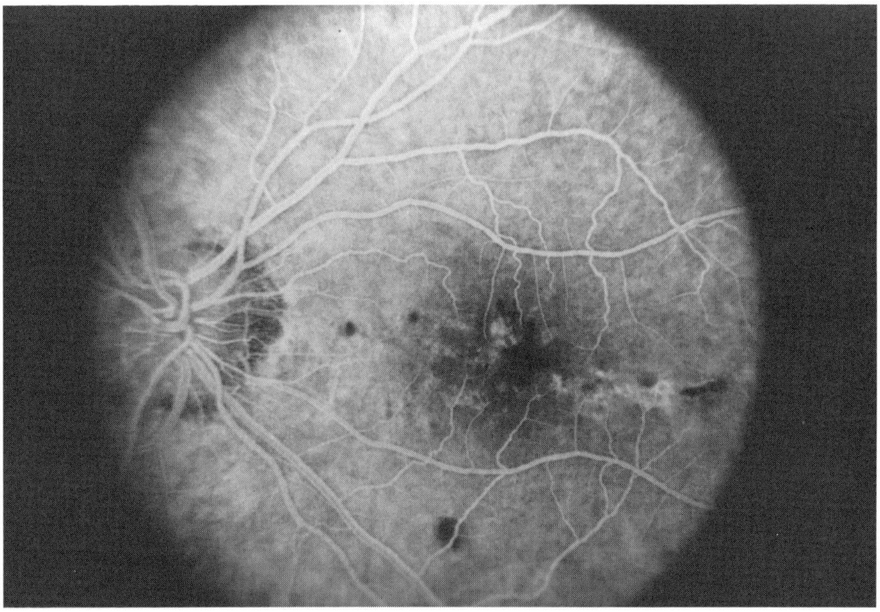

FIGURE 7-7

Fluorescein angiogram of above patient showing "lacquer cracks."

Anatomy and Physiology

These streaks represent visible cracks in Bruch's membrane.[18] It has been postulated that there may be a primary abnormality of Bruch's membrane and an increased availability of metal salts or a tendency for their pathologic deposition resulting in the brittleness of the membrane.[18]

In pseudoxanthoma elasticum, there are no normal elastic units but only abundant granulofilamentous material related to the abnormal elastic.[19] The exact biochemical alterations of pseudoxanthoma elasticum and angioid streaks have yet to be identified.

With the exception of pseudoxanthoma elasticum, which is autosomal recessive inheritance, Paget's disease and Ehlers-Danlos syndrome are autosomal dominant.

Clinical Course

Angioid streaks are gray or dark reddish lines that surround the optic disc and extend from the optic disc in radial fashion, in the second and third decade of life. There can be a speckled appearance of the fundus in patients of pseudoxanthoma elasticum.

On fluorescein angiogram, the arterial phase shows fluorescence which persists after the dye has left the veins.

Treatment

Laser treatment has been used to treat subretinal neovascularization in this disorder.

Choroidal Rupture

This entity occurs after severe blunt trauma to the globe where there is shearing forces to the affected tissue. There is then a traumatic break in Bruch's membrane that can be accompanied by subretinal neovascularization, which can occur years later. In addition, there may be the acute presentation of serous or hemorrhagic retinal detachment. Oftentimes, the choroidal rupture is filled in by scar tissue and is stable. The prognosis for good vision is excellent if the site of injury does not involve the macula.

REFERENCES

1. Leibowitz HM, Krueger HE, Maunder LR et al: The Framingham Eye Study Monograph VI. Macular Degeneration. Surv Ophthalmology 1980; *24* (suppl): 428–457

2. Hogan MJ: Role of the retinal pigment epithelium in macular disease. Trans Am Acad Ophthalmol Otolaryngol 1972; *76:* 64–80

3. Young RW: The Bowman Lecture, 1982: Biological renewal: applications to the eye. Trans Ophthalmol Soc UK 1982; *102:* 42–75

4. Grindle CFJ, Marshall J: Ageing changes in Bruch's membrane and their functional implications. Trans Ophthalmol Soc UK 1978; *98:* 172–175

5. El Baba F, Green WR, Fleischman J et al: Clinicopathologic correlation of lipidization and detachment of the retinal pigment epithelium. Am J Ophthalmol 1986; *101:* 576–583

6. Sarks SH: Ageing and degeneration in the macular region: a clinicopathological study. Br J Ophthalmol 1976; *60:* 324–341

7. Sarks SH: Drusen and their relationship to senile macular degeneration. Aust J Ophthalmol 1980; *8:* 117–130

8. Gass JDM, Jallow S, Davis B: Adult vitelliform macular detachment occurring in patients with basal laminar drusen. Am J Ophthalmol 1985; *99:* 445–459

9. Gass JDM: Pathogenesis of disciform detachment of the neuroepithelium, parts 1 and 3. Am J Ophthalmol 1967; *63:* 573–585; 617–644

10. Gass JDM: Drusen and disciform macular detachment and degeneration. Arch Ophthalmol 1973; *90:* 206–217

11. Macular Photocoagulation Study Group. Argon Laser photocoagulation for neovascular maculopathy: three-year results from randomized clinical trials. Arch Ophthalmol 1986; *104:* 694–701

12. Macular Photocoagulation Study Group. Laser photocoagulation of subfovel neovascular lesions in age-related macular degeneration. Results of a randomized clinical trial. Arch Ophthalmol 1991; *109:* 1220–1231

13. Klintworth GK, Hollingsworth AS, Lusman PA, Bradford WD: Granulomatous choroiditis in a case of disseminated histoplasmosis. Arch Ophthalmol 1973; *90:* 45–48

14. Macular Photocoagulation Study Group. Argon laser photocoagulation for ocular histoplasmosis: results of a randomized clinical trial. Arch Ophthalmol 1983; *101:* 1347–1357

15. Sperduto RD, Seigel D, Roberts J, Rowland M: Prevalence of myopia in the United States. Arch Ophthalmol 1983; *101:* 405–407

16. Curtin BJ, Karlin DB: Axial length measurements and fundus changes of the myopic eye. Am J Ophthalmol 1971; *71:* 42–53

17. Curtin BJ: The Myopias. Philadelphia, Harper & Row, 1985

18. Klein BA: Angioid streaks: a clinical and histopathological study. Am J Ophthalmol 1947; *30:* 955–965

19. Huang SN, Steele HD, Kumar G, Parker JO: Ultrastructural changes of elastic fibers in pseudoxanthoma elasticum: a study of histogenesis. Arch Pathol 1967; *83:* 108–113

CHAPTER EIGHT

Other Acquired Macular Diseases

CENTRAL SEROUS CHOROIDOPATHY

Epidemiology

Although central serous choroidopathy is a common disease for the retina specialist, it is an uncommon disease for the general ophthalmologist.

It has been associated with males more than females and it affects the younger age group of working-age Americans between the ages of 25–50 years. It has also been said that it is an entity that affects individuals in a stressful environment (Fig. 8–1).[1–3]

Anatomy and Physiology

The problem lies in the idiopathic breakdown of the retinal pigment epithelium and its ability to act as an effective barrier. There is the consequent formation of serous retinal detachments or diffuse leakage of fluid from the subretinal space.

Clinical Course

Patients complain of metamorphopsia, micropsia, central scotoma, and increasing hyperopia. Visual acuity can be in the range of 20/20 to 20/200, but oftentimes, the visual acuity levels are in the range of 20/30 to 20/60. The disease process is self-limiting and it resolves in 1 to 2 months. However, recurrences can occur in one-third to one-half of the affected patients.[4,5] The localized macular serous detachment appears to be filled with clear fluid.

Laser and Medical Treatment

Central serous choroidopathy is usually a spontaneously resolving condition requiring no treatment. Laser is considered if there is (1) persistence of serous detachments over 6 months; (2) recurrence of

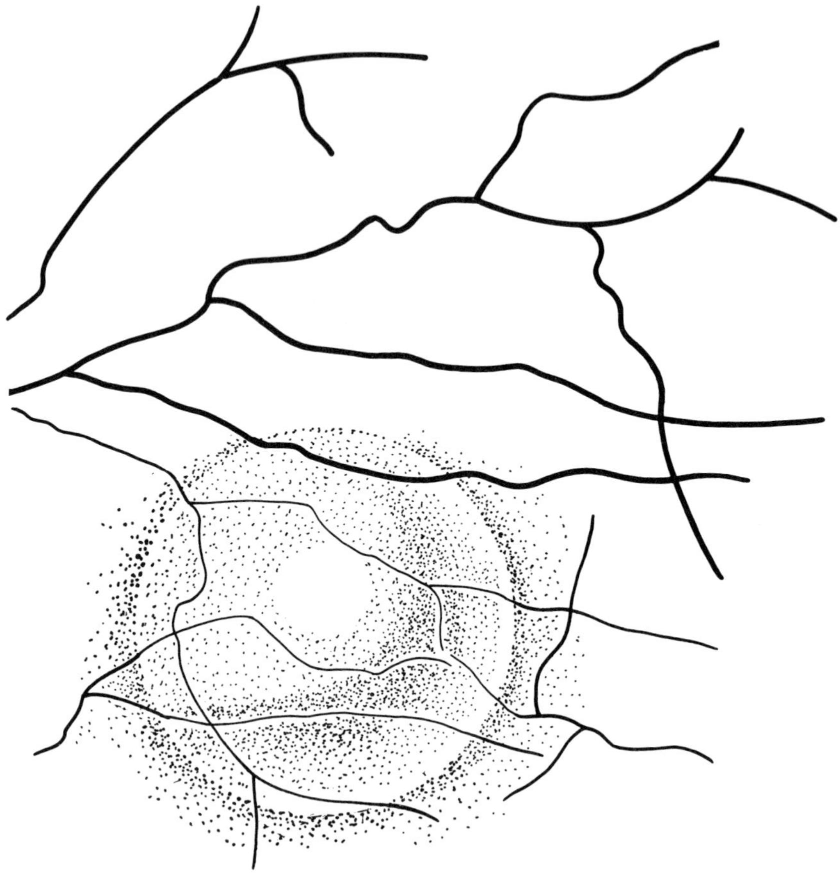

FIGURE 8–1

Central serous choroidopathy.

the same condition in an eye with a previous history of central serous choroidopathy and with resultant loss of visual function; and (3) the patient requires prompt restoration of vision because of occupational reasons.

CYSTOID MACULAR EDEMA

Irvine-Gass Syndrome[6–8]

Clinical Course

Cystoid macular edema occurs after cataract surgery, intracapsular as well as extracapsular cataract extraction. It is thought that vitreous loss plays a role and that there is localized vitreous traction. However, in cases with an intact vitreous face and an intact posterior capsule, cystoid macular edema can occur and it is postulated that release of prostaglandins during cataract surgery can cause the edema (Fig. 8–2).[9–13]

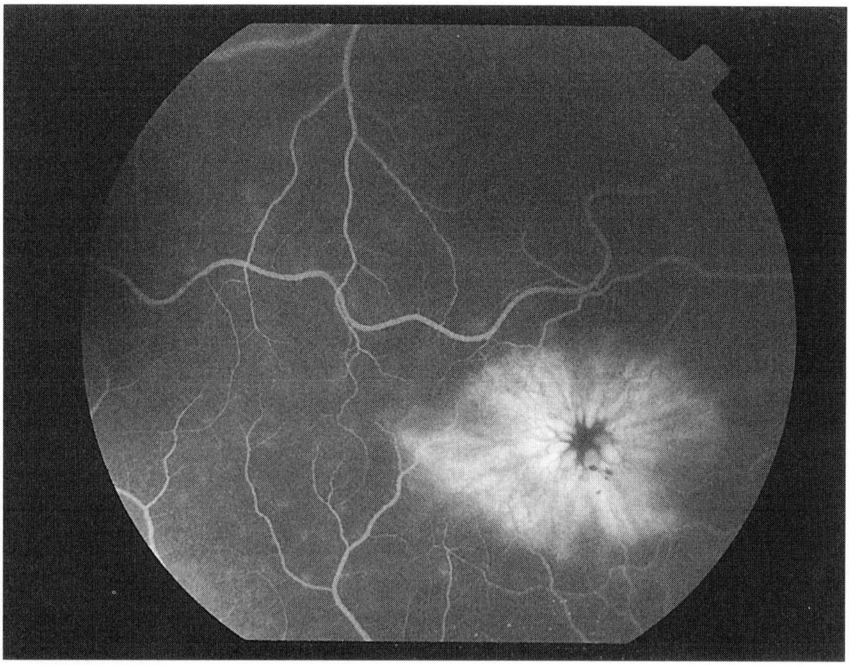

FIGURE 8-2

Cystoid macular edema, fluorescein angiogram.

Visual acuity is usually in the 20/40 to 20/100 range, occurring 1 to 3 months after surgery. There is a loss of foveal reflex in very mild cases and in some cases, there is a grainy texture to the fovea. On closer examination with a Hruby, Goldmann, or 90 diopter lenses, one can see fine cysts at the foveal area.

The prognosis for visual recovery is good. In the majority of cases, the edema will subside and the patient will achieve excellent visual acuity.[14–15] The remainder of patients will show resolution over months and years. However, a small percentage 0.5 to 2 percent of patients will not do well and have permanent visual loss from chronic cystoid macular edema.

Of course, patients with diabetes and other retinovascular disorders will be predisposed to developing cystoid macular edema.

Fluorescein Angiography

In the arterial phase of the fluorescein angiogram, there is perifoveal leakage of the capillary bed. There is also concomitant hyperfluorescence of the optic nerve suggesting abnormal vascular permeability in this entity. In the late phase of the angiogram, there is the pathognomonic formation of cysts in a flower petal-shaped pattern, hence the term, "petalloid" pattern of leakage. These cystic pockets of fluid are the accumulation of fluid in the level of the external plexiform layer.[14]

Treatment

Indomethacin topical drops, diamox, and ketorolac tromethamine have been tried with some success in decreasing the amount of cystoid macular edema postcataract surgery.[16–21]

Surgery has been useful in those cases with vitreous to the wound or chronic cystoid macular edema.[20–21]

MACULAR CYSTS AND HOLES

In the older literature, macular cysts and holes were considered different entities, however, it is now thought that macular holes and its current staging include what was previously called macular cysts.[22–23]

Macular holes occur predominantly in women in the sixth decade and beyond. They are usually idiopathic. The median visual acuity level is approximately 20/200 (Fig. 8–3).[22–23]

Stage 1 Macular Hole

Patients present with mild decrease in visual acuity or metamorphopsia only. There is clinically a decreased or absent foveal depression.

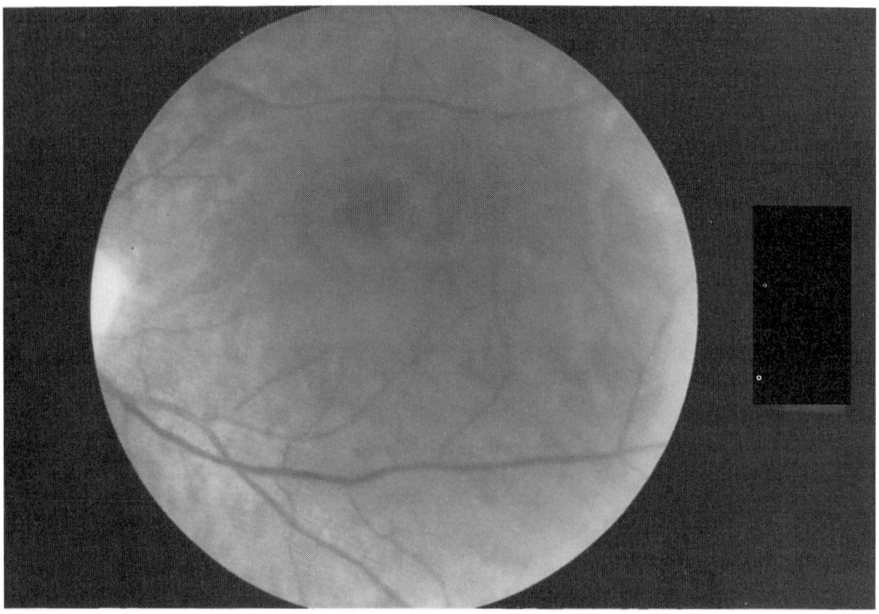

FIGURE 8–3
Macular hole, OD.

Stage 1A

The appearance of a yellow spot 100–200 μ in diameter in the center of the fovea.

Stage 1B

The appearance of a yellow ring, approximately 200–350 μ in diameter.

FLUORESCEIN ANGIOGRAPHY

There is normal or faint, central hyperfluorescence but no evidence of late staining in the areas of the yellow spot or ring.

Stage 2 Early Hole Formation

In the majority of patients, one sees the yellow ring enlarge and a full-thickness retinal dehiscence develops within several weeks or months. The retinal dehiscence begins eccentrically and as the hole enlarges, the yellow ring around it will also enlarge, becoming gray. The yellow ring will appear to coincide with the area of the hole.

Fluorescein Angiography

Focal early hyperfluorescence in the area corresponding to the macular hole. The fluorescein fades from view during later phases of angiogram. The hyperfluorescence seen in this state is more intense than in stage 1.

Stage 3 Fully Developed Macular Hole with Vitreofoveal Separation

Vision is now 20/70 to 20/400 range. Diameter of the hole is in the 500 μ range. There is an operculum suspended over the macular hole, which is visible with retroillumination (Fig. 8–3).

Fluorescein Angiography

Hyperfluorescence in the late stages of the fluorescein angiogram corresponds to the macular hole.

Stage 4 Macular Hole with Posterior Vitreous Separation

This stage happens in a small minority of cases where the overlying vitreous is fully detached from the area of the posterior pole. It is postulated that the etiology of macular holes is not only in anteroposterior vitreous traction but tangential vitreous traction.[24]

In some cases, the macular hole has been known to reverse itself. This is probably most likely secondary to Stage 1A holes where once there is a posterior vitreous detachment, the tangential traction component and anteroposterior component is removed and the fovea settles back to its original place.[25]

Surgery

Surgical treatment would be the removal of the layer of vitreous or hyaloidal membrane creating the tangential traction. Usually after such vitreous surgery, internal gas tamponade is necessary and no endolaser treatment is necessary. Improvement of visual acuity has been noted after successful surgery; however, there are complications to this type of surgery such that the macular hole could be enlarged as a result of the surgery and there would be poor postoperative visual outcome.[26–27]

MACULAR PUCKER

Epiretinal membrane formation can occur in elderly patients in the sixth and seventh decade of life. Systemic hypertension has been implicated and there is a preponderance of women to men with macular pucker. Usually surgery is performed when the level of visual acuity is 20/60 or worse. Surgical treatment is the preferred treatment of choice with excellent visual results in the hands of experienced surgeons (Fig. 8–4).[28]

PHOTIC RETINAL INJURY

Solar Retinopathy

Solar retinopathy can occur with brief solar observation during a solar eclipse because of pupillary dilation from dark adaptation. With a constricted pupil, prolonged solar observation for as seen in religious rituals or while under the influence of hallucinogenic or recreational drugs will also lead to solar retinopathy.[29–30]

Solar retinopathy presents as an acute small yellowish white foveolar lesion. Over a period of 1–2 weeks, the lesion fades and shows some retinal pigment epithelial changes. The visual complaints range from metamorphopsia, afterimage, erythropsia, blurred vision, and central scotoma. Visual acuity is reduced to 20/40 to 20/100 range.

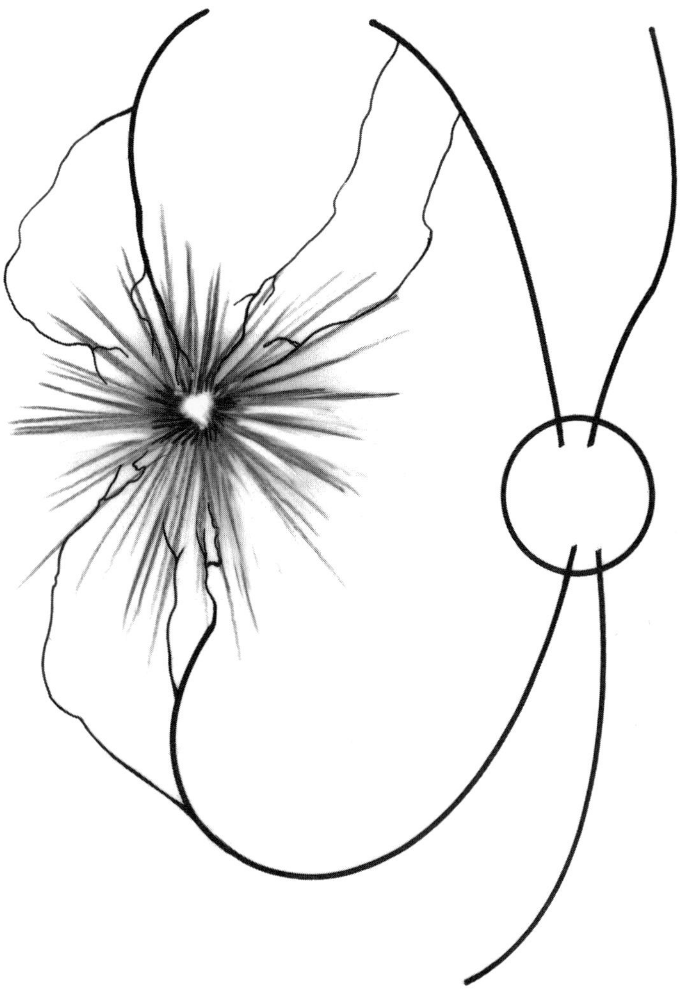

FIGURE 8–4

Macular pucker.

Fluorescein Angiography

Typically there are late transmission defects in the areas corresponding to the lesion seen ophthalmoscopically.

Photic Retinal Injury with the Operating Microscope

Photic retinal injuries with the operating microscope have been reported with cataract surgery with and without intraocular lens, and after refractive surgery in phakic patients.[31–36] Similar injuries have been found with vitreous surgery and the use of fiberoptic endoilluminators or "lightpipes."[37–38]

Operating microscope injuries are either oval lesions or they are in the shape of the rectangular filament from the operating microscope, located in the macula or adjacent to the macula. Initially, there is a yellowish white appearance of the lesion that fades over time to reveal retinal pigment epithelial disruption and irregularity. The visual loss is related to the location and the size of the lesion.

Subtle lesions of light toxicity with the operating microscope may include postoperative erythropsia that may be the clinical equivalent of damage to the blue sensitive cones—which has been observed in the primate animal model.[39–41]

Fluorescein Angiography

There is late hyperfluorescence in the areas of retinal pigment epithelial lesion.

Prevention

The duration of the patient's exposure to light should be minimized by the use of an occluder or para-axial illumination whenever coaxial illumination is not essential.

REFERENCES

1. Yannuzzi LA: Type A behavior and central serous choroidopathy. Trans Am Ophthalmol Soc 1986; *84:* 799–845

2. Gilbert CM, Owens Sl, Smith PD, Fine Sl: Long term follow-up of central serous chorioretinopathy. Br J Ophthalmol 1984; *68:* 815–820

3. Klein ML, Van Buskirk EM, Friedman E et al: Experience with non-treatment of central serous choroidopathy. Arch Ophthalmol 1974; *91:* 247–250

4. Gass JDM: Pathogenesis of disciform detachment of the neuroepithelium: I. General concepts and classification. Am J Ophthalmol 1967; *63:* 573–585

5. Gass JDM: Pathogenesis of disciform detachment of the neuroepithelium: II. Idiopathic central serous choroidopathy. Am J Ophthalmol 1967; *63:* 587–615

6. Irvine SR: A newly defined vitreous syndrome following cataract surgery: interpreted according to recent concepts of the structure of the vitreous. Am J Ophthalmol 1953; 599–619

7. Gass JDM, Norton EWD: Cystoid macular edema and papilledema following cataract extraction. A funduscopic and angiographic study. Arch Ophthalmol 1966; *76:* 646–661

8. Gass JDM, Anderson DR, Davis EB: A clinical, fluorescein angiographic and electron microscopic correlation of cystoid macular edema. Am J Ophthalmol 1985; *100:* 82–85

9. Miyake K: Presentation of cystoid macular edema after lens extraction by topical indomethacin I. A preliminary report. Graefes Arch Klin Exp Ophthalmol 1977; *203:* 81–88

10. Miyake K, Sakamura S, Miura H: Long-term follow-up study on prevention of aphakic cystoid macular edema by topical indomethacin. Br J Ophthalmol 1980; *64:* 324–328

11. Cunha-Vas JG, Travassos A: Breakdown of the blood-retinal barriers and cystoid macular edema. Surv Ophthalmol 1984; *28* (suppl.): 485–492

12. Sears ML: Aphakic cystoid macular edema: the pharmacology of ocular trauma. Surv Ophthalmol 1984; *28* (suppl.): 525–534

13. Sears ML, Neufeld AH, Jampol LM: Prostaglandins. Invest Ophthalmol 1973; *12:* 161–164

14. Gass JDM, Norton EWD: Follow-up of cystoid macular edema following cataract extraction. Trans Am Acad Ophthalmol Otolaryngol 1969; *73:* 665–682

15. Jacobson DR, Dellaporta A: Natural history of cystoid macular edema after cataract extraction. Am J Ophthalmol 1974; *77:* 445–447

16. Kraff MC, Sanders DR, Jampol LM et al: Prophylaxis of pseudophakic cystoid macular edema with topical indomethacin. Ophthalmol 1982; *89:* 885–890

17. Yannuzzi LA, Landau AN, Turtz AI: Incidence of aphakic cystoid macular edema with the use of topical indomethacin. Ophthalmol 1981; *88:* 947–954

18. Cox SN, Hay E, Bird AC: Treatment of chronic macular edema with acetazolamide. Arch Ophthalmol 1988; *106:* 1190–1193

19. Flach AJ, Jampol LM, Weinberg D et al: Improvement in visual acuity in chronic aphakic and pseudopahic cystoid macular edema after treatment with topical 0.5% ketorolac tromethamine. Am J Ophthalmol 1991; *112:* 514–519

20. Fung WE: Anterior vitrectomy for chronic aphakic cystoid macular edema. Ophthalmol 1980; *87:* 189–193

21. Fung WE, Vitrectomy-ACME group: Vitrectomy for chronic aphakic systoid macular edema: results of a national, collaborative prospective, randomized investigation. Ophthalmol 1985; *92:* 1102–1111

22. Gass JDM: Idiopathic senile macular holes: its early stages and pathogenesis. Arch Ophthalmol 1988; *106:* 629–639

23. Morgan CM, Schatz H: Idiopathic macular holes. Am J Ophthalmol 1985; *99:* 437–444

24. Akiba J, Yoshida A, Trempe CL: Risk of developing a macular hole. Arch Ophthalmol 1990; *108:* 1088–1090

25. Wiznia RA: Reversibility of the early stages of idiopathic macular holes. Am J Ophthalmol 1989; *107:* 241–245

26. Gonvers M, Machemer R: A new approach to treating retinal detachment with macular hole. Am J Ophthalmol 1982; *94:* 468–472

27. Harris MJ, De Bustros S, Michels RG: Treatment of retinal detachment due to macular holes. Retina 1984; *4:* 144–147

28. Michels RG: Vitrectomy for macular pucker. Ophthalmol 1984; *91:* 1384–1388

29. Sliney DH, Mainster MA: Potential laser hazards to the clinician during photocoagulation. Am J Ophthalmol 1987; *103:* 758–760

30. White TJ, Mainster MA, Wilson PW, Tips JH: Chorioretinal temperature increases from solar observation. Bull Math Biophys 1971; *33:* 1–17

31. Macy JL, Baerveldt G: Pseudophakic serous maculopathy. Arch Ophthalmol 1983; *101:* 228–231

32. MacDonald HR, Irvine AR: Light induced maculopathy from the operating microscope in extracapsular cataract extraction and intraocular lens implantation. Ophthalmology 1983; *90:* 945–951

33. Boldrey EE, Ho BT, Griffith RD: Retinal burns occurring at cataract extraction. Ophthalmol 1984; *91:* 1297–1302

34. Brod RD, Barron BA, Suelflow JA et al: Phototoxic retinal damage during refractive surgery. Am J Ophthalmol 1986; *102:* 121–123

35. Kwarg SG, Geohegan M, Hanscom TA: Light-induced maculopathy from the operating microscope. Am J Ophthalmol 1984; *98:* 628–630

36. Robertson DM, Reldman RB: Photic retinopathy from the operating room microscope. Am J Ophthalmol 1986; *101:* 561–569

37. Fuller D, Machemer R, Knighton RW: Retinal damage produced by intraocular fiber optic light. Am J Ophthalmol 1978; *85:* 519–537

38. Rinkoff J, Machemer R, Hida T, Chandler D: Temperature dependent light damage to the retina. Am J Ophthalmol 1986; *102:* 452–462

39. Kamel ID, Parker JA: Protection from ultraviolet exposure in aphakic erythropsia. Can J Ophthalmol 1973; *8:* 563–565

40. Sperling HG, Johnson C, Harweth RS: Differential spectral photic damage to primate cones. Vision Res 1980; *20:* 1117–1125

41. Mainster MA: Light and macular degeneration: a biosphysical and clinical perspective. Eye 1987; *1:* 304–310

CHAPTER NINE

Endophthalmitis

EPIDEMIOLOGY

The incidence of endophthalmitis is approximately 0.3–0.5 percent in the United States and Europe.[1–3] It is a devastating complication of ocular surgery, penetrating trauma, and systemic infection. The majority of cases achieve 20/400 or better vision in this present era of vitrectomy and intravitreal antibiotics.[4]

POSTOPERATIVE ENDOPHTHALMITIS

Approximately 90 percent of culture-positive postoperative endophthalmitis is from gram-positive aerobic bacteria.[5] Of this group, 20–50 percent is from *Staphylococcal aureus* and *S. epidermidis.* Common anaerobic gram-positive bacteria causing endophthalmitis include *Streptococcus, Peptostreptococcus, Propionibacterium acnes, Clostridium.* The minority (7 percent) of postoperative endophthalmitis is due to gram-negative bacteria. Most commonly, they are *Pseudomonas aeruginosa, Proteus, Hemophilus influenzae, Klebsiella pneumoniae, Escherichia coli, Enterobacter aerogenes.* Least common are fungal causes of endophthalmitis (3 percent). The most commonly cultured fungal organisms are *Cephalosporium, Paecilomyces, Candida, Aspergillus, Penicillium.*[5]

Fungal organisms are found in posttraumatic mycotic endophthalmitis. The responsible organism is a saprophytic organism found on the penetrating foreign body. Such infections indolently present in the first month postsurgery. There are varying degrees of pain and erythema. On physical examination, there is a marked anterior chamber reaction with cells, flare, and later followed by hypopyon formation. The next area affected is the anterior vitreous and then later the posterior vitreous. Satellite vitreous balls may appear. Diagnosis and treatment is the same as with all endophthalmitis (See following text) (Fig. 9–1).

ENDOGENOUS ENDOPHTHALMITIS

Endogenous endophthamitis is caused by infectious agents originating in septicemia or other remote loci of infection. The majority

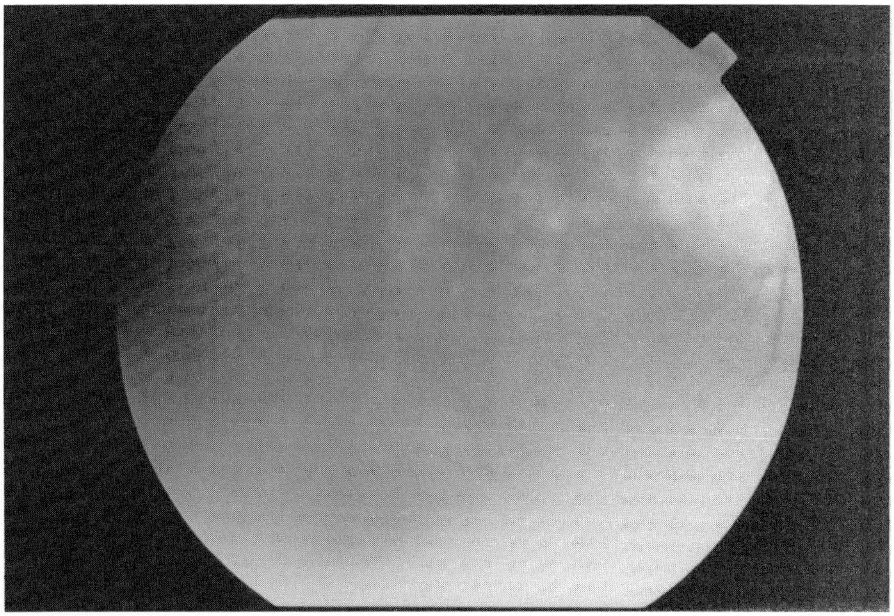

FIGURE 9–1

Endophthalmitis in an 89-year-old male 1 week after cataract surgery, OD. Vitreous haze is prominent.

of endogenous cases are from *Candida albicans*.[6,7] Second in frequency to *Candida* is *Aspergillus fumigatus*, and then *A. flavus*.[8] Endogenous fungal endophthalmitis has an insidious onset and slow progression of symptoms. In the early course of disease, the anterior segment manifests as an apparently nonspecific iridocyclitis, but hypopyon and even corneal and corneal perforation can develop eventually. Endogenous bacterial endophthalmitis is rare, and the most common cause is *S. aureus, or S. pneumoniae*.[9,10]

CHRONIC ENDOPHTHALMITIS

Chronic endophthalmitis is an endophthalmitis that appears more than 1 month postoperatively and may persist for several more months afterwards. In 1986, Meisler and colleagues reported 6 patients with chronic postoperative endophthalmitis, whose aqueous or vitreous culture was positive for *Propionibacterium* species, usually *P. acnes*.[11–14] *P. acnes* is a gram-positive, nonspore-forming pleomorphic bacillus that is ubiquitous in nature and inhabits hair follicles and sebaceous glands of the skin. It is commonly found in the anaerobic flora of the conjunctiva.

In most patients, *P. acnes* presents in the weeks or months after the initial postoperative period. There can be a gradually progressive low-grade inflammation or an abrupt onset of severe intraocular inflammation with hypopyon. Many patients will show granulomatous-appearing precipitates on the corneal endothelium or on the surfaces of the intraocular lens implant. Fibrin-beaded strands across the anterior chamber have been observed in some eyes. The patients also present with a creamy white plaque within the peripheral capsular bag or sandwiched between the intraocular lens and posterior capsule.

At time of vitrectomy, the capsular plaque needs to be cleaned and part of the capsule may be removed as a specimen. *P. acnes* is sensitive to cephalosporins, clindamycin, and penicillin. Vancomycin is an effective antibiotic against *P. acnes* and other gram-positive organisms.

Treatment failures have occurred despite intravitreal injection of appropriate antibiotics. An antibiotic injected once into the vitreous cavity may not remain in sufficiently high concentration to ensure activity during the replicative phase of the organism in the interstices of peripheral capsular bag.[11–14]

The procedure of last resort is the removal of the implant and the entire capsular bag where organisms are presumably sequestered. Injection of alpha-chymotrypsin may allow removal of the entire capsular bag and the intraocular lens complex. Additional vitrectomy surgery may be required.[15,16]

Infected Filtering Blebs

A red eye with mucoid discharge, with pain, tenderness, and photophobia occurs in patients after glaucoma filtration surgery. There can be purulence filling the filtration area. Iritis, hypopyon, and vitritis can occur as well. *Streptococcus* species can be commonly identified.[17,18]

Posttraumatic Injury

Cellular infiltration occurs around the locus of entry or injury site. Severe iritis with hypopyon is common. Tissue necrosis can occur with endophthalmitis, panophthalmitis, and cellulitis. Retained foreign material in the eye can produce a severe and aggressive endophthalmitis. Most commonly seen are *Bacillus* species-resistant to penicillin and cephalosporins, but sensitive to vancomycin or clindamycin.

HISTORY

It is important to note any systemic infectious disease, indwelling catheters, type of eye injury, or previous surgery. Ascertain the length of time between surgery or trauma and the onset of symptoms. Inquire as to prior antibiotic (topical, systemic) and steroid use. Antibiotic treatment (intravitreal, subconjunctival, systemic and topical) should be recorded as well.

DIAGNOSIS

Slit-lamp evaluation of the cornea with respect to clarity and thickness, condition of surgical wound or entry of trauma, degree of anterior chamber reaction, hypopyon are important clinical considerations. Indirect ophthalmoscopic examination of the fundus is important. The clarity of vitreous, visibility of retina, and presence or absence of a red reflex should be evaluated.

Ultrasound can define the location and degree of vitreous condensation, status of the retina (attached or detached), and presence of choroidal swelling.

Electroretinography may play a role in defining long-term visual prognosis.[19]

Vitreous Aspirate and Anterior Chamber Aspirate

The anterior chamber aspirate can be taken at the time of surgery when the patient is taken to the operating room. A 25-gauge needle on a 1 ml tuberculin syringe is introduced into the anterior chamber through a paracentesis incision. 0.1–0.2 ml of fluid is aspirated.

Posterior chamber aspirate via vitrectomy is crucial. This specimen can be collected into a small syringe (0.2–0.3 ml) for delivery to the bacteriology laboratory. This specimen is plated onto various media: blood agar, chocolate agar, thiol or other anaerobic media, brain-heart infusion, and Lowenstein's and Sabouraud's agars. The remainder of the pars plana vitrectomy specimen with the infusion fluid serving as a diluent, can be sent to the laboratory after the procedure is completed. The diluted sample can be filtered with a disposable, sterile membrane filter system. The filter is removed under sterile conditions, cut up, and innoculated onto media.

Microbiology

Culture specimens once obtained, should be sent for innoculation into both liquid and solid media, and the media should be incubated aerobically and anaerobically. *P. acnes* has been isolated in thioglycolate broth and cooked meat as well as on prereduced anaerobic blood agar.[13]

Specimens may be plated onto various media: blood agar, chocolate agar, thiol or other anaerobic media, brain-heart infusion, and Lowenstein's and Sabouraud's agars. Gram stain should be performed for appropriate antibiotic management of the patient immediately after surgery, before the final culture results are ready. At 18–24 hours, a culture diagnosis is usually available.

TREATMENT

Pars plana Vitrectomy and Intravitreal Antibiotics

Whereas vitrectomy alone has proved ineffective in sterilizing the vitreous cavity in aphakic[20] and phakic rabbit[21] models of *S. aureus* endophthalmitis, vitrectomy is useful in cases with *S. epidermidis* endophthalmitis.[20] In acute bacterial disease, vitrectomy is indicated when the vitreous is involved.[21] Pars plana vitrectomy serves to remove the high concentration of infectious organisms inside a closed system, such as the eye. If there are plaques of material on the implant, one has to consider the removal of the precipitates or plaques of material. Oftentimes, the corneal view is poor secondary to folds in Descemet's membrane or thickened cornea from inflammation. The vitrectomy is often performed under these difficult circumstances. In some eyes, the acute phase of infection may be managed successfully with salvage of the globe, but poor vision may result from persistent inflammatory opacities of the media. In these postinfectious cases, removal of the opacities may be accomplished by vitrectomy. In cases of fungal disease, vitrectomy is indicated for diagnostic and therapeutic purposes.[22,23]

Intravitreal injection of antibiotics addresses the issue of subtherapeutic levels of antibiotics when delivered through systemic and periocular routes. The use of intravitreal antibiotic injection has been advocated for almost two decades.[24,25] The intravitreal solution is usually injected with the bevel of the needle aimed towards the anterior chamber in the anterior to mid vitreous.

Some common intravitreal antibiotics are ceftazidime 2.25 mg in 0.1 ml of water, amikacin 400 μg in 0.1 ml of water, vancomycin 1000 μg in 0.1 ml of water.

Topical Antibiotics

Postoperative endophthalmitis is caused by organisms colonizing the eyelid margin and conjunctiva. Studies of antibiotic prophylaxis in nonophthalmic surgery have demonstrated that the most effective time for administration of the antibiotics is in the immediate 2-hour period prior to surgery.[26] Topical medications play a limited role in endophthalmitis. The relative concentration of medicine that reaches the anterior chamber and vitreous is low and in most cases of endophthalmitis, topical antibiotics are not used very often. However, topical medications may be used to prevent anterior chamber infection and necrosis.

Periocular Injections

Antibiotic concentrations can be effectively achieved and maintained with periocular injections. Subconjunctival injections can be given as often as every 12 hours. The conjunctiva is usually anesthetized with proparacaine or 4 percent cocaine. A preliminary injection of 0.2 ml of xylocaine can be given at the planned injection site. Approximately 0.2 ml of 2% xylocaine can be added to the antibiotic solution in the syringe. Animal studies have demonstrated the benefit of subconjunctival antibiotics.[26] There is a risk of macular infarction with subconjunctival injection of aminoglycosides such as gentamicin.[28]

Systemic Antibiotics

This is a necessary mode of antibiotic therapy for endophthalmitis. It is used in most clinical centers to provide inhibitory concentrations of the antibiotic dose. The Infectious Disease Service of the hospital staff can contribute to the overall management of the patient while on systemic intravenous antibiotics.

The combination of an aminoglycoside and cephalosporin intravenously provides broad spectrum antibiotic coverage for gram-positive and gram-negative organisms. Quinolone antibiotics, such as ciprofloxacin, is effective against many of the methicillin-resistant *Staphylococci*, in contrast to the aminoglycosides. We must be concerned about the possible emergence of resistance with routine prophylactic use of any agent. However, this is less likely within the first 24-hour course of treatment when awaiting bacterial culture results.

REFERENCES

1. Fisch A, Salvanet A, Prazuck T et al: The French collaborative Study group on Endophthalmitis. Epidemiology of infective endophthalmitis in France. Lancet 1991; *338:* 1373–1376

2. Allen HF, Mangiaracine AB: Bacterial endophthalmitis after cataract extraction. A study of 22 infections in 20,000 operations. Arch Ophthalmol 1964; *72:* 454–462

3. Allen HF: Symposium: postoperative endophthalmitis. Prevention of postoperative endophthalmitis. Ophthalmol 1978; *85:* 386–389

4. Puliafito CA, Baker AS, Haaf J, Foster CS: Infectious endophthalmitis. Ophthalmol 1982; *89:* 921–929

5. Olson JC, Flynn HW Jr, Forster RK, Culbertson WW: Results in the treatment of post-operative endophthalmitis. Ophthalmol 1983; *90:* 692–699

6. Edwards JE, Foos RY, Montgomerie JZ: Ocular manifestations of *Candida* septicemia: review of seventy six cases of hematogenous *Candida* endophthalmitis. Medicine 1974; *53:* 47–50

7. Parke DW, Jones DB, Gentry LO: Endogenous *Candida albicans* endophthalmitis among patients with candidemia. Ophthalmol 1982; *89:* 789–796

8. Doft BH, Clarkson JG, Rebell G, Forster RK: Endogenous *Aspergillus* endophthalmitis in drug abusers. Arch Ophthalmol 1980; *98:* 859–862

9. Smolin G, Tabbara K, Whitcher J: Infectious Disease of the Eye. Baltimore, Williams & Wilkins, 1984

10. Garmel J, Allansmith M: Metastatic *Staphylococcal* endophthalmitis presenting as chronic iridiocyclitis. Am J Ophthalmol 1974; *77:* 454–458

11. Jaffe GJ, Whitcher JP, Biswell R, Irvine AR: *Propionibacterium* endophthalmitis after extracapsular cataract extraction and intraocular lens implantation. Am J Ophthalmol 1986; *102:* 733–739

12. Meisler DM, Palestine AG, Vastine DW: Chronic *Propionibacterium* endophthalmitis after extracapsular cataract extraction and intraocular lens implantation. Am J Ophthalmol 1986; *102:* 733–739

13. Meisler DM, Mandelbaum S: *Propionibacterium:* associated endophthalmitis in extracapsular cataract extraction: review of reported cases. Ophthalmol 1989; *96:* 54–61

14. Roussel TJ, Culbertson WW, Jaffe NS: Chronic postoperative endophthalmitis associated with *Propionibacterium acnes.* Arch Ophthalmol 1987; *105:* 1199–2001

15. Stern GA, Engel HM, Driebe WT: Recurrent postoperative endophthalmitis. Cornea 1990; *9:* 102–107

16. Pflugfelder SC, Hernandez E, Fliesler SJ et al: Intravitreal vancomycin: toxicity, clearance, interaction with gentamicin. Arch Ophthalmol 1987; *105:* 831–847

17. Bellows R, McCulley J: Endophthalmitis in aphakic patients with unplanned filtering blebs wearing contact lenses. Ophthalmol 1981; *88:* 839-843

18. Mandelbaum S, Forster RK, Gelender H, Culbertson WW: Late onset endophthalmitis associated with filtering blebs. Ophthalmol 1985; *92:* 964–972

19. Verbraeken H, Van Laetham J: Treatment of endophthalmitis with and without pars plana vitrectomy. Ophthalmologica 1985; *191:* 1–3

20. Talley AR, D'Amico DJ, Talamo JH et al: The role of vitrectomy in the treatment of postoperative bacterial endophthalmitis. Arch Ophthalmol 1987; *104:* 1699–1702

21. Cottingham AJ Jr, Forster RK: Vitrectomy in endophthalmitis: results of study using vitrectomy, intraocular antibiotics or combination of both. Arch Ophthalmol 1976; *94:* 2078–2081

22. Forster RK, Abbott RL, Gelender H: Management of infectious endophthalmitis. Ophthalmol 1980; *87:* 313–319

23. Rowsey JJ, Newsom DL, Sexton DJ, Harms WK: Endophthalmitis: current approaches. Ophthalmol 1982; *89:* 1055–1066

24. Peyman G: Antibiotic administration in the treatment of bacterial endophthalmitis II. Intravitreal injections. Surv Ophthlamol 1977; *21:* 332–346

25. Baum J, Peyman GA, Barza M: Intravitreal administration of antibiotic in the treatment of bacterial endophthalmitis. III. Surv Ophthalmol 1982; *26:* 204–206

26. Classen DC, Evans RS, Pestonick SL et al: The timing of prophylactic administration of antibiotics and the risk of surgical wound infection. N Engl J Med 1992; *326:* 281–286

27. Shockley RK, Fishman P, Aziz M: Subconjunctival administration of ceftazidime in pigmented rabbit eyes. Arch Ophthalmol 1986; *104:* 266–268

28. Campochiaro PA, Conway BP: Aminoglycoside toxicity: a survey of retinal specialists; implications for ocular use. Arch Ophthalmol 1991: *109:* 946–950

Infectious Diseases

EPIDEMIOLOGY

Infectious diseases may affect one part of the body initially, but then present in the retina or the posterior portion of the eye. In the case of bacterial or fungal infection, a thorough history and examination of the previous medical record may be helpful in understanding the pathogenesis of visual loss. Blood cultures can be diagnostic and guide the clinician towards the ocular diagnosis. However, in some instances, the laboratory diagnostic evaluation is not helpful and the clinical picture remains perplexing.

The incidence of infectious diseases involving the retina is low in the healthy immunocompetent host. However, as more patients with acquired immunodeficiency syndrome (AIDS) are seen by ophthalmologists and other healthcare practitioners, infectious diseases affecting the eye and the retina will be of concern.

TUBERCULOSIS

Tuberculosis in the retina and choroid is seen in posterior uveitis, solitary mass lesion of the choroid, e.g., a tuberculoma and multiple choroidal infarcts.

Epidemiology

In the 1920's to the 1940's, tuberculosis and associated eye lesions were commonly diagnosed, however, it is rarely diagnosed today.

Anatomy and Pathophysiology

Tuberculosis affecting the ocular tissues can occur weeks, months, and even years after active infection. It is not clear whether the ophthalmic manifestations are a result of autoimmune phenomena or part of an active infectious process.

Diagnosis

Diagnosis is made by purified protein derivative (PPD) testing with the 1 tuberculin unit strength or in the patient with a previous history of PPD testing, the 5 tuberculin unit strength PPD may be useful. The PPD is placed intradermally and examined at 24 and 48 hours. Gastric washings and bronchial washings are useful. A chest X-ray is useful in a patient who is having his first evaluation of tuberculosis. However, a chest X-ray will not diagnose tuberculosis of the gastrointestinal system, adrenal glands, renal system, bones, or the cervical lymph nodes.

In some instances, there is a negative laboratory workup and one must rely on other clinical signs such as, old scarring of the eyelids, ectropion, and chronic draining lacrimal fistulas to the skin.

In primary tuberculosis, there may be small conjunctival ulcerations of the tarsal surface, regional lymphadenitis with caseating nodes, hypertrophic papillary conjunctivitis, and extensive granulation tissue.

Tuberculosis can rarely cause interstitial keratitis. Phlyctenular keratoconjunctivitis is thought to be the allergic response to tuberculin protein.

Granulomatous uveitis is common with associated posterior uveitis or focal or diffuse choroiditis. Choroiditis, choroidal hemorrhages and neovascularization has been documented in patients with miliary tuberculosis.[1–3]

Optic neuritis, papilledema, and papillitis has also been seen in tuberculosis.

Fluorescein Angiography

Tuberculosis affects the choroid more than the retina. In the early phase angiograms, there may be mottling of the choroid and in some cases where there is a solitary tuberculoma of the choroid, it may mimic malignant melanoma.

As in other vasculitis, the fluorescein angiogram shows leakage of the retinal vessel corresponding to the areas of vasculitis.

Management

The treatment of the primary disease process is useful in primary tuberculosis. Otherwise, in some cases where the laboratory evaluation is negative and it is assumed that the retinal and choroidal changes are immunomediated, it is important to involve the Infectious Disease specialists in your hospital or community for guidance. The patient is given isoniazid 300 mg orally every day. Adjunctive therapy of para-aminosalicylic acid (PAS) may also be given. Ethambutol 20–25 mg/kg of body weight per day for several weeks is also given.

SYPHILIS

Epidemiology

Formerly a rare entity in ophthalmologists' offices, however, as patients with AIDS are more common, syphilis is becoming more prevalent.

Anatomy and Pathophysiology

Ocular manifestations of syphilis occurs in secondary syphilis, occurring 6 weeks to 6 months after the primary infection. The infection is characterized by malaise, fever, hair loss, papular macular rash, condyloma latum, mucous patches, and generalized lymphadenopathy. Approximately 1 in 20 patients with secondary syphilis will show uveitis. Half of the cases are bilateral.

Commonly, the fundus changes seen in posterior vitritis are multiple, nonelevated yellowish gray, ill-defined chorioretinal lesions that often are confluent in the posterior pole and midperiphery of the fundus. If the lesions are seen near the optic disc, there may be associated flame-shaped hemorrhages. In addition, there is perivasculitis, occlusive arterial disease, and retinitis proliferans. Choroidal neovascularization may occur as well (Fig. 10–1).[4–7]

Congenital syphilis is characteristically the salt and pepper fundus seen in the periphery of the retina. There is narrowing of the retinal vessels, optic disc pallor, and a picture that mimicks retinitis pigmentosa, hence the name, pseudoretinitis.

Diagnosis

Venereal Disease Research Laboratory (VDRL) test is nonspecific whereas flourescent treponemal antibody absorption (FTA-ABS) test is specific, with positivity seen years after treatment. MAHA-TP should be considered. In this current age of AIDS, one might also discuss the possibility of human immunodeficiency virus testing for the patient. Some cases of luetic chorioretinitis may mimic the acute retinal necrosis syndrome.

Fluorescein Angiography

Because syphilis is largely a choroidal disease, one must look at the early stages of the angiogram for changes in the choroid. There is

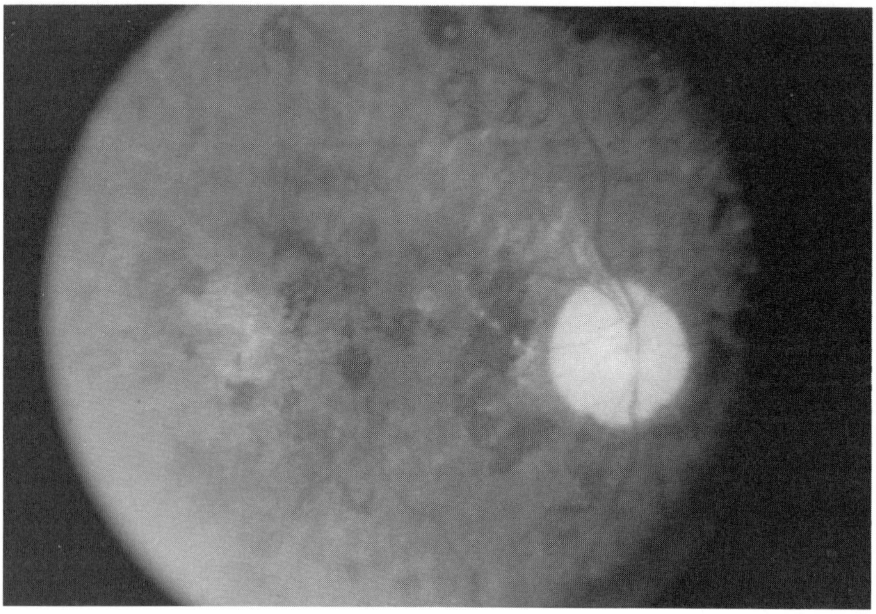

FIGURE 10–1
Syphilis.

early choroidal hypofluorescence with late staining. There can be serous retinal detachments that can progress over the course of disease and can regress with treatment.

Treatment

Intravenous penicillin G, (2.4 million U intravenously every 4 hours for 1 week) and intramuscular injection of benzathine penicillin is helpful every week for three weeks for the treatment of active disease. For congenital syphilis, there is no treatment for the reversal of the fundus changes.

LYME DISEASE

A spirochetal disease that became prominent in the mid-1980's in the United States. Usually there has been a history of a tick bite with concomitant swelling, erythema, and a characteristic ringlike lesions at the area of the tick bite.[8,9] If treated quickly, the disease subsides. If left untreated, the disease disseminates resulting in cardiac, joint, or neurologic complications. Ocular findings, especially retinal findings occur after dissemination of the disease.

Posterior pole findings were first noted in 1986.[10] Since that time, Lyme disease, as it occurs in the retina has a similar presentation as ocular syphilis. Lyme disease has been associated with pars plantis, branch retinal artery occlusion, periphlebitis, vitritis, papilledema, optic disc edema, papillitis, as well as the anterior segment changes of conjunctivitis, iritis, and corneal deposits (Figs. 10–2 and 10–3).[11–17]

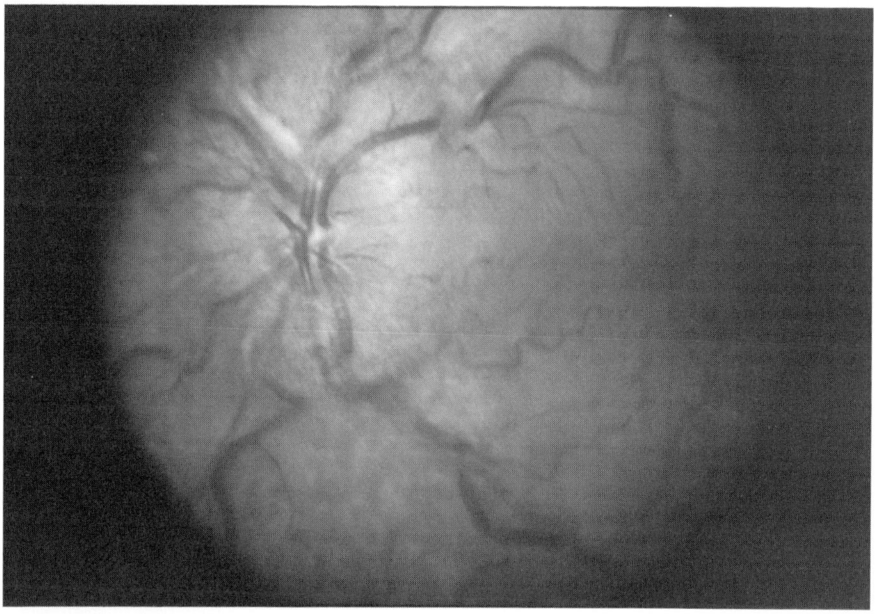

FIGURE 10–2

7-year-old male with Lyme disease, OD.

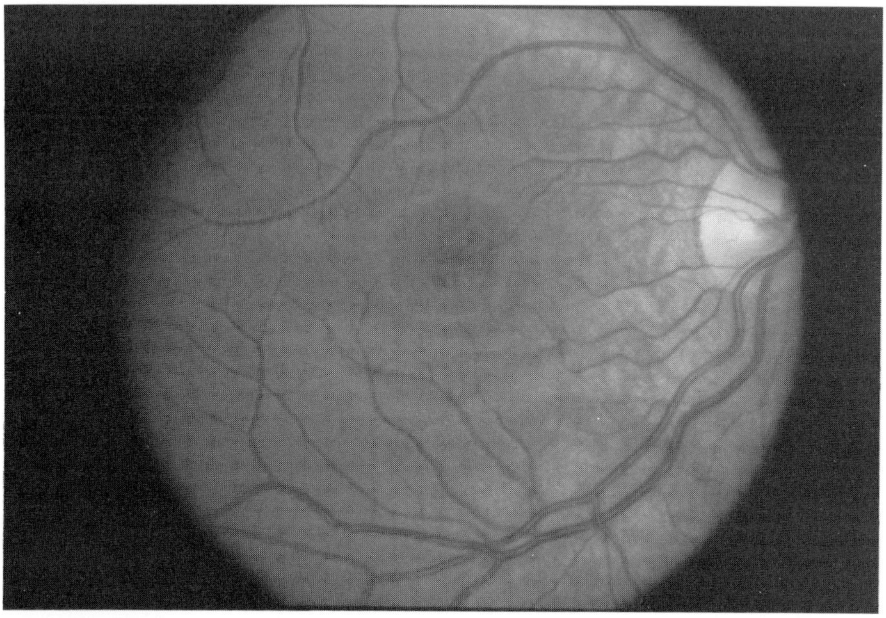

FIGURE 10–3

7-year-old male with Lyme disease and optic disc edema, OS.

Diagnosis

A specific immune response against *B. burgdorferi* is usually detectable by indirect immunofluorescence assay or enzyme-linked immunosorbent assay (ELISA) within weeks of onset of the disease. ELISA tests are preferred because of their sensitivity and reproducibility. However, the methods or serologic confirmation of Lyme disease are not standardized, and thus oftentimes, the same blood samples sent to two laboratories may yield different results.[17]

Immunoglobulin M antibody first develops within 2–4 weeks of illness, peaks after 6–8 weeks, and declines to normal range after 4–6 months. Immunoglobulin G antibody, however, is usually elevated within 6–8 weeks after the onset of the disease, peaks after 4–6 months, and remains elevated intermittently in patients with continued infection.

If clinical manifestations strongly suggest the diagnosis of Lyme disease but laboratory confirmation is lacking, the clinical judgment is given greater weight rather than a rigid adherence to a case definition. Clinical signs and symptoms should be used to direct decisions about treatment.

Fluorescein Angiography

The protean manifestations of Lyme disease is just as varied as that seen with luetic chorioretinitis. There are associated periphlebitis and choroidal lesions with early hypofluorescence and late hyperfluorescence.

Treatment[17]

EARLY LYME DISEASE

1. Doxycycline 100 mg orally twice a day for 10–21 days
2. Amoxicillin 500 mg orally three times a day for 10–21 days
3. Erythromycin 250 mg orally four times a day for 10–21 days (less effective than doxycycline or amoxicillin)

NEUROLOGIC MANIFESTATIONS INCLUDING OPTIC DISC EDEMA, PAPILLITIS

1. Ceftriaxone 2 g daily by single dose for 14–21 days, intravenously
2. Penicillin G 20 million U daily in divided doses for 10–21 days, intravenously

PREGNANT WOMEN

1. Localized early Lyme disease: Amoxicillin 500 mg three times a day for 21 days
2. Disseminated early Lyme disease, or any manifestation of late disease: Penicillin G, 20 million U daily, for 14–21 days
3. Asymptomatic seropositivity: No treatment is necessary[14]

PARASITIC DISEASE

Toxoplasmosis

This is a frequent cause of focal necrotizing retinitis. The protozoa, *Toxoplasma gondii* is transmitted to the fetus in utero or after ingestion of the organism as in contaminated meat. The organisms lie dormant encysted in parts of the retina, next to normal retina. There is a predilection for infection in the central nervous system and the retina (Fig. 10–4).[18]

Diagnosis

Clinically, the diagnosis of toxoplasmosis is a presumptive diagnosis. Oftentimes, the laboratory tests are equivocal, but the presence of a focus of active retinitis in an eye with one or more chorioretinal scars in a healthy individual will lead to this diagnosis.

Most chorioretinal scars caused by toxoplasmosis are atrophic, partly pigmented and associated with postinflammatory changes in the overlying vitreous and a nerve fiber bundle visual field defect. Localized areas of retinal necrosis associated with cells can be seen in the active disease. The different manifestations of these lesions are thought to be due to the tissue invasion of the parasite and a subsequent disruption of the chorioretinal interface. A toxoplasmosis titer is useful. Eosinophil count will be elevated.[18]

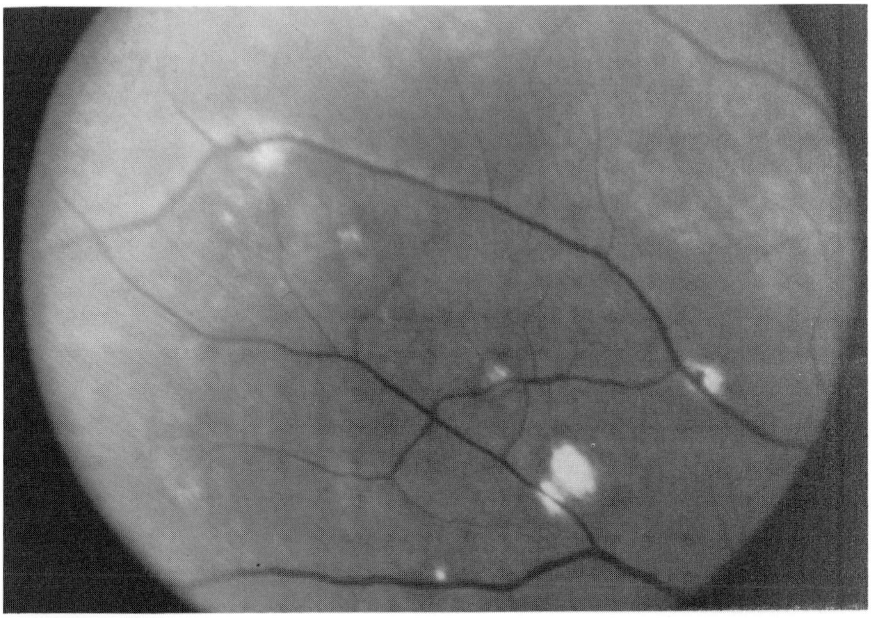

FIGURE 10–4

Toxoplasmosis.

Fluorescein Angiography

Fluorescein angiography will show nonperfusion in areas of active acute retinitis. Perivasculitis can be seen. Marked fluorescein staining can be seen in areas of active retinitis. Serous retinal detachment can occur. Periarterial plaques along the smaller arterioles and arteries can also be seen.

Treatment

Pyrimethamine (Daraprim), sulfonamide, clindamycin, minocycline, and corticosteroids in the treatment of active lesions in humans is uncertain. Treatment is only to be considered if the areas of concern are near the macular area. If there is an accompanying iridocycilitis, topical steroids and mydriatics are indicated.

TOXOCARA CANIS

Patients, typically in the first or second decade of life may experience unilateral loss of vision secondary to invasion of the eye by a single second-stage larval form of the *Toxocara canis*, a dog parasite. The human host contracts the disease by ingestion of contaminated soil. The eggs hatch in the gastrointestinal tract and enter the eye probably via the uveal tract. Bilateral ocular invasion rarely occurs.[19]

Clinically, the patients show:

Localized disciform macular detachment
Peripheral disciform retinal detachment
Papillitis
Optic nerve head tumor
Peripheral retinal mass or pars plana mass with vitritis
Retinal detachment
Endophthalmitis
Cataract
Subretinal granuloma

The ocular disease is rarely seen in the systemic manifestation of the disease, visceral larva migrans. This entity presents with coughing, wheezing, pulmonary infiltration, hepatomegaly, leukocytosis, persistent eosinophilia, elevation of isohemagglutinins, and elevated serum immunoglobulin levels (Fig. 10–5).

In laboratory diagnosis:

Eosinophilia
ELISA serum and aqueous

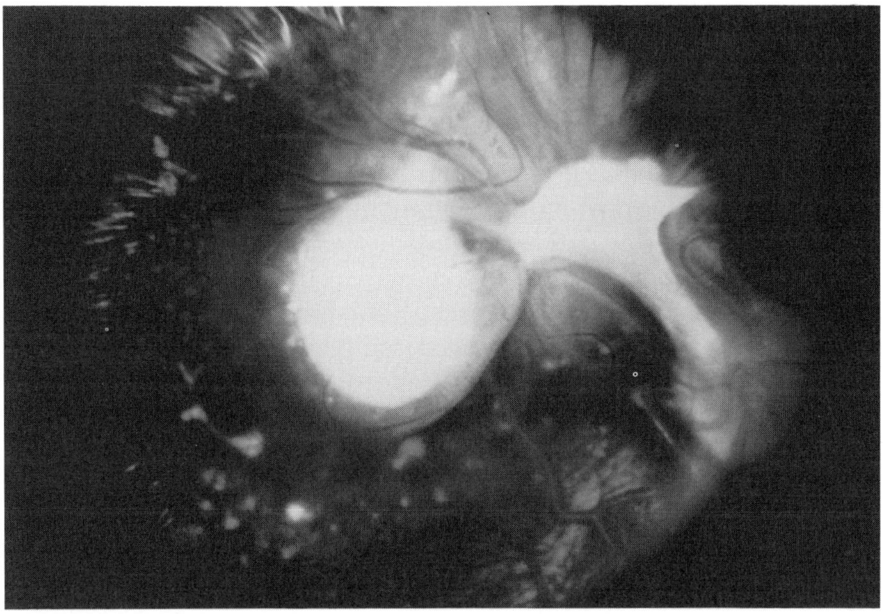

FIGURE 10–5

Toxocara canis.

Diffuse Unilateral Subacute Neuroretinitis

Diffuse unilateral subacute neuroretinitis is a very rare entity of visual loss. Vitritis, papillitis, retinal vasculitis, and recurrent crops of grayish white outer retinal lesions are seen and later characterized by progressive visual loss, optic atrophy, retinal vessel narrowing, and diffuse retinal pigment epithelial degeneration occurring in the eyes of otherwise healthy patients.[20–23] It is thought to be caused by a raccoon parasite.

Fluorescein Angiography

In the early stage of fluorescein angiography, there is leakage of dye from the optic nerve head.[20,21] The grayish white areas of active retinitis nonfluorescence early, but stain during the later phases of angiography. Prominent perivenous leakage of dye may occur in some patients in the earliest stages of the disease. Perivasculitis, extensive staining, and diffuse changes of the peripheral retinal pigment epithelium can occur.

Treatment

Laser treatment is effective in destroying the worm without causing significant intraocular inflammation.[21]

OPHTHALMOMYIASIS

The invasion of the larval form of the bot fly causes ophthalmomyiasis interna.[24] The bot fly relies on the living host of cattle, sheep, horse, deer, rodent, and humans. The eggs or larvae may be transported into the human corneal or conjunctival surface by an adult fly or by a secondary vector, such as a tick or mosquito or by the patient's hands. The maggots bore their way through the ocular coats and may live in the anterior or posterior chambers or subretinal space. Sometimes, the maggot leaves the eye, after having left crisscrossing tracts in the subretinal space of the retina. If the maggot dies inside the eye, the amount of the resultant inflammation may vary. Optic atrophy and severe visual loss can occur.

CYSTICERCOSIS

Cysticercosis is caused by the human ingestion of eggs of *Taenia solium* (pork tapeworm).[25–29] The eggs, once inside the gastrointestinal tract, leave embryos that can invade the intestinal wall and are carried throughout the body where they can develop into *Cysticercus cellulosea.* The larvae enter the eye by the central retinal artery or clilary arteries. Over a period of months, they grow into encapsulated cystic structures with a white scolex or head. At this point, it may be mistaken for a serous detachment of the retina, but the identification of the moving head inside the cyst helps with diagnosis. While encysted, there may be only a minimal reaction; however, once the death of the organism occurs, the associated secondary inflammation destroys the eye (Fig. 10–6).

FUNGAL INFECTIONS

Fungal infections in the retina and choroid are more commonly seen in the inpatient setting or in the severely immunocompromised host. However, in this era of AIDS, these infections are occurring in higher frequency in the outpatient setting.

Candida albicans occurs in hospitalized patients with postoperative complications or in the immunocompromised host, requiring the use of chronic indwelling catheters for antibiotic therapy, hyperalimentation and broviac catheters for chemotherapy.[30]

Clinical presentation involves vitreous haze, vitreous fungal balls suspended in the vitreous near the retina. The retinal findings are multiple white-centered superficial retinal hemorrhages (Fig. 10–7).

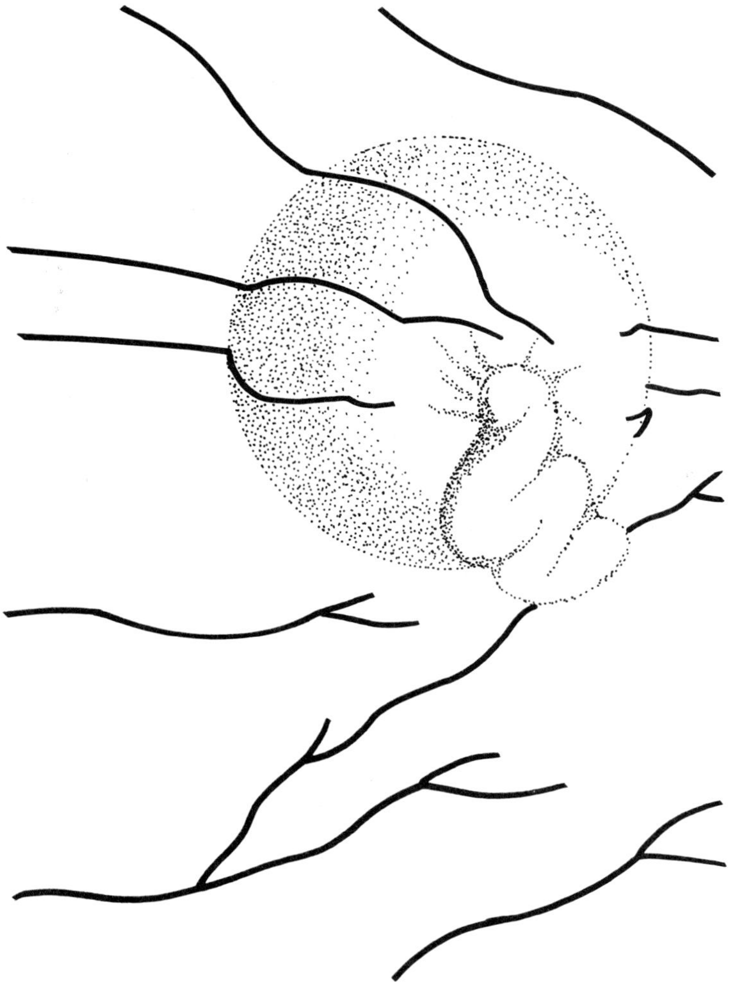

FIGURE 10–6

Cysticercosis.

Fluorescein Angiography

Vitritis presents as hazy media. There is accompanying hyperfluorescence as the retinal pigment epithelium is destroyed and the fluorescein leakage is prominent.

Diagnosis

Candida albicans can be cultured from the blood or vitreous, culturing the site of intravenous administration.

Treatment

Systemic administration of amphotericin B and/or 5-fluorocytosine can be used.

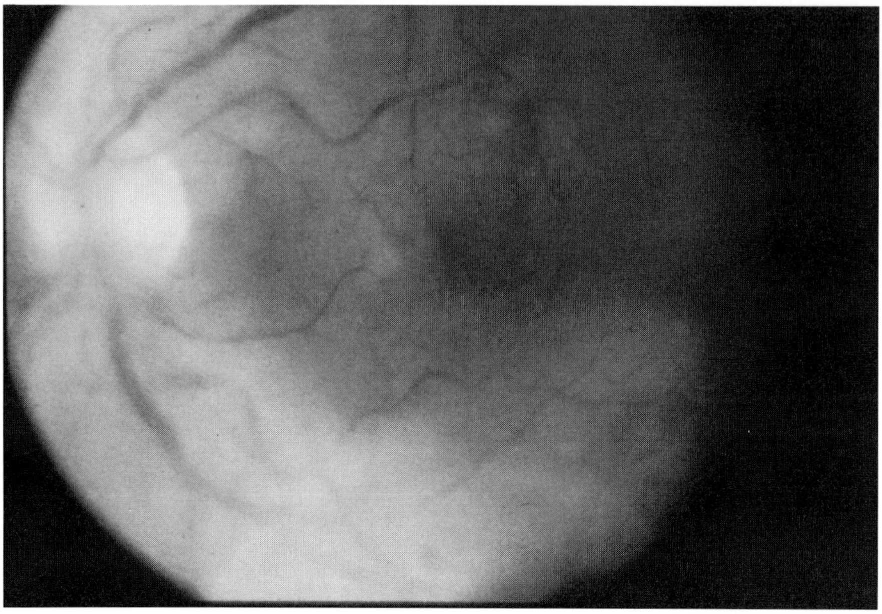

FIGURE 10-7
Candida albicans.

Intravitreal amphotericin B has been used as primary form of treatment and in combination with systemic treatment.

REFERENCES

1. Barondes MJ, Sponsel WE, Stevens TS, Plotnik RD: Tuberculous choroiditis diagnosed by chorioretinal endobiopsy. Am J Ophthalmol 1991; *112:* 460–461

2. Shiono T, Abe S, Horiuchi T: A case of miliary tuberculosis with disseminated choroidal haemorrhages. Br J Ophthalmol 1990; *74:* 317–319

3. Chung YM, Yeh TS, Sheu SJ, Liu JH: Macular subretinal neovascularization in choroidal tuberculosis. Ann Ophthalmol 1989; *21:* 225–229

4. Gass JDM, Braunstein RA, Chenoweth RG: Acute syphilitic posterior placoid chorioretinitis. Ophthalmol 1990; *97:* 1288–1297

5. McLeish WM, Pulido JS, Holland G et al: The ocular manifestations of syphilis in the human immunodeficiency virus type 1-infected host. Ophthalmol 1990; *97:* 196–203

6. Culbertson WW: Infections of the retina in AIDS. Int Ophthalmol Clin 1989; *29:* 108–118

7. de Souza EC, Jalkh AE, Trempe CL et al: Unusual central chorioretinitis as the first manifestation of early secondary syphilis. Am J Ophthalmol 1988; *105:* 271–276

8. Steere AC, Malawista SE, Hardin JA et al: Erythema chronicum migrans and Lyme arthritis: the enlarging clinical spectrum. Ann Intern Med 1977; *86:* 685–698

9. Steere AC: Medical progress: Lyme disease. N Engl J Med 1989; *321:* 586–596

10. Wu G, Lincoff H, Ellsworth RM, Haik BG: Optic disc edema and Lyme disease. Ann Ophthalmol 1986; *18:* 252–255

11. Bialasiewicz AA, Ruprecht KW, Naumann G, Blenk H: Bilateral diffuse choroiditis and exudative retinal detachments with evidence of Lyme disease. Am J Ophthalmol 1988; *105:* 419–420

12. Wiegand W: Augenbefunde bei Borreliose-bilaterale panuveitis mit exsudativer amotio. Fortschr Ophthalmol 1989; *86:* 659–662

13. Kornmehl EW, Lesser RL, Jaros et al: Bilateral keratitis in Lyme disease. Ophthalmol 1989; *96:* 1194–1197

14. Baum J, Barza M, Weinstein P et al: Bilateral keratitis as a manifestation of Lyme disease. Am J Ophthalmol 1987; *105:* 75–77

15. MacDonald AB: Lyme disease. A neuro-ophthalmologic view. J Clin Neuro-Ophthalmol 1987; *7:* 185–190

16. Zierhut M, Kreissig I, Pickert A: Panuveitis with positive serological tests for syphilis and Lyme disease. J Clin Neuro Ophthalmol 1989; *9:* 71–75

17. Rahn DW, Malawista SE: Lyme disease: recommendations for diagnosis and treatment. Ann Int Med 1991; *114:* 472–481

18. Sherman MD, Nozik RA: Other infections of the choroid and retina. Toxoplasmosis, histoplasmosis, Lyme disease, syphilis, tuberculosis and ocular toxocariasis. Infect Dis Clin North Am 1992; *6:* 893–908

19. Dernouchamps JP, Veroughstraete C, Demolder E: Ocular toxocariasis: a presumed case of peripheral granuloma. Int Ophthalmol 1990; *14:* 383–388

20. Gass JDM: Diffuse unilateral subacute neuroretinitis. Ophthalmology 1978; *85:* 521–525

21. Gass JDM, Braunstein RA: Further observations concerning the diffuse unilateral subacute neuroretinitis syndrome. Arch Ophthalmol 1983; *101:* 1689–1697

22. Price JA Jr, Wadsworth JAC: An intraretinal worm: report of a case of macular retinopathy caused by invasion of the retina by a worm. Arch Ophthalmol 1970; *83:* 768–770

23. Kazacos KR, Vestre WA, Kazacos EA, Raymond LA: Diffuse unilateral subacute neuroretinitis syndrome: probable cause. Arch Ophthalmol 1984; *102:* 967–968

24. Fitzgerald CR, Rubin ML: Intraocular parasite destroyed by photocoagulation. Arch Ophthalmol 1974; *91:* 162–164

25. Aracena T, Perez Roca F: Macular and peripheral subretinal cysticercosis. Ann Ophthalmol 1981; *13:* 1265–1267

26. Hutton WL, Vaiser A, Snyder WB: Pars plana vitrectomy for removal of intravitreous cysticercus. Am J Ophthamol 1976; *81:* 571–573

27. Malik SRK, Gupta AL, Choudhry S: Ocular cysticercosis. Am J Ophthalmol 1968; *66:* 1168–1171

28. Santos R, Chavarria M, Aguirre AE: Failure of medical treatment in two cases of intraocular cysticercosis. Am J Ophthalmol 1984; *97:* 249–250

29. Topilow HW, Yimoyines DJ, Freeman HM et al: Bilateral multifocal intraocular cysticercosis. Ophthalmol 1981; *88:* 1166–1172

30. Michelson PE, Stark W, Reeser F, Green WR: Endogenous Candida endophthalmitis. Int Ophthalmol Clin 1971; *11:* 125–147

31. Cantrill HL, Rodman WP, Ramsay RC, Knobloch WH: Postpartum Candida endophthalmitis. JAMA 1980; *243:* 1163–1165

32. Palmer EA: Endogenous Candida endophthalmitis in infants. Am J Ophthalmol 1980; *89:* 388–395

CHAPTER ELEVEN

Inflammatory (Noninfectious) Diseases

GRANULOMATOUS DISEASE

Sympathetic Ophthalmia

Sympathetic ophthalmia (sympathetic ophthalmitis or sympathetic uveitis) is a rare diffuse granulomatous uveitis that occurs within a few days to several decades after penetrating, accidental, or surgical trauma to an eye. Injury and incarceration of uveal tissue has been a feature of the majority of cases of sympathetic ophthalmia.

Epidemiology

Sympathetic ophthalmia is a rare disease, although exact figures are difficult to obtain because the onset and/or diagnosis is often delayed for months to years following the initial injury. The incidence of sympathetic ophthalmia after penetrating injury is 0.19 percent and 0.007 percent after intraocular surgery.[1] The incidence of sympathetic ophthalmia after vitrectomy is 0.01 percent.[2] The traumatized eye is considered the "exciting eye" and the fellow eye is called the "sympathizing eye." The types of surgery that can lead to sympathetic ophthalmia includes cataract extraction, iridectomy, paracentesis, cyclodialysis, retinal detachment repair, vitrectomy, and keratectomy.

Anatomy and Pathophysiology

The pathologic changes are similar in the exciting and sympathizing eyes. There are diffuse lymphocytic infiltration of the uveal tract with nests of epitheloid cells. Pigment is present within these epitheloid cells and within giant cells. The inflammatory process does not involve the choriocapillaris in the diffuse disease.

The etiology of sympathetic ophthalmia is unknown. Sixty to 70 percent of the cases are caused by accidental penetrating trauma and perforating surgical trauma accounts for nearly 30 percent. The common theme in all of these cases is the presence of a penetrating injury in which wound healing is complicated by incarceration of the iris, ciliary body, or choroid.

Clinical Course

The patient usually has had a history of penetrating accidental trauma or a history of surgery. There is complicated course of waxing and waning uveitis, followed by quiescent periods lasting several months to several years. In time, the disease becomes chronically active, eventually producing irreversible ocular damage and leading to blindness and phthisis bulbi. With the current use of corticosteroid therapy, approximately 65 percent attain a final visual acuity of 20/60 or better. Many patients become steroid dependent and with attempted discontinuation of the therapy, they experience a recurrence of the disease.

Diagnosis

The diagnosis of sympathetic ophthalmia must be differentiated from other diseases by a careful history. Other diseases which can mimic the same clinical picture include fungal and bacterial infections, posttraumatic iritis or iridocyclitis, and phacoanaphylaxis.[3,4]

Vogt-Koyanagi-Harada syndrome can mimic this disease, but its history and clinical course is very different (see below). Vogt-Koyanagi-Harada is an inflammatory uveomeningeal disorder with bilateral diffuse granulomatous uveitis, exudative retinal detachments, alopecia, vitiligo, dysacusis, and fluctuating meningeal signs and symptoms. While alopecia and vitiligo is more common in Vogt-Koyanagi-Harada syndrome, they can be seen in cases of sympathetic ophthalmia. On histopathologic study, Vogt-Koyanagi-Harada syndrome shows areas of involvement of choriocapillaris and the overlying retina, whereas sympathetic ophthalmia does not involve the choriocapillaris.

HLA-A-11 antigen[5] has been found in association with sympathetic ophthalmia.

Fluorescein Angiography

Multiple pinpoint areas of fluorescein staining are seen. These areas then enlarge during the course of the study. In sympathetic ophthalmia, the lesions may appear to be elevated. The appearance of inflammatory retinal pigment epithelial detachments on fluorescein angiography are called Dalen-Fuchs nodules.

Treatment

A combination of topical, periocular, and oral corticosteroids may be necessary.

Vogt-Koyanagi-Harada Disease

Epidemiology

Patients with Vogt-Koyanagi-Harada disease are typically, Orientals, Blacks, and darkly pigmented whites. There is a rapid loss of vision in one or both eyes caused by serous retinal detachment. There is no sex predilection.

Anatomy and Pathophysiology

Plasma cells are prominent, giant cells and lymphocytes infiltrate the choriocapillaris area. There are histologic similarities between sympathetic ophthalmia and Vogt-Koyanagi-Harada disease with the main difference in the involvement of the choriocapillaris in the latter disease.

Clinical Course

Systemic manifestations such as headache, malaise, vomiting, and occasional focal neurologic signs and symptoms may precede the onset of visual loss.

Visual loss may be gradual. Both eyes can become affected after a short period of time or the onset of symptoms could be bilateral. On examination, there are nondiscrete yellow areas of exudate or color change in the retinal pigment epithelium occurring beneath one or more isolated areas of serous retinal detachments. The affected areas can become confluent consequently forming extensive bullous serous retinal detachments that shift with positioning of the patient. In a few patients, multifocal, grayish white patches at the level of the retinal pigment epithelium are similar to but less well-defined than those seen in patients with acute posterior multifocal placoid pigment epitheliopathy. The choroid may appear thickened. The optic disc appears hypermic and swollen and there are inflammatory cells present in the vitreous (Fig. 11–1).

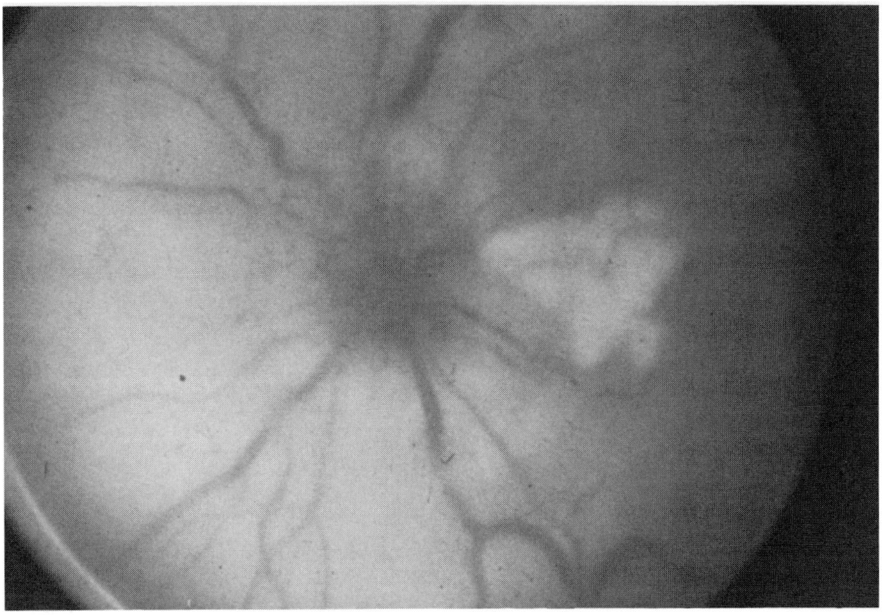

FIGURE 11-1

Vogt-Koyanagi-Harada disease. Multifocal grayish white patches are seen.

Iridocyclitis may be present in some cases. Inflammatory infiltration of the anterior choroid and ciliary body may cause some narrowing of the anterior chamber.

Laboratory Tests

The ultrasound shows a thickened choroid. The cerebrospinal fluid from a lumbar puncture shows pleocytosis, elevation of protein.

Fluorescein Angiography

Fluorescein angiography may show a patchy delay in choroidal perfusion. Many pinpoint and irregular areas of fluorescein staining develop at the level of the retinal pigment epithelium. These areas of fluorescence gradually increase in size. In some instances, the areas of hyperfluorescence look like cobblestones at the level of the retinal pigment epithelium. The subretinal exudate stains late in the angiogram.

Treatment

Intensive corticosteroid therapy appears to shorten the duration of the retinal detachment. Varying degrees of visual loss accompany the retinal pigment epithelial changes.

Sarcoidosis

Sarcoidosis is a granulomatous disorder affecting multiple systems. Ocular involvement is common and occurs in approximately 15–25 percent of patients.[6] The organs most frequently involved in sarcoidosis are the lungs, lymph nodes, spleen, skin, eyes, nervous system, and bone and joints.

Epidemiology

Sarcoidosis in the United States shows that it is a disease of early middle age, approximately three-fourths of patients being affected are under the age of 40 at the time of diagnosis. Although both sexes are affected, there is a slight female preponderance. The disease is more prevalent among African-Americans than Caucasians.[7–10]

Anatomy and Pathogenesis

There is depression of delayed type hypersensitivity, reflected by T-cell anergy and negative skin tests. Peripheral blood lymphocytes from sarcoidosis patients show decreased response to mitogens. Active T-cell driven immunologic response occurs at the target organ site and eventually leads to granuloma formation.[11,12]

Clinical Course

Ocular lesions include anterior uveitis, iris and conjunctival nodules, and corneal disease with either band keratopathy or interstitial keratitis. Posterior segment findings include chorioretinitis, periphlebitis, chorioretinal nodules, vitreous inflammation, retinal neovascularization, and orbital disease including involvement of the lacrimal gland, optic nerve, and orbital granuloma. The periphlebitis show white debris, called candle wax drippings or *tache de bougie.* In the vitreous, findings include accumulation of vitreous debris, "snowballs" or string of pearls. Exudative retinal detachments are rare (Figs. 11–2 and 11–3).

Fluorescein Angiography

Fluorescein angiography can show serous retinal detachment, choroidal neovascularization, and subretinal fibrosis.

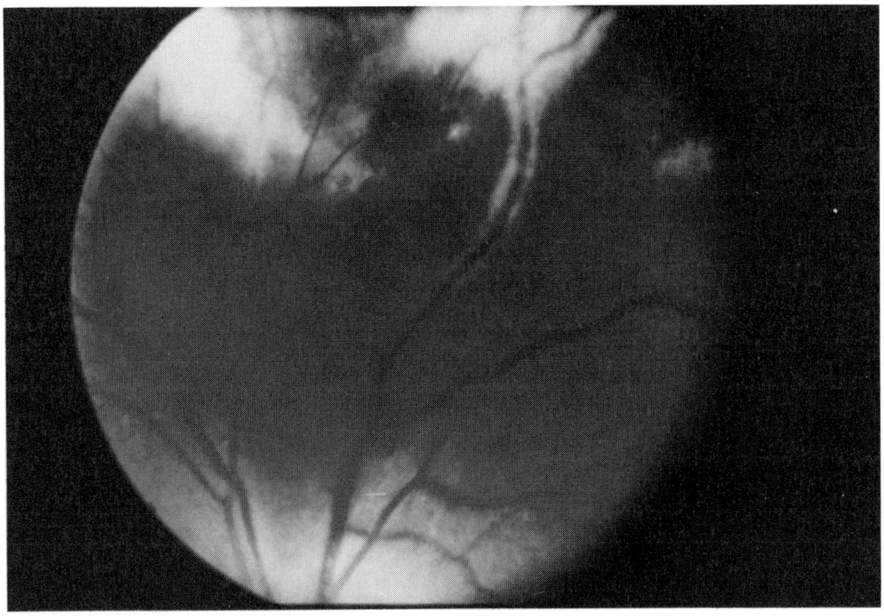

FIGURE 11-2

Sarcoid periphlebitis.

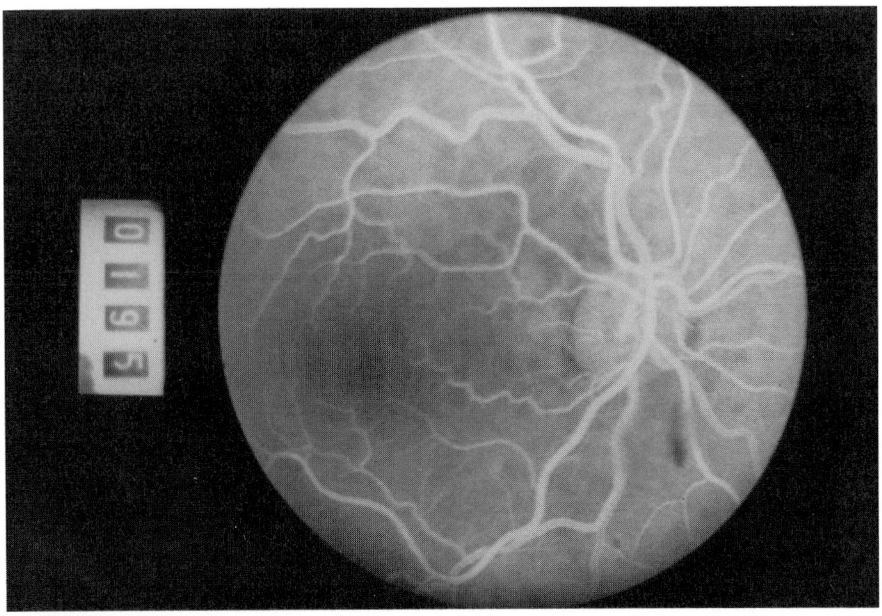

FIGURE 11-3

Fluorescein angiogram of optic nerve involvement in sarcoidosis. Hyperfluorescence temporally at optic disc, OD.

Laboratory Diagnosis

Chest X-ray

Histologic confirmation can be obtained by tissue biopsy of the conjunctival nodules and transconjunctival biopsy of the lacrimal gland

Serum angiotensin converting enzyme

Gallium scan of the spleen.

The Kveim test is used occasionally. It uses human sarcoid tissue prepared from spleen of patients suffering from sarcoidosis. The saline suspension is injected intradermally and the site is inspected for nodule formation. After 3–6 weeks, a palpable nodule is biopsied. If the biopsy shows noncaseating granuloma, the diagnosis of sarcoid is established.

Treatment

Intensive topical corticosteroids and oral corticosteroids may be necessary in refractory cases.

OTHER INFLAMMATORY DISEASES (NONINFECTIOUS)

Uveal Effusion

See Chapter 21.

Scleritis

Scleritis is a range of acute necrotizing granuloma to a low-grade chronic granulomatous inflammation. Many patients have anterior sclera affected with foci of posterior affected. There can be associated exudative retinal detachment. There can be associated vitritis.

Epidemiology

It is a rare inflammatory disorder of the sclera.

Anatomy and Pathophysiology

Adjacent to the sclera lies a deep vascular plexus that is primarily involved with scleritis. Pathology studies have shown fibrinoid necrosis with destruction of the collagen.[14,15] The cellular infiltrate is composed of polymorphonuclear leukocytes, plasma cells, lymphocytes, and macrophates. These cells and multinucleated giant cells surround the central granulomatous lesion. Thrombosed vessels are seen with vaculitis, i.e., medial necrosis and perivascular cuffing with lymphocytes.

Clinical Course

Patients present with ocular pain or tenderness, injection of the conjunctival and episcleral vessels, evidence of intraocular inflammation, and a history of rheumatoid arthritis.

Conditions associated with scleritis:

Systemic: Rheumatoid arthritis, Wegener's granulomatosis, polyarteritis nodosa, systemic lupus erythematosus, Behçet's syndrome, pyoderma gangrenosum, sarcoidosis, dermatomyositis, relapsing polychondritis, spondyloarthritis, atopy.

Local and systemic: *Pseudomonas,* herpes zoster, tumors, chemical injury, metabolic disorders such as gout, following cataract extraction.[13–15]

Fluorescein angiographic findings are chorioretinal folds and cystoid macular edema.

Ultrasonography shows thickened choroid if the disease is diffuse. Otherwise, the scleritis can present as a mass and may be difficult to differentiate from choroidal melanoma (see Chapter 20).

Laboratory Diagnosis

Laboratory diagnosis includes complete blood count, erythrocyte sedimentation rate, immunoglobulin levels, complement levels, antinuclear antibody, rheumatoid factor, serum immune complexes, chest X-ray and sinus films. Some potentially treatable diseases are systemic lupus erythematosus, Wegener's granulomatosis, and polyarteritis nodosa.

Uveitis

Uveitis (See also other sections in this chapter and chapters 7, 10) includes all intraocular inflammation caused by a wide variety of infective agents and noninfective agents. In the sections above and in this chapter, we discuss some of the different entities causing posterior segment disease and uveitis.

Pars planitis

Pars planitis is a relative common uveitis in children and young adults. It can occur at any age and affects both sexes equally. Eighty percent of the patients develop bilateral disease. The etiology is unknown.[16]

Clinical Course

The clinical findings are floaters and hazy vision due to cells in the vitreous. If the macula is affected, there is cystoid macular edema. There is no pain, redness, or photophobia and rarely is there any sign of severe iridocyclitis (Fig. 11–4).

Although one eye is symptomatic, the other eye can have signs of the disease, i.e., cells in the vitreous cavity, a few cells in the aqueous, and low-grade cystoid macular edema.

The affected eye shows inferior vitreous base exudate, called "snowbanking." There can be patchy periphlebitis as well.

The clinical course and visual prognosis has been categorized in several ways:

1. Self-limiting course characterized by gradual improvement (10 percent)[16]
2. Prolonged course but without exacerbations (59 percent)
3. Chronic smoldering course with one or more episodes with exacerbations (31 percent).

The prognosis for good vision lies in the absence of less severe inflammation and absence of cystoid macular edema. The major cause of visual loss is macular damage.

Other observers such as Brockhurst, Schepens, and Okamura divide the pars planitis patients into five groups[17]:

1. Benign course (28 percent)
2. Chronic smoldering form (46 percent)

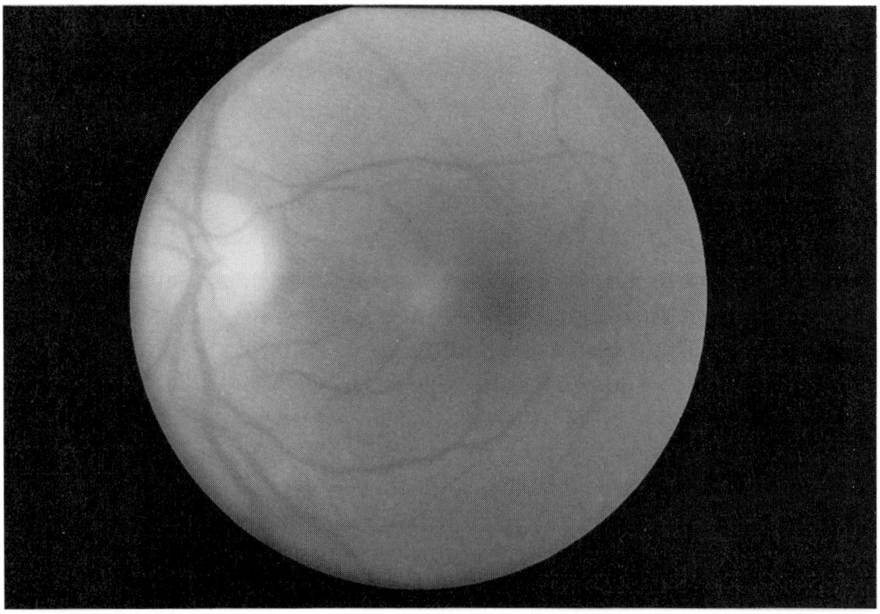

FIGURE 11–4

Pars planitis with hazy view of vitreous.

3. Choroidal and retinal detachments (12 percent)
4. Malignant course with development of organizing membranes and exudate in the vitreous cavity (6 percent)
5. Occlusion of the peripheral retinal veins, worsening of the disease in the posterior pole and optic atrophy (8 percent)

Laboratory Diagnosis

Serum lysozyme
Angiotensin-converting enzyme
Chest X-ray
Tuberculin skin test to examine for tuberculosis
Fluorescent treponemal antibody absorption test (FTA-ABS), MHA-TP for syphilis

Fluorescein Angiography

The presence of cystoid macular edema guides the clinician towards treatment with steroids. Perivasculitis is seen with hyperfluorescence during midtransit.

Treatment

Topical and oral steroids and periocular corticosteroids are used for treating patients whose vision is threatened. There is a role for periocular steroids for patients with vision less than 20/40 and severe disease (macular edema, peripheral venous sheathing, and retinoschisis).

Behçet's Disease

Behçet's disease is a triad of oral and genital ulcers and hypopyon uveitis. It is most common in the Middle East, Far East, and Japan. In these places, the disease is associated with HLA-Bw51.[18] The disease is most often bilateral.[19]

Pathology

Perivascular infiltrate with lymphocytes and plasma cells is associated with retinal necrosis and with Behçet's disease. Later lesions show loss of retinal architecture with neovascularization.

The endstage of the disease shows secondary glaucoma, rubeosis, and retinal detachment associated with pain and loss of vision.

Clinical Course

Oral ulcers are the most common manifestation, genital ulcers the next most common, and ocular disease is third most common. Ocular disease occurs as anterior uveitis, hypopyon uveitis, and retinal vasculitis.

Posterior pole lesions include occlusive disease of the arteries, vasculitis of the veins and arteries, and retinal necrosis. Secondary retinal neovascularization and retinal detachment will develop.

Skin lesions can occur—erythema nodusum, superficial thrombophlebitis, pyoderma, or presence of a pustule after breaking the skin by a needle. The arthritis is asymmetric, nondeforming, with large joint polyarthritis that is steroid responsive.

Cranial nerve palsies, papilledema, and ischemic optic neuropathy are seen as well.[20,21]

The visual prognosis of Behçet's disease is poor. Most of the patients will suffer from severe visual loss within 5 years. The clinical impression of most authors has been that steroids delay the progression of the disease but do not alter the ultimate outcome.[22]

Treatment

Indications for treatment are ocular or neurologic manifestation of Behçet's. Chlorambucil (0.1–0.2 mg/kg/day)[23–26] is administered under the supervision of an ophthalmologist and internist or rheumatologist. Cyclophosphamide 1–2 mg/kg/day can be administered as well. The dose is adjusted to maintain the white blood cell count over 3000/mm^3.[26] The use of immunosuppressive drugs has frequently resulted in an arrest of the disease process and many studies have suggested that a long-term remission can be induced with 1–2 years of treatment.[25,26] Cyclosporin can be given up to 10/mg/kg/day. Nephrotoxicity, however, has been reported with cyclosporin.[26–27] Colchicine has been reported to be useful, effective in oral and genital disease but ineffective in ocular disease.[28]

Acute Multifocal Placoid Pigment Epitheliopathy

In 1968, Gass described a condition of multiple pale lesions deep to the retina, at the level of the retinal pigment epithelium, with acute loss of central vision and spontaneous resolution in 2–3 weeks.[29] Acute multifocal placoid pigment epitheliopathy affects 20–50-year-olds and is bilateral in nature. As a late sequela there are pigment epithelial scars. There can be recurrent attacks.[30–32] The cause is unknown, although some researchers believe that the disorder has followed after viral infections (Fig. 11–5).[33]

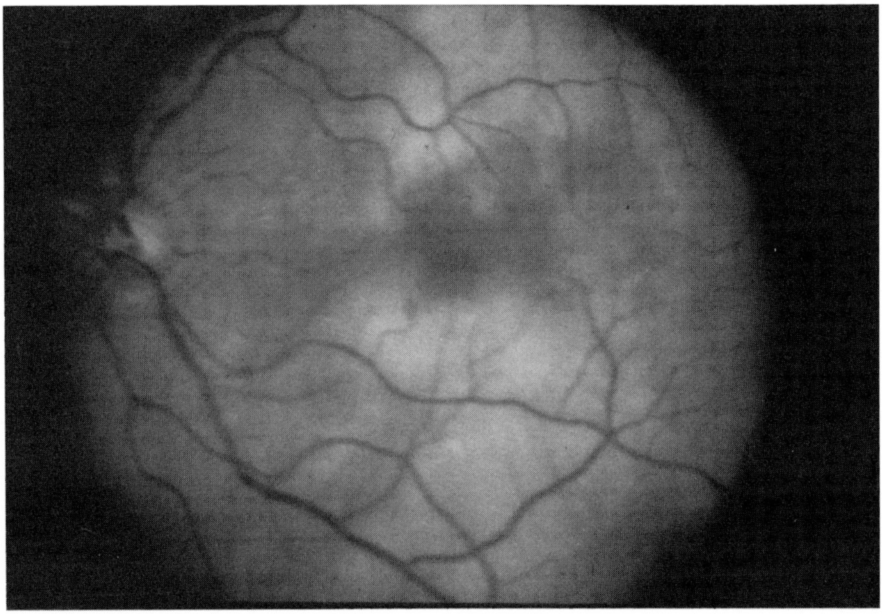

FIGURE 11-5

Acute multifocal placoid pigment epitheliopathy with multiple pale lesions deep in the retina.

Fluorescein Angiography

Fluorescein angiography shows the lesions to be dark during the initial dye transit but become hyperfluorescent later in the study. Occasionally, large choroidal vessels can be seen in the depths of the lesion. In large areas of confluent involvement, solitary choriocapillaris lobules may be perfused. In many cases, the filling phase of the choroid is prolonged (Fig. 11–6).

Some patients have the same appearance as described by Gass, but also there are those patients with serous detachments. However, these cases fall in the category of Harada's disease and therefore, acute multifocal placoid pigment epitheliopathy may represent a limited form of Harada's disease.

Treatment

Because the disease is self-limited and the visual prognosis is good, there is no treatment.

Serpiginous Choroiditis

Serpiginous choroiditis or geographic helicoid peripapillary choroidopathy is a rare, bilateral, inflammatory disease affecting the choroid and retinal pigment epithelium, having unknown etiology.[34–38] Most patients are middle-aged or older, and there is

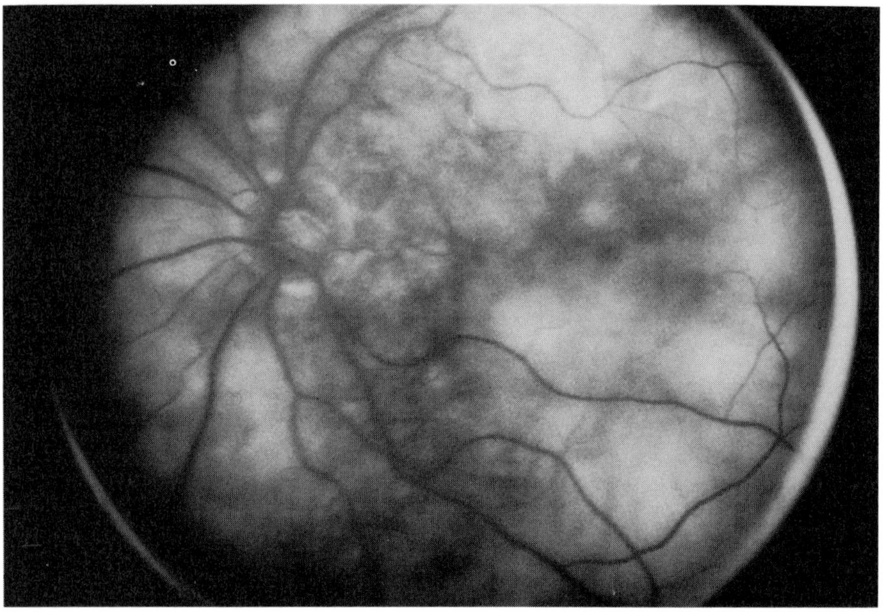

FIGURE 11–6

Fluorescein angiogram of acute multifocal placoid pigment showing lobules of choriocapillaris.

no race or sex predilection. The histopathology of geographic helicoid peripapillary choroidopathy is unknown.

Clinical Course

The patient is usually asymptomatic until the lesion affects the macula. The acute lesion is grayish white. Active lesions may arise from the optic nerve head. The spread of the disease is through contiguous patches of advancing inflammation. The pattern in the fundus looks like fingerlike projections. However, the macula rarely is affected initially. Within a few weeks, the active gray lesion becomes pale and eventually atrophies. Fibrous scar tissue and loss of choroidal tissue ensues. Anterior cells and posterior vitreous cells can be seen.[39] Subretinal neovascularization occurs. The visual prognosis is poor (Fig. 11–7).

Fluorescein Angiography

Acute lesions show hypofluorescence. Hypofluorescence occurs because the choriocapillaris and choroid have been destroyed. Later in the transit, the area becomes slowly hyperfluorescent, beginning at the edge of the lesion and spreading inward. Late hyperfluorescent staining of fibrous scar tissue within the old lesions is common.

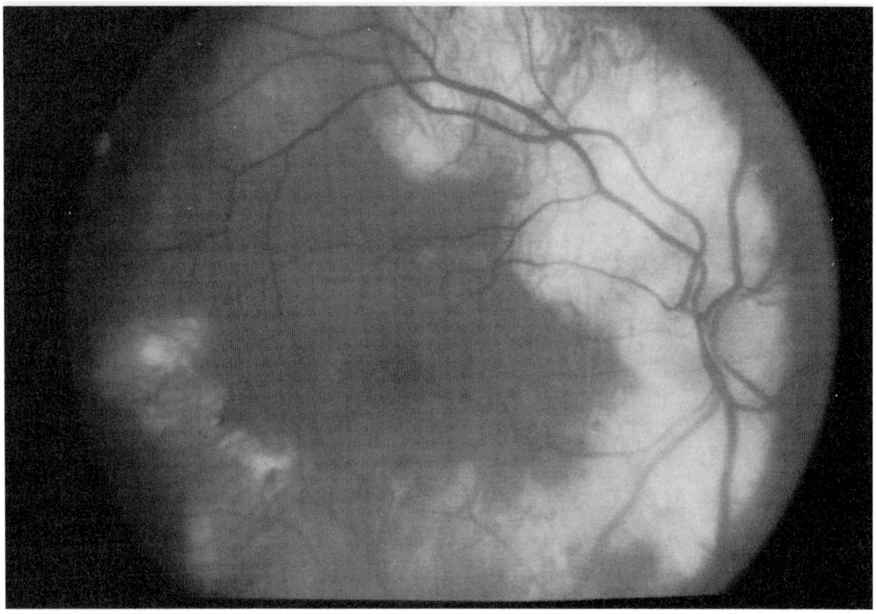

FIGURE 11–7

Serpiginous choroiditis with contiguous patches of advancing inflammation emanating from optic disc.

Treatment

There is no treatment known to be beneficial. Steroids (oral and periocular) have been used.[35,38] Laser has been tried.[40] However, the active border of the lesion can grow beyond areas of photocoagulation.

Birdshot Retinochoroidopathy

In 1975, Ryan and Maumenee[41] described birdshot retinochoroidopathy as a rare disease. It is acquired, chronic, bilateral and symmetric. It presents as intraocular inflammation. It has multiple discrete cream-colored areas of depigmentation scattered diffusely throughout the fundus. These deep hypopigmented lesions often have a vascular orientation. The course of the disease is characterized by exacerbations and remissions. The disorder may lead to reduced visual acuity.

The most common presenting symptoms are decreased vision from cystoid macular edema, floaters and vitreous cells and debris. Some eyes have keratitic precipitates, anterior chamber cell, and flare. However, all eyes have vitreous cells and debris. At the level of the choroid, there are spots of depigmentation, approximately a quarter of a disc diameter (Fig. 11–8).

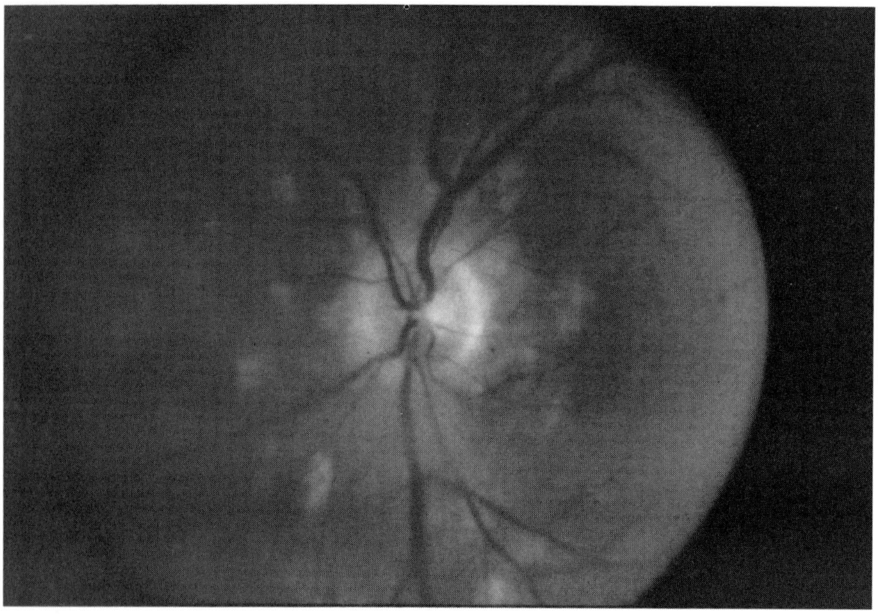

FIGURE 11-8

Birdshot retinochoroidopathy with spots of depigmentation.

Retinal findings include diffuse narrowing of retinal arterioles. Perivascular hemorrhages in the nerve fiber layer and tortuosity of vessels are also common findings. Optic disc swelling is noticed as well.

Fluorescein Angiography

Hypofluorescence in the early phase with slight diffuse hyperfluorescence in the late phase. It is important to note that many of the depigmented lesions show no fluorescein findings and thus, the lesions are more prominent on ophthalmoscopy than angiography. The retinal circulation demonstrates marked leakage and accumulation of dye as well as cystoid macular edema on fluorescein angiography. Some patients have subretinal neovascularization.

Electroretinography

Diminished rod b-wave amplitudes, cone and rod b-wave implicit times, and cone a- and b-wave amplitudes are borderline ranging from low normal.

Laboratory Diagnosis

HLA-A-29[42] has been found in some patients with birdshot retinochoroidopathy.

Punctate Inner Choroidopathy

In 1984, Watzke et al.[43] described myopic women with blurred vision, light flashes, and paracentral scotomas associated with yellow lesions of the inner choroid and retinal pigment epithelium as suffering from punctate inner choroidopathy. The etiology of this disease is unknown.

Clinical Course

Patients with punctate inner choroidopathy usually present with poor central vision. Most do not have vitreous cells or anterior chamber cells. The visual acuity ranges from 20/200 to 20/400.

The lesions are discrete, yellow, opaque spots 100–300 μ in diameter and are scattered throughout the posterior pole and periphery. In chronic lesions, the lesions show atrophy and associated hyperpigmentation. Occasionally there are associated serous detachments and subretinal neovascular membranes (Fig. 11–9). Only in cases of subretinal neovascular membranes is the visual prognosis poor. Most of these patients have spontaneous resolution with good final visual acuity.

Fluorescein Angiography

The acute lesions are hypofluroescent; then gradually, there is associated hyperfluorescence.

Treatment

In those cases with extrafoveal neovascular membranes and decreasing visual acuity, laser can be used with positive results. However, it is uncertain whether laser is better than the natural history of the disease.

Multiple Evanescent White Dot Syndrome

Multiple evanescent white dot syndrome affects one eye of young females, is associated with blurred vision, and multiple paracentral scotomata occurring in approximately 50 percent of patients after a flu-like illness. It rarely occurs in both eyes and late recurrences are also possible.[44–46]

Clinical Course

There are multiple grayish white patches each comprised of small white dots at the level of the retinal pigment epithelium and outer

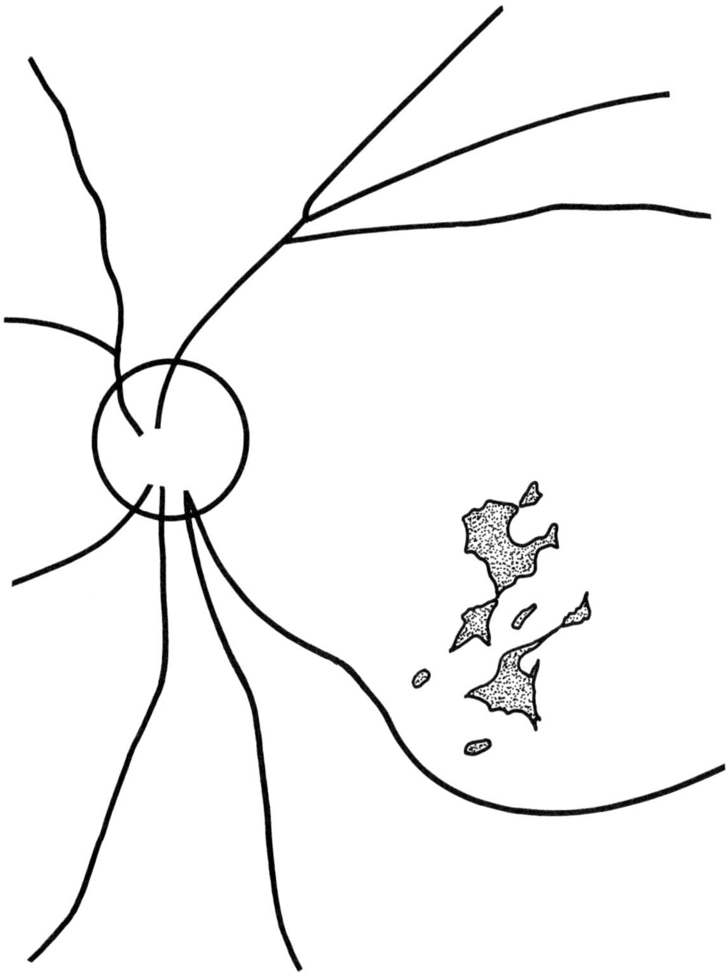

FIGURE 11-9
Punctate inner choroiditis.

retina at the center of the macula. Vitreous cells can be present as well (Fig. 11–10).

Fluorescein Angiography

Early punctate hyperfluorescence of the grayish white patches occur in early transit, but in later transit there is a cluster or wreath-shaped pattern. There is late staining of these lesions and the optic nerve (Fig. 11–11).

Electroretinography

There is a decrease in the a-wave and early receptor potentials. These changes can return to normal in 7–10 weeks as the fundus and fluorescein changes return to normal.

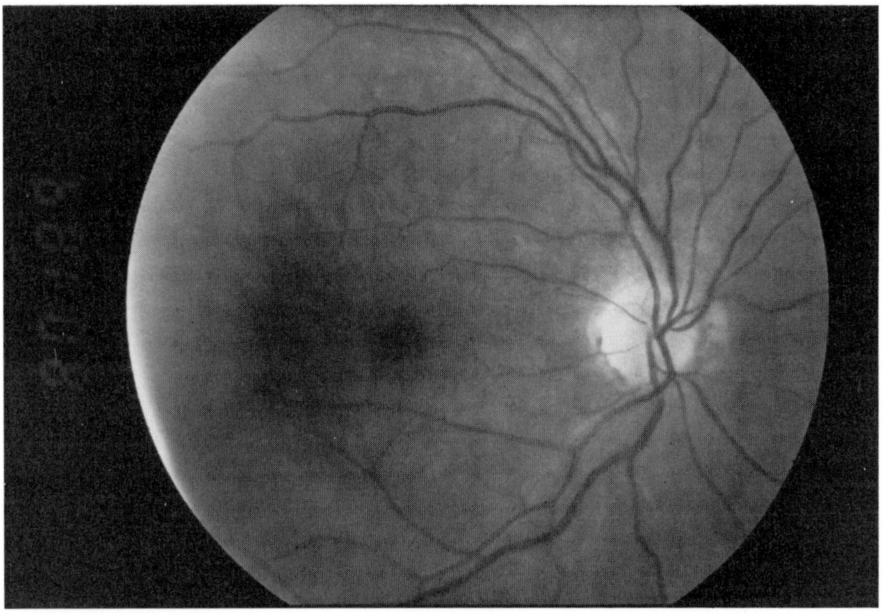

FIGURE 11-10

Multiple evanescent white dot syndrome, OD. Courtesy of Dr. Ann Bidwell, Gurnee, IL.

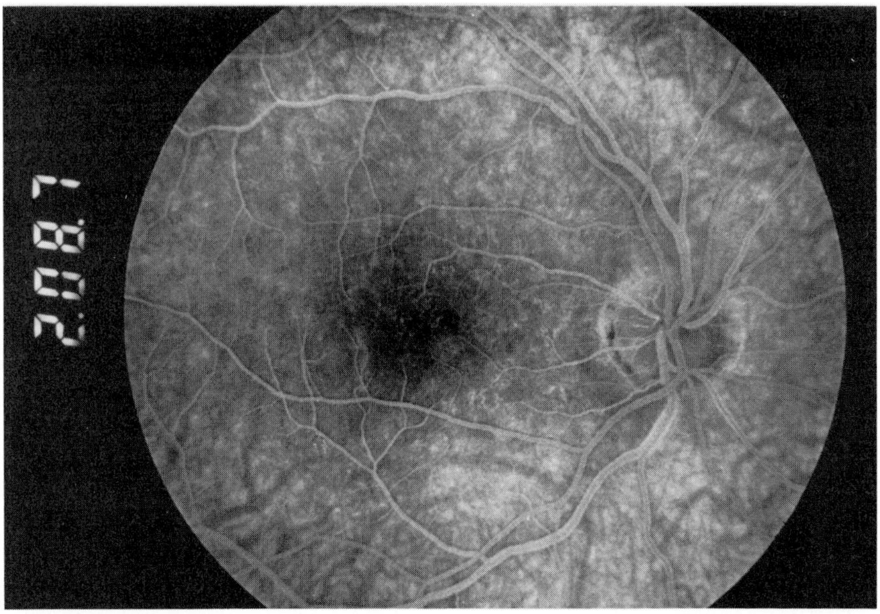

FIGURE 11-11

Fluorescein angiogram of multiple evanescent white dot syndrome with wreath-shaped pattern. Courtesy of Dr. Ann Bidwell, Gurnee, IL.

Acute Macular Neuroretinopathy

Acute macular neuroretinopathy is an entity that shows clover-leaf or wedge-shaped gray lesions in the macular region of both eyes of young patients who complain of rapid vision loss of central and paracentral vision. Usually, there is a preceding flu-like illness. The macular lesion can resemble a dark flower petal. There are no associated vitreous cells.[47,48]

Fluorescein Angiography

There is faint hypofluorescence corresponding to the lesion.

Electroretinography

Electroretinogram shows early receptor potential changes.[49]

Acute Retinal Pigment Epithelitis

Acute retinal pigment epithelitis is a rare entity where there is an acute onset of visual disturbance in one or both eyes of young adults followed by gradual and almost complete recovery in 7–10 weeks.[50] One to 2 weeks after the onset of symptoms, there are multiple clusters of round, dark spots surrounded by depigmented halo-like areas present at the level of the retinal pigment epithelium in the macula and paramacular area. These lesions are usually ¼ disc diameter in size.

Fluorescein Angiography

The fluorescein angiogram shows a halo of hyperfluorescence surrounding the dark spot seen ophthalmoscopically. In some cases the fluorescein angiogram is normal. The visual loss is more than one would expect with the fundus findings.

Treatment

There is no treatment since this is a self-limited disease and spontaneous resolution occurs within 7–10 weeks.

REFERENCES

1. Liddy BSL, Stuart J: Sympathetic ophthalmia in Canada. Can J Ophthalmol 1972; *7:* 157–159

2. Gass JDM: Sympathetic ophthalmia following vitrectomy. Am J Ophthalmol 1982; *93:* 552–558

3. Eason HA, Zimmerman LE: Sympathetic ophthalmia and bilateral phacoanaphylaxis: a clinicopathologic correlation of the sympathogenic and sympathizing eyes. Arch Ophthalmol 1964; *72:* 9–15

4. Blodi FC: Sympathetic uveitis. p. 417. In Freeman HM (ed.): Ocular Trauma. New York, Appleton-Century-Crofts, 1979, pp 417-428

5. Reynard M, Shulman IA, Azen SP, Minckler DS: Histocompatibility antigens in sympathetic ophthalmia. Am J Ophthalmol 1983; *95:* 216–220

6. James DG, Neville E, Siltzbach LE et al: A worldwide review of sarcoidosis. Ann NY Acad Sci 1976; *278:* 321–334

7. Jabs DA, Johns CJ: Ocular involvement with chronic sarcoidosis. Am J Ophthalmol 1986; *102:* 297–301

8. Johns CJ, Schonfeld SA, Scott PP et al: Longitudinal study of chronic sarcoidosis with low-dose maintenance corticosteroid therapy: outcome and complications. Ann NY Acad Sci 1986; *465:* 702–712

9. Mayock RL, Bertrand P, Morrison CE, Scott JH: Manifestations of sarcoidosis: analysis of 145 patients with a review of nine series selected from the literature. Am J Med 1963; *35:* 67–89

10. Obenauf CD, Shaw HE, Sydnor CF, Klintworth GK: Sarcoidosis and its ophthalmic manifestations. Am J Ophthalmol 1978; *86:* 648–655

11. Crystal RG, Roberts WC, Hunninghake GW et al: Pulmonary sarcoidosis: a disease characterized and perpetuated by activated lung T-lymphocytes. Ann Intern Med 1981: *94:* 73–94

12. Hunninghake GW, Crystal RG: Pulmonary sarcoidosis: a disorder mediated by excess helper T-lymphocyte activity at sites of disease activity. N Engl J Med 1981: *305:* 429–434

13. McGavin DDM, Williamson JV, Forrester JV et al: Episcleritis and scleritis: a study of their clinical manifestations and association with rheumatoid arthritis. Br J Ophthalmol 1976; *60:* 192–226

14. Watson PG: The diagnosis and management of scleritis. Ophthalmol 1980; *87:* 716–720

15. Watson PG, Hayreh SS: Scleritis and episcleritis. Br J Ophthalmol 1976; *60:* 163–191

16. Smith RE, Godfrey WA, Kimura SJ: Chronic cyclitis. I. Course and visual prognosis. Trans Am Acad Ophthalmol Otolaryngol 1973; *77:* 760–768

17. Brockhurst RJ, Schepens CL, Okamura ID: Uveitis II. Peripheral uveitis: clinical description, complications and differential diagnosis. Am J Ophthalmol 1960; *49:* 1257–1266

18. Ohno S, Ohguchi M, Hirose S et al: Close association of HLA-Bw5 1 with Behçet's disease. Arch Ophthalmol 1982; *100:* 1455–1458

19. Dinning WJ, Perkins ES: Immunosuppressives in uveitis. A preliminary report of experience with chlorambucil. Br J Ophthalmol 1975; *59:* 397–403

20. Kalbian VV, Chaliis MT: Behçet's disease: report of 12 cases with three manifesting as papilledema. Am J Med 1970; *49:* 823–829

21. Scouras J, Koutroumanos J: Ischaemic optic neuropathy in Behçet's syndrome. Ophthalmologica 1976: *173:* 11–18

22. Mamo JG: The rate of visual loss in Behçet's disease. Arch Ophthalmol 1970; *84:* 451–452

23. Mamo JG: Treatment of Behçet's disease with chlorambucil. Arch Ophthalmol 1970; *84:* 446–450

24. Mamo JG: Treatment of Behçet's disease with chlorambucil: a follow-up report. Arch Ophthalmol 1976; *94:* 580–583

25. Michelson JB, Chisari FV: Behçet's disease. Surv Ophthalmol 1982; *26:* 190–203

26. Nussenblatt RB, Palestine AG, Chan CC: Effectiveness of cyclosporin therapy for Behçet's disease. Arthritis Rheum 1985; *28:* 671–679

27. Palestine AG, Austin HA, Balow JE et al: Renal histopathologic alterations in patients treated with cyclosporine for uveitis. N Eng J Med 1986; *314:* 1293–1298

28. Atkulga E, Altac M, Muftuoglu A et al: A double blind study of colchicine in Behçet's disease, Haematologica 1980; *65:* 399–402

29. Atkulga E, Altac M, Muftuoglu A et al: A double-blind study of colchicine in Behçet's disease.

30. Damato BE, Nanjiani M, Foulds WS: Acute posterior multifocal placoid pigment epitheliopathy: a follow-up study. Trans Ophthalmol Soc UK 1983; *103:* 517–522

31. Fishman GA, Rabb MF, Kaplan J: Acute posterior multifocal placoid pigment epitheliopathy. Arch Ophthalmol 1974; *92:* 173–177

32. Lewis RA, Martonyi CL: Acute posterior multifocal placoid pigment epitheliopathy: a recurrence. Arch Ophthalmol 1975; *93:* 235–238

33. Azar P Jr, Gohd RS, Waltman D, Gitter KA: Acute posterior multifocal placoid pigment epitheliopathy associated with an adenovirus 5 infection. Am J Ophthalmol 1975; *80:* 1003–1005

34. Blumenkranz MS, Gass JDM, Clarkson JG: Atypical serpiginous choroiditis. Arch Ophthalmol 1982; *100:* 1773–1775

35. Chisolm IH, Gass JDM, Hutton WL: The late stage of serpiginous (geographic) choroiditis. Am J Ophthalmol 1976; *82:* 343–351

36. Gass JDM: Stereoscopic Atlas of Macular Disease: Diagnosis and Treatment. 3rd ed. St Louis, The CV Mosby, Co, 1987, pp. 136-143

37. Hamilton AM, Bird AC: Geographical choroidopathy. Br J Ophthalmol 1974; *58:* 784–787

38. Hardy RA, Schatz H: Macular geographic helicoid choroidopathy. Arch Ophthalmol 1987; *105:* 1237–1242

39. Masi RJ, O'Connor GR, Kimura SJ: Anterior uveitis in geographic or serpiginous choroiditis. Am J Ophthalmol 1978; *86:* 228–232

40. Jampol LM, Orth D, Daily MJ, Rabb MF: Subretinal neovascularization with geographic serpiginous choroiditis. Am J Ophthalmol 1979; *88:* 683–689

41. Ryan SJ, Maumenee AE: Birdshot retinochoroidopathy. Am J Ophthalmol 1980; *89:* 31–45

42. Priem HA, Kijlstra A, Noens L et al: HLA typing in birdshot chorioretinopathy. Am J Ophthalmol 1988; *105:* 182–185

43. Watzke RC, Packer AJ, Folk JC et al: Punctate inner choroidopathy. Am J Ophthalmol 1984; *98:* 572–584

44. Jampol LM, Sieving PA, Pugh D: Multiple evanescent white dot syndrome. Am J Ophthalmol 1985; *100:* 29–34

45. Sieving PA, Fishman GA, Jampol LM, Pugh D: Multiple evanescent white dot syndrome. II. Electrophysiology of the photoreceptors during retinal pigment epithelial disease. Arch Ophthalmol 1984; *102:* 675–680

46. Aaberg TM, Campo RV, Joffe L: Recurrences and bilaterality in the multiple evanescent white dot syndrome. Am J Ophthalmol 1985; *100:* 29–33

47. Bos PJM, Deutman AF: Acute macular neuroretinopathy. Am J Ophthalmol 1975; *80:* 573–579

48. Gass JDM: Stereoscopic Atlas of Macular Disease: Diagnosis and Treatment. 2nd ed. St. Louis, The CV Mosby, Co, 1977, p. 304

49. Sieving PA, Fishman GA, Salzano T, Rabb MF: Acute macular retinopathy: early receptor potential changes suggests photoreceptor pathology. Br J Ophthalmol 1984; *68:* 229–235

50. Krill AE, Deutman AF: Acute retinal pigment epithelitis. Am J Opththalmol 1972; *74:* 193–198

CHAPTER TWELVE

Acquired Immunodeficiency Syndrome

Epidemiology

It is thought that 1 to 2 million people in the United States have the serologic evidence of previous infection of human immunodeficiency virus (HIV).[1] By the end of 1991, there were 200,000 patients with acquired immunodeficiency syndrome (AIDS) and two-thirds of these patients have died.[2] With AIDS, the five-year mortality rate is 85 percent. With longer intervals, the rate approaches 100 percent. Most are asymptomatic and some will have mild lymphadenopathy. The virus appears to be transferred by the exchange of body fluids during intimate sexual contact, parenteral innoculation (sharing infected needles), and passage from infected mothers to fetuses or newborns.

Risk Groups

In the United States, there are five major risk groups:

1. Homosexual or bisexual males (70 percent of the cases)
2. Intravenous drug abusers without history of homosexual contact (20 percent of the cases)
3. Hemophiliacs—especially those who received large amounts of pooled factor VIII before 1985 (1 percent of the cases)
4. Blood component recipients excluding hemophiliacs (2.5 percent of the cases). Transmission can occur with as little as one unit of whole blood with an efficieny rate approaching 90 percent
5. Heterosexual contacts (4 percent) and approximately 3.7 percent of the cases, the mode of transmission is unknown.[3]

Heterosexual transmission is now beginning to outpace other modes of transmission in the United States. HIV is not transmitted by casual sexual contact. Outside the United States and Europe, male to female transmission, mostly via vaginal intercourse, is the most common mode of spread.

The risk of seroconversion after an accidental needle stick from HIV infected blood is 0.3 percent.[4]

Pathogenesis

The human immunodeficiency virus, type 1 (HIV-1 virus) is thought to be part of the human type C retrovirus in the same family as the human T-cell leukemia virus-1 (HTLV-1) and is closely related to the HIV-2 virus which causes a similar disease primarily in West Africa. HIV-1 is a cytopathic retrovirus inducing immune destruction of target T-cells with the cell surface antigen of T_4 or CD_4.[5,6] This particular T-cell phenotype is usually referred to as the T-helper phenotype, but also includes subgroups of T-cells responsible for suppressor induction and cytotoxicity.[7] HIV infection will damage or kill the T_4 helper cells, resulting in a reversal of the T-cell helper to suppressor ratio (normal = 1.0 to 2.0 in normal individuals; AIDS patients show ratios < 1.0). The reversal of the helper to suppressor ratio leads to a cell-mediated immunologic incompetence which then causes opportunistic infections and unusual neoplasms.

Clinical Course

Systemic Involvement

Patients have a severe depression of cellular immune function characterized by decreased numbers of circulating T-helper cells and a relative increase in circulating T-suppressor cells. There is an associated elevated circulating immune complexes and elevated serum immunoglobulin A (IgA) and immunoglobulin G (IgG) levels.

After a variable prodromal period, the following signs and symptoms are observed:

1. Acute viral-like illness in 30–50 percent of patients with changes reminiscent of mononucleosis.
2. Persistent generalized lymphadenopathy with mild constitutional symptoms. Minimal CD_4+ T-cell depletion.
3. AIDS-related complex is characterized by persistent fever for 3 months, weight loss, and diarrhea. CD_4+ T-cells are greatly reduced in numbers and there is anemia, thrombocytopenia, and hypergammaglobulinemia. Approximately

30 percent of HIV-positive patients will progress to AIDS, over 55 percent of patients with an AIDS-related complex will progress to AIDS.[8]

4. Full-blown AIDS

a. Opportunistic infections with cytomegalovirus, *Candida albicans*, pneumocystic carinii, *Mycobacterium avium, M. intracellulare, Cryptococcus neoformans,* herpes simplex virus, *Cryptosporidium* sp., *Toxoplasma gondii,* Varicella zoster virus are common in AIDS patients.[9,10]

b. Pyogenic bacterial infections occur, reflecting altered humoral immunity in these patients.

c. Malignant neoplasms: Kaposi's sarcoma occurs in 25 percent of the patients. For unknown reasons, Kaposi's sarcoma is more common in homosexuals than in other risk groups.[11]

d. Neurologic involvement: Acute aseptic meningitis, subacute encephalitis, vacuolar myelopathy, and peripheral neuropathy.

Ocular Involvement

Ocular findings occur in 50–70 percent of the AIDS patients.

1. Cotton wool spots: This is the most common manifestation of AIDS. Up to 60–70 percent of the patients have cotton wool patches.[12] Patients are visually asymptomatic when diagnosed with cotton wool spots. These are focal areas of retinal ischemia and are histologically similar to those cotton wool spots seen in diabetic retinopathy. Histologically, the cotton wool spot is a cytoid body representing a local area of axoplasmic accumulation in the nerve fiber layer resulting from interruption of axoplasmic flow. Cotton wool spots are seen for 4–8 weeks, are not infectious in origin, and no treatment is indicated. Cotton wool spots may just represent a sign of systemic immunosupression (Fig. 12–1).[4]
2. Retinal hemorrhages: These have been seen in up to 30 percent of the AIDS patients, up to 40 percent of patients in autopsy.[13,14] Retinal hemorrhages have also been seen in association with cotton wool spots and cytomegalovirus retinitis.
3. Cranial nerve palsies: These are seen as a result of the meningitis and neurologic involvement of AIDS.
4. Kaposi's sarcoma of adnexa, conjunctiva: One-fifth of the patients have Kaposi's sarcoma which can be seen in the ocular adnexa and on the face (Fig. 12–2).[15] Purplish vascularized lesions are seen in the conjunctival cul-de-sac.

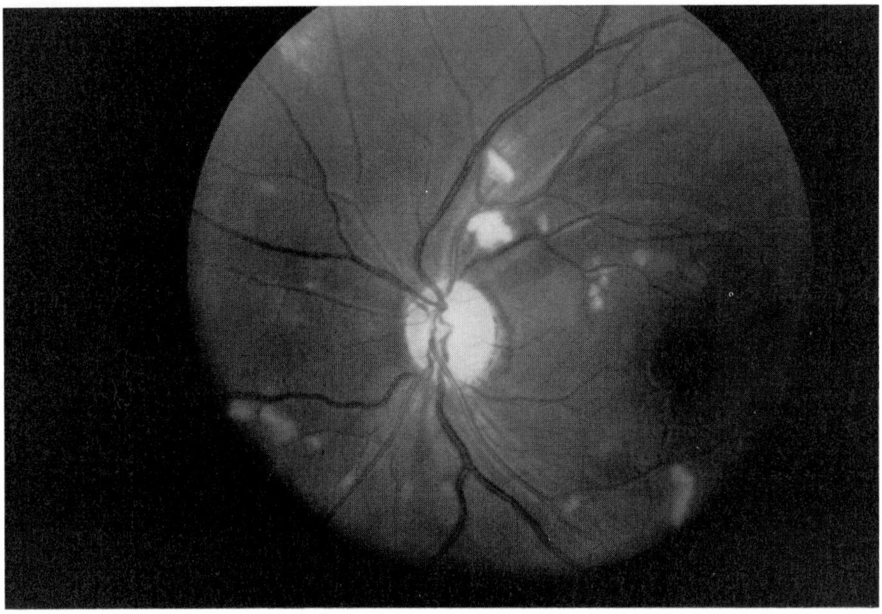

FIGURE 12-1

Cotton wool spots in the immunosuppressed host.

Also seen as small grapelike clusters of vascular tumors appearing around the eyelids. Kaposi's sarcoma can be mistaken for subconjunctival hemorrhages in AIDS patients. Periorbital lymphedema secondary to Kaposi's

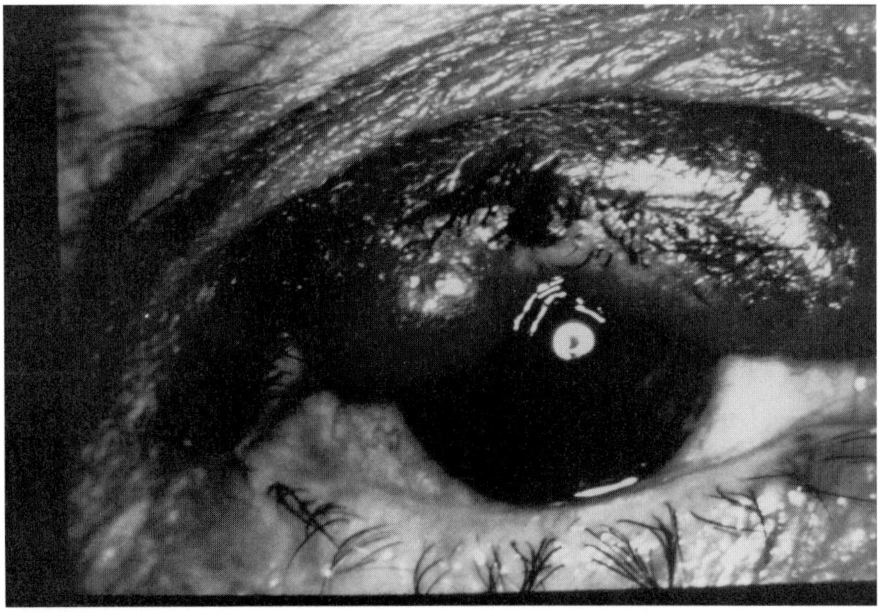

FIGURE 12-2

Kaposi's sarcoma.

sarcoma has been reported.[16] Treatment is directed at local palliation with local irradiation. Interferon alpha has been used with 30–40 percent success, but the side effects of interferon alpha include high fevers, rigors, nausea, vomiting, myalgia, headache, fatigue, and weight loss.[17]

5. Motility defects: See no. 3 above.
6. Conjunctivitis: Look for Kaposi's sarcoma which can be mistaken for conjunctivitis by the primary care physician.
7. Corneal involvement: Corneal changes can occur from herpes zoster ophthalmicus with associated keratitis and uveitis.[18,19] There has been reported chronic active infection of the corneal epithelium by varicella zoster virus after herpes zoster ophthalmicus active infection is treated with high-dose oral or intravenous acyclovir.[20] Chronic bilateral diffuse corneal epitheliopathy has been described with microsporidiosis.[21,22]
8. Vitritis: Can be associated with various opportunistic infections of the eye, e.g., *Candidiasis, Toxoplasmosis* and syphilitic chorioretinitis.
9. Retinitis: See section below on cytomegalovirus retinitis.
10. Choroiditis: Pneumocystis carinii infection can present with yellowish white lesions that are located in the choroid. The lesions are usually in the posterior pole, approximately ½ to ⅓ disc diameter in size.[23]
11. Papilledema: Related to neurologic findings (item no. 1). In cases of various brain abscesses from opportunistic infections, there is increased intracranial pressure and papilledema is present.
12. Optic neuropathy and optic atrophy: Optic neuropathy can be the only presenting eye problem in HIV-positive patients.[24] Optic atrophy can be seen in hospitalized AIDS patients with systemic infections. This can be the sequela of cytomegalovirus retinitis or opportunistic infections of the central nervous system, or part of the HIV infection.[25,26]

Fluorescein Angiography

Fluorescein angiography of these lesions are indistinguishable from those seen from other causes.

CYTOMEGALOVIRUS RETINITIS

Twenty to 25 percent of all AIDS patients have cytomegalovirus retinopathy. Of the numerous opportunistic infections that can be seen in AIDS patients, cytomegalovirus infection occurs commonly.

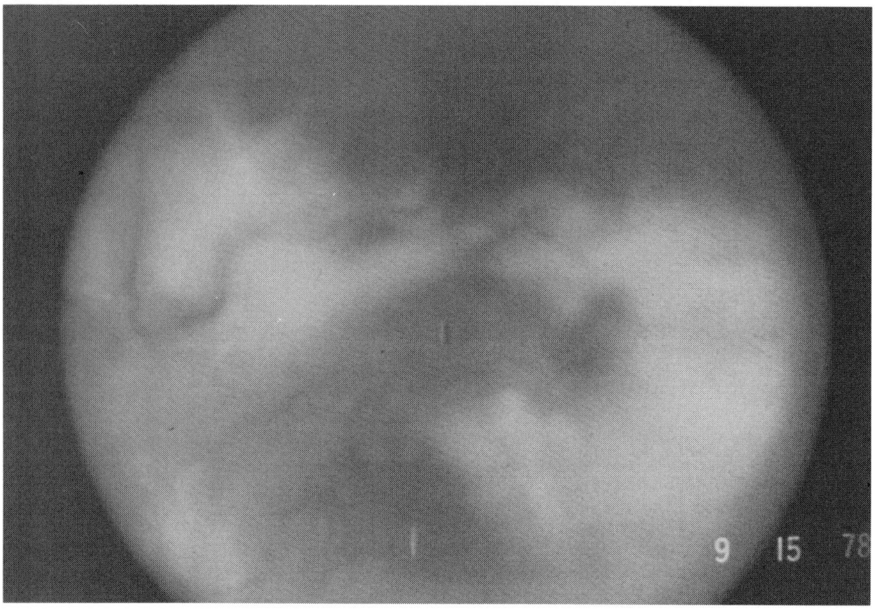

FIGURE 12–3

Cytomegalovirus retinitis.

This usually develops in patients with the most severe immunosuppression and it is part of the current Centers for Disease Control Criteria for diagnosis of AIDS (Fig. 12–3).[3]

Clinical Course

The patient with cytomegalovirus retinitis complains of floaters or visual field deficit. The retina shows a dry, white, granular lesion, near the retinal vessels. Over weeks to months, the lesions show full-thickness retinal necrosis with hemorrhages. Perivascular sheathing is present also. However, there is a minimal overlying vitreous reaction. There is an abrupt transition between necrotic retina and normal retina. Cytomegalovirus does not cross over to the pars plana to involve the ora serrata. There is a slow enlargement of the lesions and lack of prominent intraocular inflammatory reaction. Cytomegalovirus can invade the optic nerve head and present as papillitis with decreased vision.

In the late stage of cytomegalovirus retinitis, there is retinal atrophy, retinal pigment epithelial atrophy, and chorioretinal scarring. Visual loss can occur over a period of months. Regression is associated with a decrease in the number of satellite lesions, disappearance of venous sheathing, and a stable border to the retinal lesions. The areas of viral retinitis will change in color from white to gray to yellow. It will then evolve into a thin, translucent retinal scar with retinal pigment epithelial hyperpigmentation and mottling. In areas of resolved retinitis, there is arteriolar narrowing.

Cytomegalovirus retinitis is most easily confused with toxoplasmic retinochoroiditis, varicella-zoster virus retinitis, and syphilitic retinitis. Varicella-zoster retinitis is rapidly progressive, but cytomegalovirus retinitis is slowly progressive. Toxoplasmic retinochoroiditis and syphilitic retinitis are characterized by marked vitreous inflammatory reaction, severe iridocyclitis, and photophobia.

Treatment

The Food and Drug Administration (FDA) has approved the treatment of cytomegalovirus retinopathy in immunosuppressed patients with ganciclovir (formerly known as dihydroxypropoxymethyl guanine [DHPG] and foscarnet (trisodium phosphonoformate). Both are intravenously delivered and once initiated, the patient must maintain the regimen for life.

For ganciclovir, use a loading dose of 2.5 mg/kg every 8 hours for 10 days followed by a maintenance dose of 5.0 mg/kg every day for 5 days a week. If the drug is discontinued, retinitis often recurs within 10–21 days, continuing its progression at the edges of the healed areas. Recurrences have occurred on maintenance therapy, occurring in 30–40 percent of the patients, usually from 3 weeks to 5 months after institution of therapy. Then it is important to restart the loading dose regimen.[27–31]

The loading dose for foscarnet is 40–60 mg/kg intravenously every 8 hours for 10 days.[32] Maintenance dose of 90–120 mg/kg intravenous infusion over 2 hours everyday.[33]

Both drugs are associated with life-threatening complications. Ganciclovir causes bone marrow supression, with neutropenia and thrombocytopenia. Foscarnet causes renal failure and electrolyte abnormalities and severe hypocalcemia with cardiac disturbances.

In 1988, The National Eye Institute conducted a clinical trial regarding the efficacies and toxicities of ganciclovir and foscarnet. There was no apparent difference between the treatment groups for such major ophthalmic outcome variables as to final visual acuity.[34] The study found that foscarnet-treated patients lived 12.6 months after treatment whereas the ganciclovir-treated patients lived 8.5 months. Thus the study's Policy and Data Monitoring Board suspended randomization of treatment assignments. The choice of treatment with ganciclovir or foscarnet is best left to the patient and the primary care provider. Together, they will make a decision based on the risk of systemic complications and mortality from the drugs.

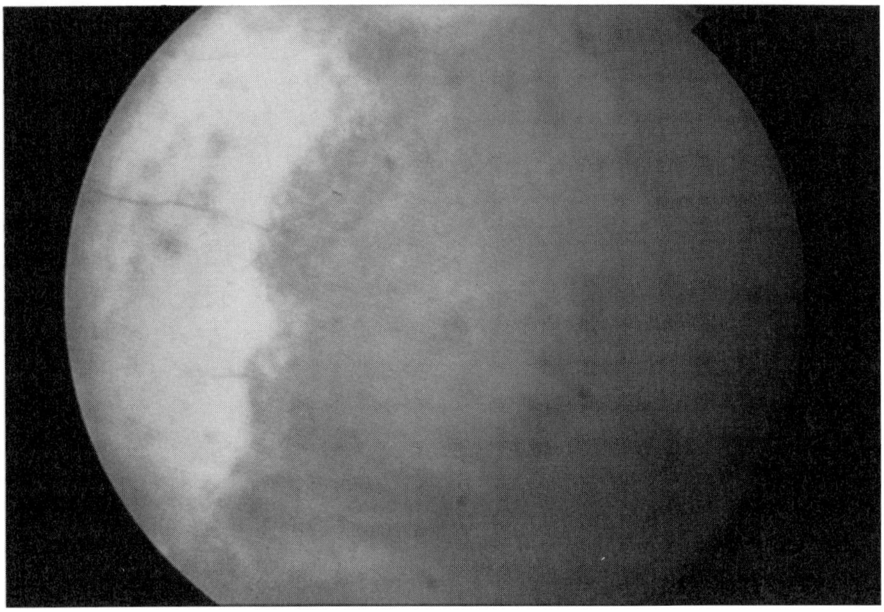

FIGURE 12–4
Acute retinal necrosis.

ACUTE RETINAL NECROSIS

In AIDS patients, acute retinal necrosis is characterized by fulminant panuveitis with confluent, well-demarcated areas of retinitis. Within days, vision deteriorates to the light perception level. There is widespread retinitis up to the far periphery with retinal breaks and subsequent retinal detachment. Retinal atrophy with severe proliferative vitreoretinopathy is seen in the late stages. It is thought that the herpes virus and varicella virus are responsible etiologic agents (Fig. 12–4).[35,36]

Treatment

Treatment of retinal detachments and proliferative vitreoretinopathy in acute retinal necrosis has involved scleral buckle surgery, vitrectomy, the use of perfluorocarbon gases, and silicone oil. Although surgical reattachment is successful, the visual results are disappointing after surgery.[37–39]

REFERENCES

1. Palca J: The sobering geography of AIDS. Science 1991; *252:* 372–374

2. Centers for Disease Control: Human immunodeficiency virus/AIDS surveillance report. 1991; November: 1–18

3. Centers for Disease Control: Revision of the CDC surveillance case definition for acquired immunodeficiency syndrome. MMWR 1987; *36* (suppl. 1)

4. Holland GN: Acquired immunodeficiency syndrome and ophthalmology: the first decade. Am J Ophthalmol 1992; *114:* 86–95

5. Broder S, Gallo RC: Pathogenic retrovirus (HTLV-III) linked to AIDS. N Engl J Med 1984; *311:* 1292–1297

6. Dalgleish AG, Beverley PCL, Clapham PR et al: The CD4 (T4) antigen is an essential component of the receptor for the AIDS retrovirus. Nature 1984; *312:* 763–767

7. Seligmann M, Chess L, Fahey JL et al: AIDS: An immunologic reevaluation. N Engl J Med 1984; *311:* 1286–1292

8. Kaplan JE, Spira TJ, Fishbein DB et al: Lymphadenopathy syndrome in homosexual men: evidence for continuing risk of developing the acquired immunodeficiency syndrome. JAMA 1987; *257:* 335–337

9. Centers for Disease Control: Revision of the case definition of acquired immunodeficiency syndrome for national reporting—United States. MMWR 1985; *3:* 373–375

10. Centers for Disease Control: Update: Acquired immunodeficiency syndrome—United States. MMWR 1986; *35:* 757–766

11. Centers for Disease Control: Update: acquired immunodeficiency syndrome—United States MMWR 1985; *35:* 17–21

12. Pepose JS, Holland GN, Nestor MS et al: Acquired immunodeficiency syndrome: pathogenic mechanisms of ocular disease. Ophthalmol 1895; *92:* 472–484

13. Holland GN, Pepose JS, Pettit TH et al: Acquired immunodeficiency syndrome: ocular manifestations. Ophthalmol 1983; *90:* 859–853

14. Newsome DA, Green WR, Miller ED et al: Microvascular aspect of acquired immunodeficiency syndrome retinopathy. Am J Ophthalmol 1984; *98:* 590–601

15. Centers for Disease Control: Update: acquired immunodeficiency syndrome—United States. MMWR 1985; *35:* 17–21

16. Freeman WR, Lerner CW, Mines, JA et al: A prospective study of the ophthalmologic findings in the acquired immunodeficiency syndrome. Am J Ophthalmol 1984; *97:* 133–142

17. Kaplan LD, Wofsy CB, Volberding PA: Treatment of patients with acquired immunodeficiency syndrome. JAMA 1987; *257:* 335–337

18. Cole EL, Meisler DM, Calbrese LH et al: Herpes zoster ophthalmicus and acquired immune deficiency syndrome. Arch Ophthalmol 1984; *102:* 1027–1029

19. Sandor EV, Millman A, Croxson TS, Mildvan D: Herpes zoster ophthalmicus in patients at risk for the acquired immune deficiency syndrome (AIDS). Am J Ophthalmol 1986; *101:* 153–155

20. Engstrom RE, Holland GN: Chronic herpes zoster virus keratitis associated with the acquired immunodeficiency syndrome. Am J Ophthalmol 1988; *105:* 556–558

21. Lowder CY, Meisler DM, McMahon JT et al: Microsporidia infection of the cornea in a man seropositive for human immunodeficiency virus. Am J Ophthalmol 1990; *109:* 242–244

22. Friedberg DN, Stenson SM, Orenstein JM et al: Microsporidial keratoconjunctivitis in acquired immunodeficiency syndrome. Arch Ophthalmol 1990; *108:* 504–508

23. Dugel PU, Rao NA, Forster DJ et al: Pneumocystis carinii choroiditis after longterm aerosolized pentamidine therapy. Am J Ophthalmol 1990; *110:* 113–116

24. Newman NJ, Lessell S: Bilateral optic neuropathies with remission in two HIV-positive men. J Clin Neuro-Ophthalmol 1992; *12:* 1–5

25. Shaw GM, Harper ME, Hahn BH et al: HTLV-III infection in brains of children and adults with AIDS encephalopathy. Science 1985; *227:* 177–181

26. Brodie SE, Friedman AH: Retinal dysfunction as an initial ophthalmic sign in AIDS. Br J Ophthalmol 1990; *74:* 49–51

27. Bach MC, Bagwell SP, Knapp NP et al: 9-(1,3-dihydroxy-2-propoxymethyl) guanine for cytomegalovirus infections in patients with the acquired immunodeficiency syndrome. Ann Intern Med 1985; *103:* 381–382

28. Collaborative DHPG Treatment Study Group. Treatment of serious cytomegalovirus infections with 9-(1,3-dihydroxy-2-propoxymethyl)guanine in patients with AIDS and other immunodeficiencies. N Engl J Med 1986; *314:* 801–805

29. Felsenstein D, D'Amico DJ, Hirsch MS et al: Treatment of cytomegalovirus retinitis with 9-(2-hydroxy-1-(hydroxymethyl) ethoxymethyl) guanine. Ann Intern Med 1985; *103:* 377–380

30. Palestine AG, Stevens G Jr, Lane HC et al: Treatment of cytomegalovirus retinitis with dihydroxy propoxymethyl guanine. Am J Ophthalmol 1986; *101:* 95–101

31. Rosecan LR, Stahl-Bayliss CM, Kalman CM, Laskin OL: Antiviral therapy for cytomegalovirus retinitis in AIDS with dihydroxypropoxymethyl guanine. Am J Ophthalmol 1986; *101:* 405–418

32. Safrin S, Crumpacker C, Chatis P et al: AIDS clinical trials group. A controlled trial comparing foscarnet with vidarabine for acyclovir-resistant mucocutaneous herpes simplex in the acquired immunodeficiency syndrome. N Engl J Med 1991; *325:* 551–555

33. Abramowicz M (ed): Handbook of Antimicrobial Therapy. New Rochelle: The Medical Letter, 1992, p. 68

34. Studies of ocular complications of AIDS (SOCA) research group in collaboration with the AIDS Clinical trials group (ACTG): Mortality in patients with the acquired immunodeficiency syndrome with either patients with the acquired immunodeficiency syndrome with either foscarnet or ganciclovir for cytomegalovirus retinitis. N Engl J Med 1992; *326:* 213–220

35. Freeman WR, Thomas EL, Rao NA et al: Demonstration of herpes group virus in acute retinal necrosis syndrome. Am J Ophthalmol 1986; *102:* 701–709

36. Ludwig IH, Zegarra H, Zakov ZN: The acute retinal necrosis syndrome: possible herpes simplex retinitis. Ophthalmol 1984; *91:* 1659–1664

37. Sidikaro Y, Silver L, Holland GN, Kreiger AE: Rhegmatogenous retinal detachments in patients with AIDS and necrotizing retinal infections. Ophthalmol 1991; *98:* 129–132

38. Jabs DA, Enger C, Haller J, De Bustros S: Retinal detachments in patients with cytomegalovirus retinitis. Arch Ophthalmol 1991; *109:* 794–797

39. Holland GN: The management of retinal detachments in patients with acquired immunodeficiency syndrome. (editorial) Arch Ophthalmol 1991; *109:* 791–793

CHAPTER THIRTEEN

Retinal Vein Occlusion

BRANCH RETINAL VEIN OCCLUSION

Epidemiology

Branch retinal vein occlusion is the second most common retinal vascular disease entity after diabetic retinopathy.[1] Males and females are equally affected, with the common age in the sixth and seventh decade of life. Increased incidence of branch retinal vein occlusion occurs with hypertension,[2–4] history of cardiovascular disease, and history of glaucoma.[4]

Anatomy and Pathophysiology

On histopathologic examination, arteriosclerotic changes have been found in the eyes of patients with branch retinal vein occlusions.[5] The common sheath at the site of crossing between the branch artery and vein predisoposes this site as a region for branch retinal occlusions. Clinically, the artery crossing the vein lies anteriorly (towards the vitreous cavity) in the site of the branch retinal vein occlusions.[6–8] The superotemporal veins are most frequently involved.[2]

Associated Diseases

Associated disorders of branch retinal vein occlusion[1–5] are hypertension, carotid artery disease, diabetes mellitus, open-angle glaucoma, hyperlipidemia, Crohn's disease,[9] and systemic inflammatory disease.

Clinical Course

The patient presents with sudden visual loss in the central visual axis or a peripheral visual field deficit. In early and mild cases of branch retinal vein occlusion, reading visual acuity could be affected. The prognosis for good vision depends on the extent of involvement, associated macular edema, and retinal vascular changes.

Diagnosis

A classic branch retinal vein occlusion occurs at an arteriovenous crossing, usually superotemporally. This is usually at the disc or in the posterior pole. There are superficial hemorrhages, retinal edema, and soft exudates. The vein, peripheral to the site of occlusion is usually distended. Usually, the changes are limited to one side of horizontal raphe. The hemorrhages are most obvious at the nerve fiber layer (Fig. 13–1).

The diagnosis is made with slit-lamp biomicroscopy and indirect ophthalmoscopy. It is important to check the intraocular pressure and check the angle of neovascularization. In addition, it is important to look at the anatomic sites, because the patient may develop neovascular glaucoma later on.

Classification[1]

Major branch retinal vein occlusion at disc margin (with and without macular edema)

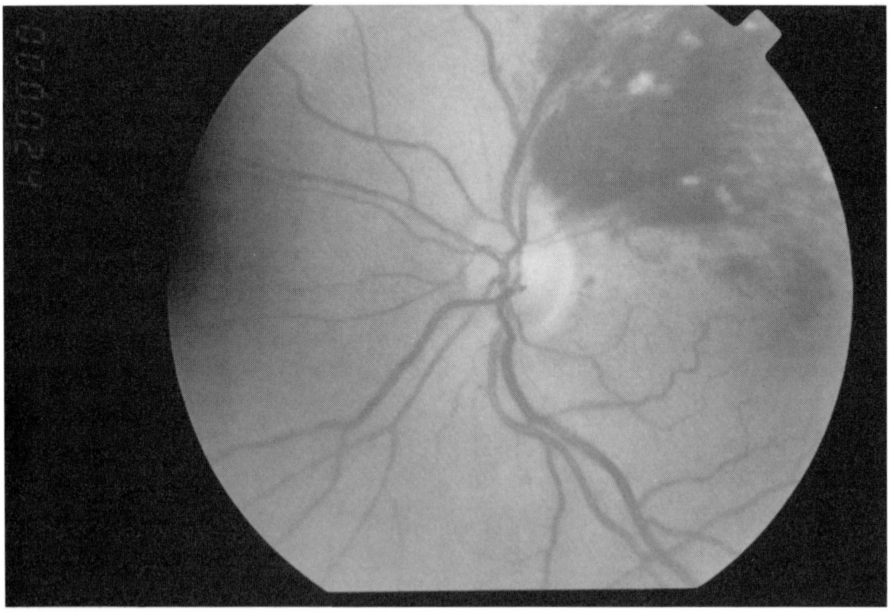

FIGURE 13–1

Branch retinal vein occlusion, OS.

Major branch retinal vein occlusion away from the disc margin (with and without macular edema)

Macular branch vein occlusion

Peripheral branch vein occlusion

Branch vein occlusion with neovascularization at the optic disc

Branch retinal vein occlusion with neovascularization elsewhere

Complications include chronic macular edema (cystoid macular edema, circinate ring of hard exudate, and associated retinal edema in the macula). Macular changes include retinal pigment epithelial atrophy or hypertrophy, macular hole, persistent macular hemorrhages. The vasculature changes include dilated pre-existing vascular channels, arteriolosclerosis, abnormal iris vascular patterns, iris neovascularization, and retinal neovascularization. Vitreous hemorrhage, serous detachments of the sensory retina, rhegmatogenous retinal detachment, and retinal holes can also occur.

Fluorescein Angiography

Acute

There is obscuration of background choroidal fluorescence caused by intraretinal hemorrhage. There can be areas of capillary nonperfusion. In addition, there is diffuse intraretinal leakage of fluorescein dye.

Chronic

There is the presence of collaterals and shunt vessels, microaneuryms and large areas of capillary loss, macular edema, progressive arteriolar obliteration through nonperfused areas, staining of venous walls associated with occasional faint leakage of fluorescein into the retina, fluorescein leakage from neovascularization on the disc or elsewhere in the retina, and serous detachment of the sensory retina.

Treatment

Branch Retinal Vein Occlusion Study

In 1984, the Branch Retinal Vein Occlusion Study[10] examined eyes with macular edema and branch retinal vein occlusion and vision worse than 20/40. These eyes were considered for laser treatment. The percentage of eyes gaining two or more lines of vision was 65 percent in the treated group and 37 percent in the untreated group. This difference was found to be statistically significant. Since that time, this has been the accepted level of care for the treatment of macular edema in branch retinal vein occlusion patients.

Laser

Argon laser is used to perform a grid pattern over the areas of capillary nonperfusion seen on fluorescein angiography, photocoagulation extending up to the foveal avascular zone, and not extending peripherally to the major vascular arcade.[10]

CENTRAL RETINAL VEIN OCCLUSION

Epidemiology

Central retinal vein occlusion is the second leading cause of retinal vascular disease after diabetic retinopathy.[1] Central retinal vein occlusion is associated with hypertension, diabetes[11–14] and an elevated erythrocyte sedimentation rate.[14] Ischemic heart disease is another risk factor.[12] Open-angle glaucoma and elevated intraocular pressure is associated more with central vein occlusion than branch retinal vein occlusion.[14–16] Although the mechanism is unclear, collagen vascular disease, malignancies, infections, and tuberculosis may cause changes in blood viscosity and changes in the flow or hemodynamics which can lead to central retinal vein occlusion.

Anatomy and Pathophysiology

The central retinal vein narrows as it passes through the lamina cribosa in the normal eye. Conditions that lead to the narrowing or increased turbulence of flow through this partial barrier may predispose to central retinal vein occlusion.[17,18] Thrombosis of the central retinal vein is the inciting event.[19] A fresh or recanalized thrombus is seen in the central retinal vein in all 29 eyes reported by Green and coworkers.[19] Chronic inflammation was seen in the area of the thrombus and/or wall or perivenular area in many of the eyes examined.[19]

Associated Diseases

Predisposing ophthalmic diseases are glaucoma,[20] papilledema, subdural hemorrhage, optic nerve hemorrhage,[21] optic nerve drusen.[22] Associated systemic diseases are hypertension,[23] cardiovascular[24] and cerebrovascular diseases, diabetes mellitus, and leukemia with thrombocytopenia.[19] The use of oral contraceptives has also been associated with central retinal vein occlusion.[25]

Clinical Course

Although the classification of central retinal vein occlusion in the past had been divided into the ischemic and nonischemic varieties, pathologic studies[19] do not really support this differentiation. In addition, both groups of eyes are found to have a high rate of neovascularization of the iris. Ongoing studies such as the Central Retinal Vein Occlusion Study is trying to further delineate the natural history of this disease.[12]

Diagnosis

The diagnosis of central retinal vein occlusion occurs with the sudden loss of vision in one eye. The retinal examination shows hemorrhages in four quadrants. Most prominently, there are dilated veins emanating from the optic disc. In the posterior pole, there are different caliber of veins associated with intraretinal hemorrhages.

In early stages of central retinal vein occlusion, there are just dilated veins at the optic disc and in the next few days, hemorrhages and widespread venous engorgement appears. At the earliest stages of a central retinal vein occlusion, the vision may be only mildly impaired. With increased retinal hemorrhages, the vision decreases markedly (Fig. 13–2).

The diagnosis of central retinal vein occlusion is made with the indirect ophthalmoscope which permits viewing of the posterior pole as well as the periphery. Using slit-lamp biomicroscopy, the optic nerve vasculature can be seen. In addition, with 90 diopter or Hruby lenses, early macular edema can be identified. Examination of the retinal periphery is useful to note any retinal neovascularization, areas of thrombotic vessels, or marked arteriolosclerotic changes. Gonioscopy of the angle will highlight any areas of iris neovascularization, a harbinger of neovascular glaucoma. Examination of the fellow eye is useful to determine open-angle glaucoma as an associated condition.

Electroretinography

The Central Vein Occlusion Study examined the usefulness of the electroretinogram.[12] The electroretinogram has been used to evaluate overall retinal ischemia of the eye since the retinal examination and fluorescein angiography is limited when massive hemorrhages exist. Sabates, Hirose, and McMeel found that if the

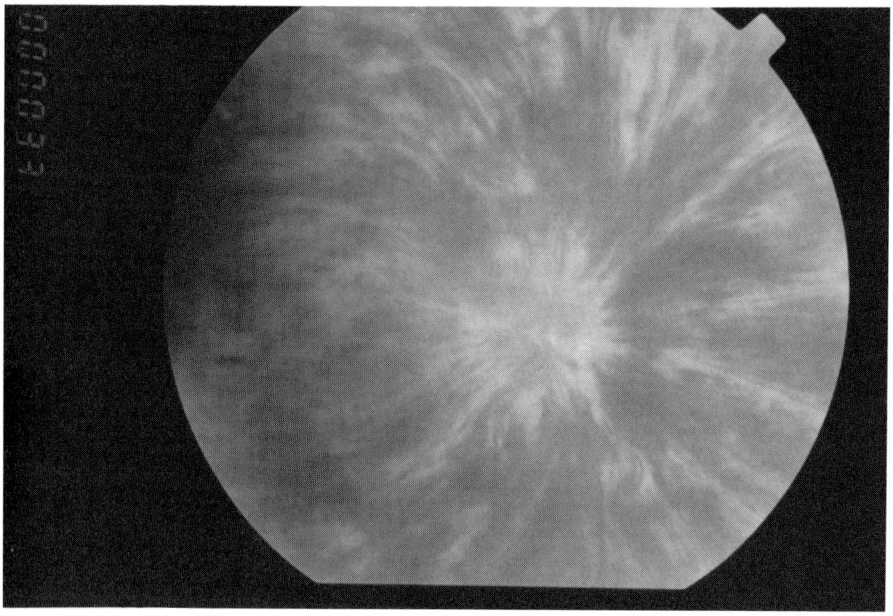

FIGURE 13-2

Central retinal vein occlusion, OD.

b/a wave ratio is less than 1, there is a high risk for the development of neovascular glaucoma.[13]

Fluorescein Angiography

With massive retinal hemorrhages, there is obscuration of much of the fluorescein detail in the choroidal phase of the angiogram. In later phases of the angiogram, there is profuse intraretinal leakage and concomitant hyperfluorescence of the fluorescein dye. However, in areas with fewer hemorrhages, as in the periphery, the fluorescein angiogram is helpful in determining areas and extent of capillary nonperfusion. In eyes with large areas of capillary nonperfusion and ischemia, one needs to monitor closely for the development of neovascular glaucoma.

Treatment

Medical

There is no medical treatment available for central retinal vein occlusion. However, the treatment of the underlying systemic disease is helpful, i.e., control of systemic hypertension, diabetes mellitus, or open-angle glaucoma. There has been previous attempts at anticoagulation or antithrombolytic therapy; however, their efficacy has remained unproven at this point. However, patients with central retinal vein occlusion appear to be at no greater risk for mortality compared with a United States population-based mortality rate and no less healthier (except for hypertension) than age-matched institutional controls.[13]

Laser

The evolution of laser treatment for areas 5 disc diameters or more of capillary nonperfusion began with the Branch Retinal Vein Occlusion Study in 1984.[12] Physicians began treating similar changes in patients with central retinal vein occlusion. However, controversy exists about the efficacy of laser photocoagulation in central retinal vein occlusion.[27–31] The ongoing Central Retinal Vein Occlusion Study will discuss some of the these treatment parameters in future publications.[12]

REFERENCES

1. Orth DH, Patz A: Retinal vein occlusion. Surv Ophthalmol 1978; *22:* 357–376

2. Blankenship GW, Okun E: Retinal tributary vein occlusion: history and management by photocoagulation. Arch Ophthalmol 1973; *89:* 363–368

3. Gutman FA, Zegarra H: The natural course of temporal retinal branch vein occlusion. Trans Am Acad Ophthalmol Otolaryngol 1974; *78:* 178–192

4. The Eye Disease Case–Control Study Group. Risk factors for branch retinal vein occlusion. Am J Ophthalmol 1993; *116:* 286–296

5. Bowers DK, Finkelstein D, Wolff SM, Green WR: Branch retinal vein occlusion: a clinicopathologic case report. Retina 1987; *7:* 252–259

6. Duker J, Brown GC: Anterior location of the crossing artery in branch retinal vein obstruction. Arch Ophthalmol 1989; *107:* 998–1000

7. Weinberg D, Dodwell DG, Fern SA: Anatomy of arteriovenous crossings in branch retinal vein occlusion. Am J Ophthalmol 1990; *109:* 298–302

8. Feist RM, Ticho BH, Shapiro MJ, Farber M: Branch retinal vein occlusion and quadrantic variation in arteriovenous crossings. Am J Ophthalmol 1992; *113:* 664–668

9. Ruby AJ, Jampol LM: Crohn's disease and retinal vascular disease. Am J Ophthalmol 1990; *110:* 349–353

10. The Branch Vein Occlusion Study Group. Argon laser photocoagulation for macular edema in branch vein occlusion. Am J Ophthalmol 1984; *98:* 271–282

11. Zegarra H, Gutman FA, Conforto J: The natural course of central retinal vein occlusion. Ophthalmol 1979; *86:* 1931–1939

12. The Central Retinal Vein Occlusion Study Group: Baseline and early natural history report: The central retinal vein occlusion study. Arch Ophthalmol 1993; *111:* 1087–1095

13. Elman MJ, Bhatt AK, Quinlan PM, Enger C: The risk for systemic vascular diseases and mortality in patients with central retinal vein occlusion. Ophthalmol 1990; *97:* 1543–1548

14. Sabates R, Hirose T, McMeel JW: Electroretinography in the prognosis and classification of central retinal vein occlusion. Arch Ophthalmol 1983; *101:* 232–235

15. Appiah AP, Trempe CL: Differences in contributory factors among hemicentral, central, and branch retinal vein occlusions. Ophthalmol 1989; *96:* 364–366

16. Vannas S, Tarkkanen A: Retinal vein occlusion and glaucoma: Tonographic study of the incidence of glaucoma and of its prognostic significance. Br J Ophthalmol 1960; *44:* 583–589

17. Frucht J, Shapiro A, Merin S: Intraocular pressure in retinal vein occlusion. Br J Ophthalmol 1984; *68:* 26–28

18. Ring CP, Pearson TC, Sanders MD, Wetherley-Mein G: Viscosity and retinal vein thrombosis. Br J Ophthalmol 1976; *60:* 397–410

19. Hayreh SS: Pathogenesis of occlusion of the central retinal vessels. Am J Ophthalmol 1971; *72:* 998–1011

20. Green WR, Chan CC, Hutchins GM, Terry JM: Central retinal vein occlusion: a prospective histopathologic study of 29 eyes in 28 cases. Retina 1981; *1:* 27–55

21. Dryden RM: Central retinal vein occlusion and chronic simple glaucoma. Arch Ophthalmol 1965; *73:* 659–663

22. Broderick JD: Drusen of the disc and retinal haemorrhages. Br J Ophthalmol 1973; *57:* 299–306

23. Boyce SW, Platia EV, Green WR: Drusen of the optic nerve head. Ann Ophthalmol 1978; *10:* 695–704

24. Paton A, Rubinstein K, Smith VH: Arterial insufficiency in retinal venous occlusion. Trans Ophthalmol Soc UK 1964; *84:* 559–586

25. Rubinstein K, Jones EB: Retinal vein occlusion: Longterm prospects—10 years follow-up of 143 patients. Br J Ophthalmol 1976; *60:* 148–150

26. Stowe GC, Zakov ZN, Albert DM: Central retinal vascular occlusion associated with oral contraceptives. Am J Ophthalmol 1978; *86:* 798–801

27. Magargal LE, Brown GC, Augsberger JJ, Donoso LA: Efficacy of panretinal photocoagulation in preventing neovascular glaucoma following ischemic central retinal vein obstruction. Ophthalmol 1982; *89:* 780–784

28. Hayreh SS, Klugman MR, Podhajsky P et al: Argon laser panretinal photocoagulation in ischemic central retinal vein occlusion. Graefes Arch Clin Exp Ophthalmol 1990; *228:* 281–296

29. May DR, Klein ML, Peyman GA, Raichand M: Xenon arc panretinal photocoagulation for central vein occlusion: a randomized prospective study. Br J Ophthalmol 1979; *63:* 725–734

30. Laatkainen L, Kohner EM, Khoury D, Blach RK: Panretinal photocoagulation in central vein occlusion: a randomomized controlled clinical study. Br J Ophthalmol 1977; *61:* 741–753

31. Central Vein Occlusion Study: Photocoagulation for ischemic central retinal vein occlusion. Arch Ophthalmol 1991; *109:* 1218–1219

CHAPTER FOURTEEN

Ocular Ischemia Syndrome

Ocular symptoms and signs attributable to severe carotid artery obstruction or other ischemic coronary artery disease is called the ocular ischemia syndrome.

EPIDEMIOLOGY

Ocular ischemia syndrome is an underreported disorder since this syndrome mimicks other disorders such as diabetic retinopathy or arterial and venous obstructive diseases (see Chapters 4, 6, 13, respectively) (Fig. 14–1). There has been one English report of 6 patients who had this disease, found over a two-year period in a hospital serving a population of 400,000.[1]

The age of presentation is usually in the fifth and sixth decade of life when carotid artery and coronary artery diseases are prevalent. Although usually unilateral, 20 percent of the time, it is bilateral.[2] There is a male preponderance in this disease entity again reflecting the same population as those who have carotid artery and coronary artery diseases.

ANATOMY AND PATHOPHYSIOLOGY

It is postulated that those who have carotid disease with stenosis of the carotid artery, the eye ipsilateral to the internal or common carotid artery stenosis experiences a markedly reduced flow, and hence, ischemia to the eye. A 90 percent stenosis of the carotid artery diminishes retinal arterial perfusion pressure by 50 percent.[3,4]

CLINICAL COURSE

There is a mild loss of vision to severe loss of vision that occurs gradually. The symptom of pain is found in 40 percent of patients

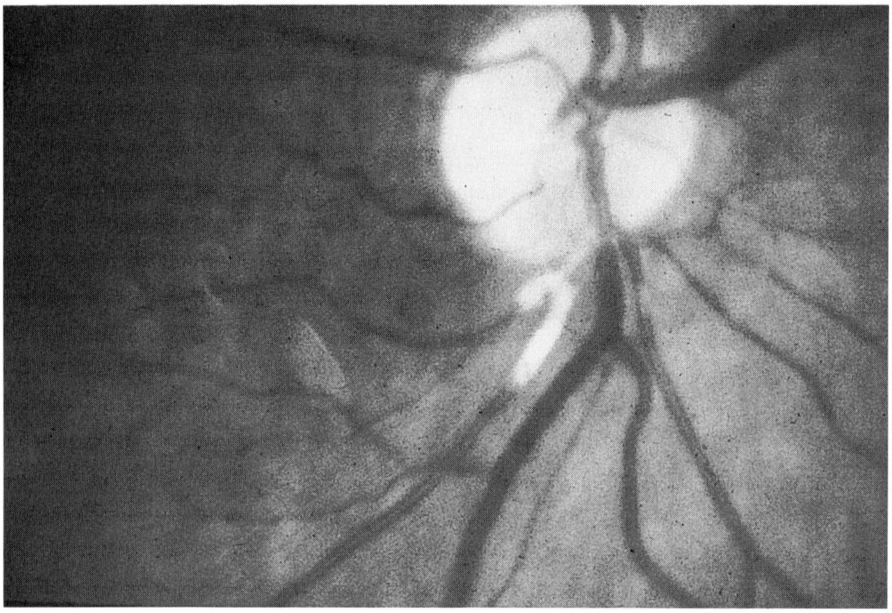

FIGURE 14–1

Cholesterol plaque in arterial system.

with ocular ischemia. When pain occurs, there may be ischemia to the globe and neovascular glaucoma.

DIAGNOSIS

In the anterior segment, neovascularization of the iris is observed in two-thirds of the cases. The pupillary border or the angle was a good place to look for rubeosis iridis. When rubeosis was present, flare was also present in the anterior chamber. Neovascular glaucoma is also present in this syndrome. Iritis can be the presenting complaint in one-fifth of the cases. Retinal findings show narrowed retinal arteries and dilated but not tortuous retinal veins. Midperipheral retinal hemorrhages are common. Posterior retinal neovascularization is seen in one-third of the cases. Rarely is a cherry-red spot seen. In diabetic patients, there is marked asymmetry of the diabetic retinopathy.

FLUORESCEIN ANGIOGRAPHY

Delayed choroidal and delayed arteriovenous filling can be seen. Patchy or delayed choroidal filling pattern, staining of the retinal vessels, macular edema, microaneurysms in nondiabetic individuals, retinal capillary nonperfusion is evident as well.

ELECTRORETINOGRAPHY

There is an overall reduction in amplitude of both a- and b-waves.

ASSOCIATED DISEASES

Hypertension and diabetes are commonly associated with ocular ischemia, as well as atherosclerotic cardiovascular disease, previous cerebrovascular accident, and amaurosis fugax. The following is a list of various procedures:

Medical consultation
Medical laboratory diagnostic evaluation
Carotid artery ultrasound
Protein C to look for hypercoagulable state
Electroretinogram
Electrocardiogram
Echocardiogram of the heart
Holter monitoring of the heart

TREATMENT

Because ocular ischemia syndrome is rather rare, there are no large clinical trials evaluating the long-term effects of treatment for these patients. The visual prognosis of untreated eyes with ocular ischemia is poor.

Mild ocular ischemia is probably underdiagnosed. In patients with known carotid artery stenosis, but less than 90 percent, and the above signs and symptoms are noted, it is important for the patient to consult an internist or cardiologist. Use of daily dose of 325 mg of aspirin may be indicated for treatment of underlying cardiovascular disease. It is unclear about the efficacy of this treatment long term.

In patients with rubeosis iridis and/or neovascular glaucoma, panretinal photocoagulation should be considered.[5,6] Regression of these neovascular vessels occur over a longer period of time than in patients with diabetic retinopathy and central retinal vein occlusion.

In patients with obvious ocular ischemia, evaluating the severity of carotid stenosis is important. Noninvasive studies such as carotid ultrasonography, oculoplethysmography, and periorbital doppler scanning can detect lesions. Carotid arteriography is the most sensitive test for detecting stenosis; however, it carries a higher risk than the noninvasive studies.

In complete obstruction of the carotid artery, successful endarectomy may lead to stabilization of the vision in some cases only. There is no guarantee of return of good vision for the patient.

REFERENCES

1. Surrock GD, Mueller HR: Chronic ocular ischemia. Br J Ophthalmol 1984; *68:* 716–723
2. Brown GC, Magargal LE: The ocular ischemic syndrome. Int Ophthalmol 1988; *11:* 239–251
3. Kearns TP: Ophthalmology and the carotid artery. Am J Ophthalmol 1979; *88:* 714–722
4. Kobayashi S, Hollenhorst RW, Sundt TM Jr: Retinal arterial pressure before and after surgery for carotid artery stenosis. Stroke 1971; *2:* 569–575
5. Carter JE: Panretinal photocoagulation for progressive ocular neovascularization secondary to occlusion of the common carotid artery. Ann Ophthalmol 1984; *16:* 572–576
6. Eggleston TF, Bohling CA, Eggleston HC, Hershey FB: Photocoagulation for ocular ischemia associated with carotid artery occlusion. Ann Ophthalmol 1980; *12:* 84–87

CHAPTER FIFTEEN

Pregnancy

PATHOPHYSIOLOGY

The pregnant woman undergoes many physiologic changes in the course of a normal pregnancy. There is an average weight gain of 11 kg during pregnancy with retention of an average of 6.5 L of water. Serum osmolality is decreased. Pregnancy can be diabetogenic because of an increase of human placental lactogen, increased levels of estrogen, progesterone, and insulinase activity of the placenta.[1]

The blood volume averages about 45 percent above nonpregnancy levels with an increase in plasma volume as well as 33 percent increase in circulating erythrocytes.[1] Consequently, an iron deficiency is present and there is an increase in the level of clotting factors and clotting activity.[1] There is an increase in the resting pulse rate and a decrease in arterial blood pressure which reaches a minimum during the second or early third trimester. Cardiac output is increased and there is decreased vascular resistance.[1]

Pregnancy has been assumed to be associated with suppression of humoral and cellular-mediated immunologic functions in order to tolerate the "foreign" semiallogenic fetal graft. It is possible that altered immunity status of pregnant women may account for their observed improvement with certain autoimmune diseases and increased susceptibility to certain infections.[1]

RETINAL CHANGES

Central Serous Choroidopathy

Proposed causes of central serous choroidopathy in pregnancy include hormonal alterations of increased blood flow, increased cardiac output, and changes in permeability along with decreased colloid osmotic pressure.[2,3] The presenting complaints of women with central serous choroidopathy is the same as in the male patients, i.e., decreased central vision, central scotoma, and metamorphopsia. Central serous choroidopathy can occur at any time during pregnancy, and in most cases, symptomatic visual recovery occurs in the postpartum period.[4] The postpartum course shows mottling and clumping of the retinal pigment epithelium. In some cases, recurrent central serous choroidopathy has occurred in the same eye in successive pregnancies. However, with other patients, during their subsequent pregnancies, they do not have repeat episodes of central serous choroidopathy.[4]

Diagnosis (See Chapter 8)

The diagnosis, in pregnant patients, is often made on clinical findings. The patient usually complains of a central relative scotoma and metamorphopsia. On physical examination, there is a clear blisterlike pocket of fluid in the center of the macula area. Usually just under the superior half of the retinal detachment is an area of retinal pigment epithelial mottling, demarcating the area of the retinal pigment epithelial detachment. The retinal pigment epithelium may be best seen with slit-lamp biomicroscopy with retroillumination techniques.

Fluorescein Angiography

Although no harm has been reported to the pregnant woman or her fetus, fluorescein angiography is not universally used in the management of pregnant patients.[5,6]

The fluorescein angiographic characteristics are the same as those in nonpregnant patients (see Chapter 8). There is the classic hyperfluorescence seen at the choroidal phase of the fluorescein angiogram. Usually this is followed by slow filling of the hyperfluorescent fluorescein dye into the bleb of the serous elevation of the retina.

Treatment

Since central serous choroidopathy is a self-limiting disease, usually no treatment is necessary.

HYPERTENSIVE CHANGES IN THE RETINA

Pregnancy-induced hypertension is hypertension that occurs in a pregnant woman who was previously normotensive in the non-pregnant state. In this same category is pre-eclampsia—hyper-tension, edema, and proteinuria—present in the twentieth week of pregnancy (Fig. 15–1).

Pre-eclampsia in the otherwise healthy women occurs in 5 percent of pregnant patients, a disease of first pregnancies. Very young, older, or multiparous women with multifetal pregnancy are

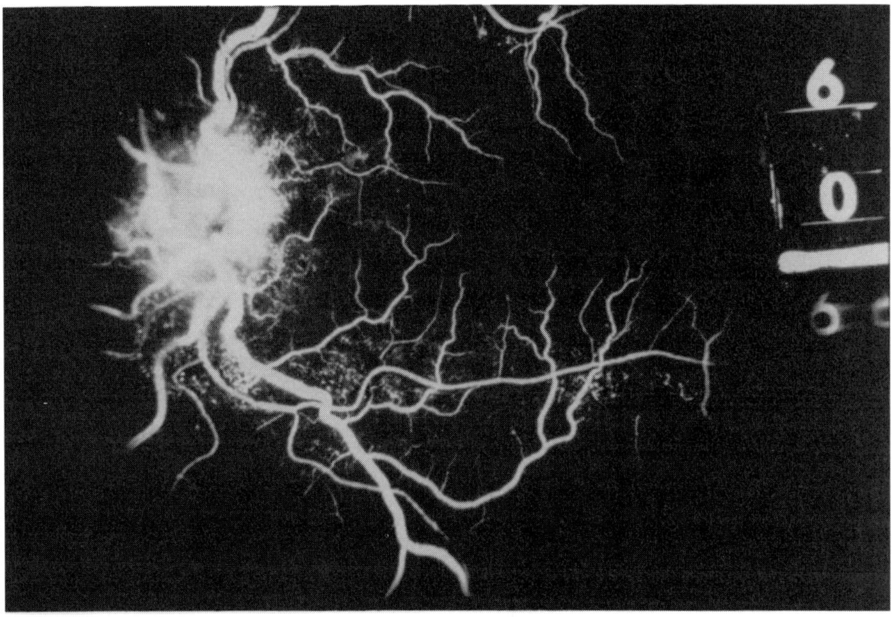

FIGURE 15–1

Severe hypertension in pregnancy. Fluorescein angiogram of optic disc edema and tortuous vessels.

at increased risk. Other groups at risk are diabetic pregnant women with chronic hypertension and renal disease.[7]

The presenting complaint is scotoma, diplopia, and dimness of vision seen in 30–50 percent of the patients with eclampsia and 20–25 percent of patients with severe pre-eclampsia and hypertension. Clinically, the patients present with retinal edema, hemorrhages, and optic disc edema.[8]

Treatment is aimed toward the control of hypertension during the pregnancy and postpartum periods.[9]

RETINOPATHY IN TOXEMIA

Toxemia occurs in 2–3 percent of all pregnancies.[9,10] The changes in toxemia are those of hypertensive retinopathy; however, the physician has the added responsibility of considering the viability of the fetus and the success of the pregnancy in making the correct diagnosis. For example, the absence or regression or retinopathy has been used as a sign to allow a pregnancy to continue.[11]

The changes seen in toxemia are (1) segmental, focal, arteriolar spasm (reversible after pregnancy); (2) hemorrhages, hard exudates; (3) diffuse retinal edema; (4) optic disc edema; (5) retinal detachment; and (6) choroidal infarct. If significant hypertensive changes, listed above, are seen accompanying diabetes mellitus and renal disease, there is the risk of fetal mortality.[12]

Fluorescein Angiography

Choroidal hyperfluorescence can be seen in the early transit along with marked constriction of arterioles. In the late transit, there can be pooled hyperfluorescence in the subretinal space.

Diagnosis

Bilateral arteriolar constriction is usually seen; however, one eye can be more severely affected than the other. Small localized serous elevations of the retina can be seen. Beneath the retinal vessels, there can be associated hemorrhages and exudates. Small fibrinous subretinal exudates can be seen and these exudates may look like dotlike precipitates.[13]

DIABETIC RETINOPATHY (SEE CHAPTER 4)

There usually is an exacerbation of the existing level of diabetic retinopathy during pregnancy and a regression of the retinopathy after parturition. If the patient has good glycemic control 6 months prior to pregnancy and continues to maintain this control during pregnancy, the level of retinopathy may proceed from level 20 (microaneuryms only) to level 30 (microaneurysms, questionable soft exudates, venous beading) and regress in the postpartum course. However, many juvenile onset diabetic patients during pregnancy will have short, transient periods of poor control, despite best efforts, and they need to be closely monitored. Macular edema and preproliferative diabetic retinopathy can be exacerbated within the 9 months of pregnancy and early treatment with laser may be required.

RARE COMPLICATIONS OF PREGNANCY

Rare complications of pregnancy include disseminated intravascular coagulopathy, associated with complex obstetric cases, such as abruptio placentae, retained dead fetus, and severe systemic disease. This entity above shows thrombotic occlusion of the choriocapillaris with subsequent retinal pigment epithelial changes.

Thrombotic thrombocytopenia purpura can occur in pregnancy associated with serous retinal detachments, retinal hemorrhages, and exudates. The etiology is unknown.

Amniotic fluid emboli which can occur during labor, delivery or, postpartum, is a catastrophic event. There is associated chills, convulsions, and cardiopulmonary collapse. Retinal arteriolar occlusions has been reported in one case, presumably from widespread systemic entrapment of particulate matter from the amniotic fluid.

REFERENCES

1. Cunningham FG, MacDonald PC, Grant NF et al: Williams Obstetrics. E Norwalk, CT: Appleton & Lange. 1993; pp. 213–214, 216–226

2. Sunness JS: The pregnant woman's eye. Surv Ophthalmol 1988; *32:* 219–238

3. Chumbley LC, Frank RN: Central serous retinopathy and pregnancy. Am J Ophthalmol 1974; *77:* 158–160

4. Sunness JS: Chorioretinopathy and pregnancy. Arch Ophthalmol 1993; *111:* 360–364

5. Halperin LS, Olk RJ, Soubrane G, Coscas G: Safety of fluorescein angiography during pregnancy. Am J Ophthalmol 1990; *109:* 563–566

6. Yannuzzi LA, Roher KT, Tindel LJ et al: Fluorescein angiography complications survey. Ophthalmol 1986; *93:* 611–617

7. Dieckmann WJ: The Toxemias of Pregnancy. 2nd ed. St Louis: CV Mosby, 1952, pp. 240–249

8. Gitter KA, Houser BP, Sarin LK, Justice J: Toxemia of pregnancy. An angiographic interpretation of fundus changes. Arch Ophthalmol 1968; *80:* 449–454

9. Sadowsky A, Serr DM, Landau J: Retinal changes and fetal prognosis in toxemias of pregnancy. Obstet Gynecol 1956; *8:* 426–431

10. Landau J, Koran Z, Sadowsky A: Detachment of retina in eclampsia of pregnancy in a severely anemic patient. Obstet Gynecol 1960; *15:* 231–234

11. Mussey RD, Mundell BJ: Retinal examinations: a guide in the management of the toxic hypertensive syndrome of pregnancy. Am J Obstet Gynecol 1939; *37:* 30–36

12. Landesman R, Douglas RG, Snyder SS: Retinal changes in the toxemias of pregnancy. Am J Obstet Gynecol 1952; *63:* 16–27

13. Gass JDM: Central serous chorioretinopathy and white subretinal exudation during pregnancy. Arch Ophthalmol 1991; *109:* 677–681

14. Chang M, Herbert WNP: Retinal arteriolar occlusions following amniotic fluid embolism. Ophthalmol 1984; *91:* 1634–1637

CHAPTER SIXTEEN

Peripheral Retinal Degenerations

POSTERIOR VITREOUS DETACHMENT

Anatomy and Pathophysiology

The vitreous body has several points of adherence at the optic disc, the vessels, at the macula, vitreous base, and ora serrata area. At these various points, the vitreous can spontaneously detach when the vitreous becomes syneretic with age. The aging process causes the lattice network of the vitreous body to change and collapse and subsequently, there is a subtle spontaneous detachment of the vitreous fibrils from its points of attachment. With blunt trauma to the orbit or globe, the vitreous can be avulsed from its points of attachment and a posterior vitreous detachment can result.

Epidemiology

The incidence is approximately 28 percent in all age groups, 53 percent incidence in persons over 50 years of age.[1] In patients with an acute symptomatic posterior vitreous detachment, the incidence of retinal tears varies from 8–15 percent.[2–5] High-risk characteristics for the development of retinal tear in the setting of a posterior vitreous detachment include vitreous cells, vitreous blood, and diffuse dots. In such eyes with one or more high-risk factors, there is a 52.8 percent incidence of retinal tears.[6]

Clinical Course

Posterior vitreous detachment is most commonly encountered in ophthalmologists' offices as flashes, floaters of sudden duration, or gradually over a period of days. Occasionally, the patient may have happened to have noticed it for the first time, when he or she covered one eye.

Examination of this entity requires the examination of the vitreous. This can first be performed at the slit lamp using 60 diopter or Hruby lenses to view its attachment at the optic disc, macula, or retinal vessels. Another method is to tilt the optical column of the slit lamp (Haag-Streit models) towards the patient to direct the beam of the slit posteriorly towards the vitreous. These two methods allow the visualization of the vitreous fibrils and the actual posterior vitreous detachment. With the use of 60 or 90 diopter lenses, one can make the slit beam extremely small and narrow then one can see the actual vitreous interface at the macular internal limiting membrane interface.

The next part of the examination is careful viewing of the ora serrata to look for retinal breaks in that area. This is done with scleral depression.

Finally, the Goldmann contact lens is useful to identify questionable areas if the examiner suspects peripheral pathology.

If the only diagnosis is posterior vitreous detachment, the only clinical finding will be the small ring of the vitreous as it detaches from the optic nerve. Other clinical findings include clumps of vitreous slightly off-center from the visual axis (Fig. 16–1). Finally, when the eye moves, one can identify the vitreous fibrils in movement. These fibrillar movements also can be seen with B-scan ultrasound. However, it is not necessary to have ultrasonagraphy if the view of the retina is clear.

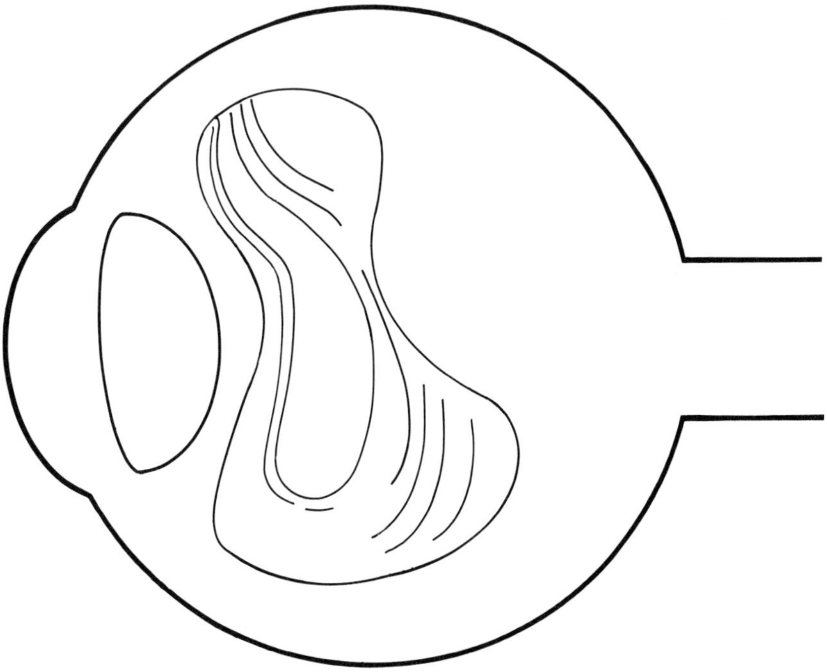

FIGURE 16–1

Posterior vitreous detachment.

Rarely, in acute posterior vitreous detachment, is there a small preretinal hemorrhage. Most commonly, the hemorrhage is small and flame-shaped in the direction of the nerve fiber layer. Careful examination of the ora serrata is necessary. However, if the hemorrhage is in the vitreous, it is imperative that the eye be carefully examined for a retinal hole. Sometimes, it may be necessary to bring the patient back in 24 hours, after the settling of the vitreous hemorrhage to re-examine for a retinal hole.

Management

The management of a posterior vitreous detachment is reassurance and the explanation of warning signs for a retinal detachment. It is important to stress that in times of an acute posterior vitreous detachment, there is a period when a retinal detachment can occur.

The warning signs for the patient are (1) flashes and floaters which continue and increase in frequency, number, and size, (2) "curtain coming downwards, upwards, or sideways," and (3) decrease of vision. Any or all of these signs should lead the patient to see his or her ophthalmologist.

LATTICE DEGENERATION

The incidence of lattice degeneration is 6–8 percent in the general public.[7] There is no racial predilection.[8] Males and females are equally affected.[9,10] Lattice degeneration is frequently associated with retinal detachment, occurring in 20 percent to 35 percent of patients with retinal detachment. Lattice degeneration is found in myopic eyes with the incidence becoming the greatest (up to 15 percent) in those eyes with the longest axial lengths.[11] The genetics of lattice degeneration is unclear. There may be polygenic or multifactorial inheritance.[12]

In the areas of lattice, there is liquefaction of the vitreous overlying the area of the involved retina. The lesions are characterized by prominent vitreoretinal attachments.[10,13]

Clinical Course

Usually there may be no symptomatic complaints by the patient. However, there can be complaints of floaters.

On ophthalmoscopy, there are small atrophic, round holes, retinal thinning, with retinal pigment epithelial atrophy and hypertrophy, white lines suggesting sclerosed vessels. It can be associated with retinal tears in the ends of the lattice area or the posterior edge of the lattice (Fig. 16–2).

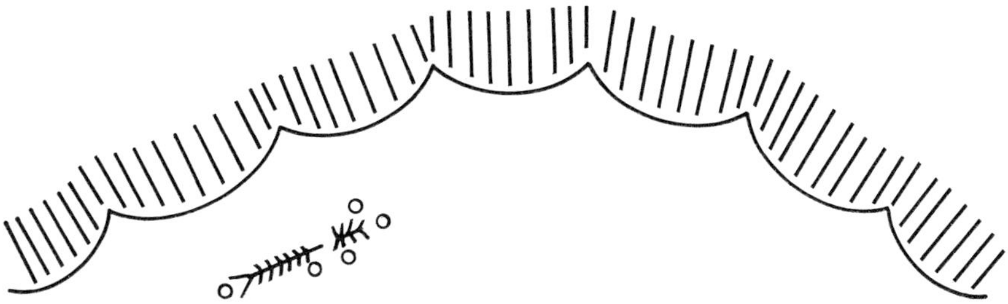

FIGURE 16-2

Lattice degeneration with retinal holes.

Usually the areas of lattice are located near the ora serrata. Radially oriented lattice may occur in severely myopic eyes and are along blood vessels or the vortex vein areas.

Diagnosis

Indirect ophthalmoscopy and scleral depression will allow for the evaluation of these areas. The use of the Goldmann contact lens will enable the clinician to see the areas in question with magnification and allow for the checking of retinal holes. The fellow eye usually has lattice degeneration in a symmetrical location or a mirror image location.

Management

When lattice degeneration is present with retinal holes and the patient is symptomatic, i.e., the patient sees floaters, treatment is indicated. Laser photocoagulation treatment of these retinal holes can be performed.

Atrophic retinal holes have a 37 percent risk of retinal detachment.[10,13] Thus, the mere presence of round atrophic holes without symptoms should not mean treatment automatically.

Other Risk Factors

Extenuating circumstances that would lead to treatment include (1) retinal detachment in the fellow eye, (2) strong family history of retinal detachment, and (3) myopia and aphakia or pseudophakia are all conditions that have been thought to be associated with higher risk of retinal detachments. In patients with lattice degeneration, these risks may be additive.[14,15]

Cryotherapy is usually considered for the anterior lesions and laser for the posterior lesions; however, with the advent of the

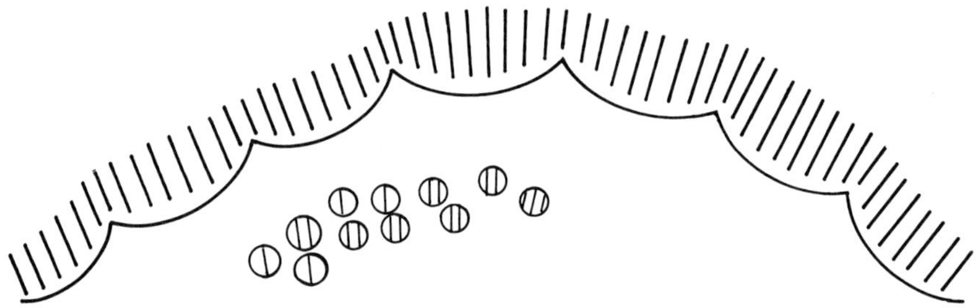

FIGURE 16–3

Pavingstone degeneration.

indirect laser, the very peripheral lesions can be treated with laser as well.

Complications of laser and cryopexy include (1) new tears, (2) retinal detachment, (3) macular pucker, (4) vitreous hemorrhage, and (5) cystoid macular edema.

PAVINGSTONE DEGENERATION

Pavingstone degeneration describes peripheral retinal changes at the area of the ora serrata. The lesions show punched-out atrophy of the retinal pigment epithelium and atrophy of choroid. The large choroidal vessels are then exposed (Fig. 16–3).[16,17]

WHITE WITH AND WITHOUT PRESSURE

In White with pressure, the retina shows a whitish sheen and these light reflexes move along with scleral depression. The area of White with pressure lacks discrete contours. The borders of White with pressure are reminiscent of a map. Some degree of White with pressure is found in 30 percent of normal eyes, with bilateral manifestation; two-thirds of patients over 70 years, will show White with pressure.[18]

White without pressure is a vitreoretinal interface that changes in the ora serrata area showing a bright iridescent sheen. These are changes of interface between the internal limiting membrane and the vitreous. Presumably this change suggests that there are more dense bundles of vitreous collagen present.

Both of these notations suggest some association with posterior vitreous detachment. There may be an increased risk for giant retinal tears in fellow eyes with White without pressure at the vitreous base.[19]

RETINAL BREAKS

Retinal tears (See Chapter 23) occur when the vitreous detaches posteriorly and pulls on the surrounding retina. The traction then causes an acute posterior vitreous detachment and the additional traction causes a retinal tear. Such a tear is called a horseshoe tear, where the posterior aspect of the retinal flap has vitreous adherent to it. The open end of the horseshoe is facing in the direction of the ora serrata.

The incidence of retinal tears is higher than the incidence of retinal detachment. Whereas the incidence of retinal detachment is only 24 per 100,000,[20] the incidence of retinal tears is approximately 7.3 percent in a study that involved 2,334 cases.[8] In postmortem eyes, the incidence is slightly less than 4 percent.[21] Thus, some patients with retinal breaks do not develop retinal detachments. The incidence of retinal tears developing into retinal detachment ranges from 2–18 percent.[22,23]

Usually retinal tears are accompanied by symptoms secondary to the vitreous traction. The most common complaints are floaters or scintillating lights. The other complaint is decreased vision from a mild vitreous hemorrhage caused by traction and subsequent avulsion of a retinal vessel that bridges the retinal tear.

The treatment is usually cryotherapy or laser photocoagulation. In cases of a large tear with a small area of fluid and overlying vitreous traction, the above treatment modalities may be insufficient and a small scleral buckle may be necessary.

RETINAL TUFTS AND MERIDIONAL COMPLEXES

Retinal tufts are internal projections of peripheral retinal tissue located within the area of the vitreous base and have been classified as cystic, noncystic, and zonular traction.[24]

Meridional complexes are anatomic variations of the ora serrata bays and teeth. A meridional retinal fold is a permanent fold of developmental origin and is a posterior extension of ora serrata teeth. It is not associated with retinal detachment. It measures 0.5 to 1.5 disc diameter in length and involves all retinal layers.[25]

Retinal tags are seen in early states of vitreoretinal traction where the internal limiting membrane area may be tented-up, causing a taglike appearance. Tags are usually found in the posterior border of the detached vitreous at the vitreous base. In autopsy cases, there is an 11.8 percent incidence in autopsy eyes (Fig. 16–4).[24]

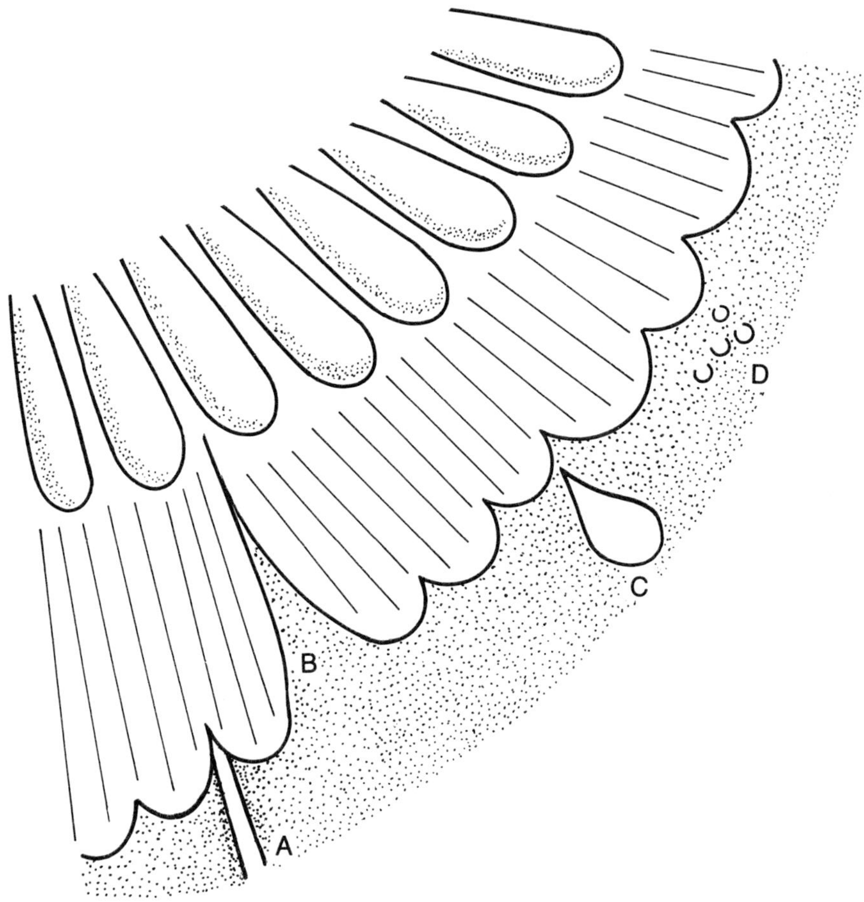

FIGURE 16-4

A. Meridional fold; B. Meridional complex; C. Enclosed oral bay; D. Retinal tag.

ACQUIRED RETINOSCHISIS

Acquired retinoschisis is found in the elderly in the inferotemporal quadrants of the retina. This entity is usually bilateral. This can occur without change for many years. Females are more affected than males.[26]

Early cases of acquired retinoschisis occur at the ora serrata. The inner layer is elevated and appears translucent and smooth. Sometimes broken columns of grayish white glial tissue protrude into the cystic cavity of the anterior border of the retinoschisis.

In early acquired retinoschisis, there may be some venules and arterioles with a sclerosed appearance to the vessels. In more advanced cases of acquired retinoschisis, there is extensive retinal vessel sheathing and small white vitreous condensates thought to be a product of degeneration between the inner layer of the retina and the cortical vitreous (Figs. 16–5 and 16–6).

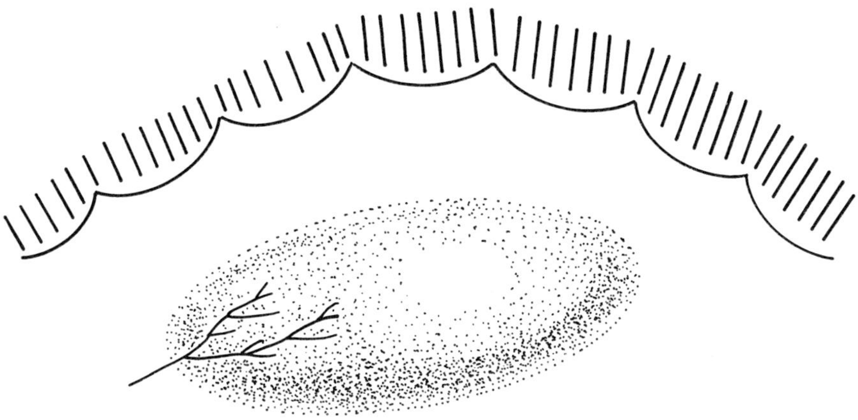

FIGURE 16-5

Schisis, acquired. Note that there is an area of normal retina at the ora serrata.

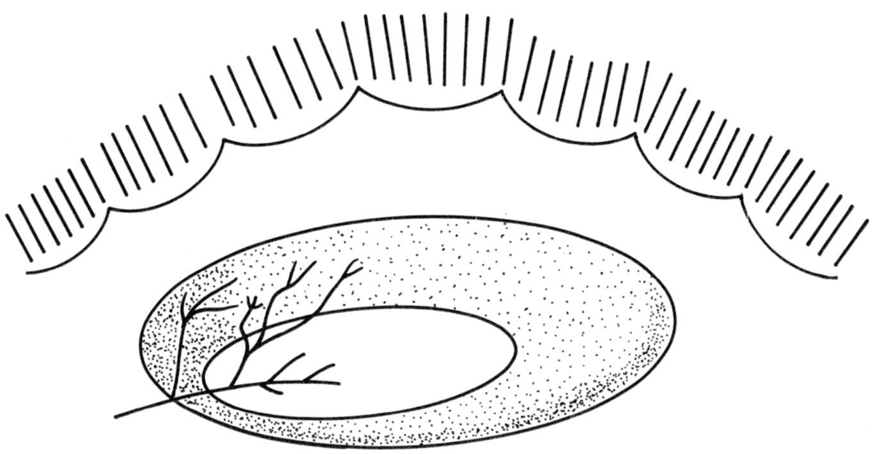

FIGURE 16-6

Schisis, acquired. There is a partial hole and there are sclerosed vessels on both flaps of the schisis cavity.

Examination with indirect ophthalmoscopy and Goldmann contact lens to examine the periphery is necessary to observe the above details.

Acquired retinoschisis may change slowly over time and occasionally develops full-thickness retinal holes. Then, scleral buckling surgery would have to be performed.

REFERENCES

1. Pishel DK: Detachment of the vitreous base as seen with slit lamp examination. Trans Am Ophthalmol Soc 1952; *50:* 329–346

2. Jaffe NS: Complications of acute posterior vitreous detachment. Arch Ophthalmol 1968; *79:* 568–571

3. Novak MA, Welch RB: Complications of acute symptomatic posterior vitreous detachment. Am J Ophthalmol 1984; *97:* 308–314

4. Tabotabo MM, Karp LA, Benson WE: Posterior vitreous detachment. Ann Ophthalmol 1980; *12:* 59–61

5. Tasman WS: Posterior vitreous detachment and peripheral retinal breaks. Trans Am Acad Ophthalmol Otolaryngol 1968; *72:* 217–224

6. Boldrey EE: Risk of retinal tears in patients with vitreous floaters. Am J Ophthalmol 1983; *96:* 783–787

7. Byer N: Lattice degeneration of the retina. Surv Ophthalmol 1979; *23:* 213–248

8. Foos RY, Simons KB, Wheeler NC: Comparison of lesions predisposing to rhegmatogenous retinal detachment by race or subjects. Am J Ophthalmol 1983; 644–649

9. Byer NE: Clinical study of lattice degeneration of the retina. Trans Am Acad Ophthalmol Otolaryngol 1965; *69:* 1064–1081

10. Straatsma BR, Zeegan PD, Foos RY et al: Lattice degeneration of the retina. Am J Ophthalmol 1974; *77:* 619–649

11. Karlin DB, Curtin BJ: Peripheral chorioretinal lesions and axial length of the myopic eye. Am J Ophthalmol 1976; *81:* 625–635

12. Murakami F, Ohba N: Genetics of lattice degeneration of the retina. Ophthalmologica 1982; *185:* 136–140

13. Foos RY, Simons KB: Vitreous in lattice degeneration of the retina. Ophthalmol 1984; *91:* 452–457

14. Benson WE, Morse PH: The prognosis of retinal detachment due to lattice degeneration. Ann Ophthalmol 1978; *10:* 1197–1200

15. Folk JD, Burton TC: Bilateral phakic retinal detachment. Ophthalmol 1982; *89:* 815–820

16. O'Malley P, Allen RA, Straatsma BR, O'Malley CC: Pavingstone degeneration of the retina. Arch Ophthalmol 1965; *73:* 169–182

17. Rehsteiner K: Ophthalmoskopische Untersuchungen uber Veranderungen der Fundersperipherie in myopen und senilen Augen. Arch Ophthalmol 1928; *120:* 282–316

18. Schepens CL: Diagnostic and prognostic factors as found in preoperative examination. Trans Am Acad Ophthalmol Otolaryngol 1952; *56:* 398–418

19. Freeman HM: Fellow eyes of giant retinal tears. Trans Am Ophthalmol Soc 1978; *76:* 343–382

20. Byer NE: Clinical study of retinal breaks. Trans Am Acad Ophthalmol Otolaryngol 1967; *71:* 461–473

21. Foos RY: Tears of the peripheral retina: pathogenesis, incidence and classification in autopsy eyes. Mod Probl Ophthalmol 1975; *15:* 68–81

22. Neumann E, Hyams S: Conservative management of retinal breaks: a follow-up of subsequent retinal detachment. Br J Ophthalmol 1972; *56:* 482–486

23. Davis MD: Natural history of retinal breaks without retinal detachment. Arch Ophthalmol 1974; *92:* 183–194

24. Foos RY, Allen RA: Retinal tears and lesser lesions of the peripheral retina. Am J Ophthalmol 1967; *64:* 643–655

25. Spencer LM, Foos RY, Straatsma BR: Meridional complexes and associated abnormalities of the peripheral retina. Am J Ophthalmol 1970; *70:* 697–713

26. Rutnin U, Schepens CL: Fundus appearance in normal eyes III. Peripheral degenerations. Am J Ophthalmol 1967; *64:* 1042–1062

CHAPTER SEVENTEEN

Retinal Degenerations

PRIMARY RETINAL DEGENERATIONS AND DYSTROPHIES

Primary retinal degenerations and dystrophies include many disorders that are usually hereditary, progressive, bilateral, and symmetrical. Many of these diseases were first discovered and described in the nineteenth century and are rare. They exhibit a sporadic nature of these diseases, and research has been limited. Consequently, the exact pathophysiologic or genetic mechanism of many of these entities is still unclear.

Retinitis Pigmentosa

Retinitis pigmentosa (RP) describes a group of diseases characterized by progressive visual field loss, night blindness, and abnormal or nonrecordable electroretinogram. There is no uniformly accepted classification of many pigmented retinopathies. In addition, reliable consistent methods of differentiating the subcategory of RP by etiology and/or pathophysiology has not been well-developed.

Another classification breaks down RP into type I RP where rod disease is present and type II RP where rod disease is not present.[1] However, in Great Britain, type I is diffuse rod disease and type II describes regional areas of cone and rod loss.[2]

The pigmented retinopathies can be divided into two groups: group 1, the degeneration affects the eye only and group 2, the degeneration affects the eye and other organs (Table 17–1).

Anatomy and Pathophysiology

Histologic studies suggest that the source of the pigmentary clumpings is at the site of the retinal pigment epithelium.[3] The retinal degenerative process is intrinsic to the disease process and does not appear to be related to pigment deposition process.

TABLE 17-1 Retinitis Pigmentosa Associated wth Systemic Disease

Autosomal Dominant RP

1. Arterioheptic Dysplasia (Alagille Syndrome): Intrahepatic cholestatic syndrome, congenital heart disease, flattened facies and bridge of nose, bony abnormalities, posterior embryotoxon, axenfeld anomaly, myopia, pigmentary retinopathy.
2. Charcot-Marie-Tooth Disease: Degeneration of lateral horn spinal cord, optic, atrophy, and pigmentary retinopathy.
3. Flynn-Aird Syndrome: Nerve deafness, ataxia, skin atrophy, baldness, cystic bone changes, cataract, myopia, atypical pigmentary retinopathy.
4. Myotonic Dystrophy (Steinert's disease): Muscle wasting, "Christmas tree" cataract, retinal degeneration, may have pigmentary deposits, electroretinogram findings subnormal to abnormal.
5. Oculodentodigital Dysplastic Syndrome: Thin nose with hypoplastic alae, narrow nostrils, abnormality of fourth and fifth fingers, hypoplastic dental enamel, congenital cataract, colobomas.
6. Olivopontocerebellar Atrophy: Cerebellar ataxia, external ophthalmoplegia may occur, retinal degeneration (peripheral and/or macular involvement).
7. Paget's Disease: Occasionally angioid streaks, one family tree of pigmentary retinopathy.
8. Pierre-Marie Syndrome: Disturbed hair growth, pachyacria, bitemporal hemianopia, choked disc, code-rod degeneration.
9. Stickler Syndrome (arthro-ophthalmopathy): Joint hypermobility, arthritis, progressive myopia with myopic retinal degeneration, radial perivascular retinal atrophy, cataract, retinal detachment common, electroretinogram findings are subnormal to abnormal; visual field is consistent with myopia.
10. Wagner's Hereditary Vitreoretinal Degeneration: Overlaps with Stickler syndrome which is characterized by retinal detachment; narrow and sheathed retinal vessels, pigmented spots in the retinal periphery and along retinal vessels, choroidal atrophy and optic atrophy, extensive liquefaction and membranous condensation of the vitreous body.
11. Waardenburg Syndrome: White forelock, poliosis, hypertelorism, wide bridge of nose, cochlear deafness, heterochromia iridis, pigmentary retinopathy; electroretinogram findings are normal to subnormal.

Autosomal Recessive RP

1. Abetalipoproteinemia (Bassen-Kornzweig disease): Secondary vitamin A deficiency, acanthocytosis, anemia, celiac syndrome.
2. Alström's Disease: Diabetes, obesity, normal IQ, neurosensory deafness, pigmentary retinopathy.
3. Batten's-Mayou Disease
   Haltia-Santavuori Disease: Occurs in infancy with rapid deterioration, fine granular inclusions.
   Jansky-Bielschowsky Disease: Children—onset, age 2–4 years, rapid central nervous system deterioration, curvilinear body inclusions.
   Spielmeyer-Sjögren Disease: Children—onset 6–8 years, slowly progressive, "fingerprint" inclusions.
4. Bardet-Biedl Syndrome (also see Laurence-Moon syndrome): Mild mental retardation, polydactyly, obesity, hypogenitalism, pigmentary retinopathy; electroretinogram findings are barely recordable; progressive visual field loss.
5. Carotenemia (familial): Failure of absorption or cleavage of beta-carotene, retinal degeneration for vitamin A deficiency.
6. Cerebrohepatorenal (Zellweger Syndrome) syndrome: Muscular hypotonia, high forehead and hypertelorism, hepatomegaly, deficient cerebral myelination, nystagmus, cataract, microphthalmia, retinal degeneration; electroretinogram is nonrecordable.
7. Cockayne's Syndrome: Optic atrophy, deafness, cachetic dwarfism, characteristic facies, mental retardation, pigmentary degeneration.
8. Cystinosis II (late onset, nephropathic variety): Proteinuria due to glomerulonephritis, late pigmentary retinopathy.
9. Friedreich's Ataxia: Spinocerebellar degeneration, limb incoordination, nerve deafness, optic atrophy and retinal degeneration.
10. Hallgren's Syndrome (Usher III, Merin classification): Congenital deafness, vestibulocerebellar ataxia, psychoses, pigmentary retinopathy.
11. Homocystinuria: Marfanoid appearance, cardiovascular abnormalities (thromboses), mental retardation, myopia, subluxated or dislocated lenses, glaucoma, fine pigmentary or cystic degeneration of the retina.
12. Hyperostosis corticalis deformans juvenilis (Juvenile Paget's Disease): Large head, expanded and bowed extremities, chronic idiopathic hyperphosphatasemia, angioid streaks, occasional retinal degeneration.
13. Jeune's syndrome: Dwarfing skeletal dysplasia, respiratory insufficiency, renal disease, liver fibrosis, pigmentary retinopathy.
14. Mannosidosis: Resembles Hurler's syndrome; macroglossia, flat nose, large head and ears, skeletal abnormalities, hepatosplenomegaly, storage material in the retina.
15. Marinesco-Sjögren Syndrome: Oligophrenia, cerebellar ataxia, congenital cataract, retinal degeneration.
16. Microphthalmos with hypermetropia and retinal degeneration.

TABLE 17-1. Retinitis Pigmentosa Associated wth System Disease, continued

17. Mucopolysaccharidosis I (Hurler's syndrome): Gargoyle facies, deafness, mental retardation, dwarfism, skeletal abnormalities, hepatosplenomegaly, early corneal clouding, optic atrophy, pigmentary retinopathy; electroretinogram findings are subnormal.
18. Mucopolysaccharidosis IS (Scheie's syndrome): Coarse facies, aortic regurgitation, stiff joints, early clouding of the cornea, normal life span, normal IQ, pigmentary retinopathy.
19. Mucopolysaccharidosis III (Sanfilippo's syndrome): Severe mental retardation, little corneal clouding, pigmentary retinopathy, optic atrophy, retinal vascular narrowing; electroretinogram findings are subnormal to nonrecordable.
20. Osteopetrosis (Albers-Schönberg Disease): Defective absorption of immature bone, macrocephaly, progressive deafness, hepatosplenomegaly, anemia, retinal degeneration; electroretinogram findings are abnormal or extinguished.
21. Pallidal Degeneration and RP: Extrapyramidal rigidity, dysarthria, destruction of the pallida and substantia nigra, progressive pigmentary retinopathy.
22. Polycystic kidney, cataract, congenital blindness: Hypoplastic retina, absence of ciliary body, persistent fetal angle structures may occur, small pupil.
23. Progressive external ophthalmoplegia, ptosis, pigmentary retinopathy, heart block (Kearns-Sayre syndrome). Electroretinogram findings are normal to abnormal.
24. Pseudoxanthoma elasticum (Grönblad-Standberg syndrome): Characteristic plaquelike skin lesions on skin of neck, axilla, areas of flexion of limbs, gastrointestinal bleed, angioid streaks, focal fine exudates in equatorial retina.
25. Refsum's Disease: Elevation of phytanic acid level, partial deafness, cerebellar ataxia, ichthyosis, pigmentary retinopathy.
26. Renal dysplasia and retinal aplasia: Kidney developmental abnormalities, congenital blindness, pigmentary retinopathy.
27. Usher's syndrome (Merin classification)
    Type I: Congenital total deafness, no vestibular function, pigmentary retinopathy.
    Type II: Partial deafness, normal vestibular function, pigmentary retinopathy.
28. Wolfram Syndrome: Juvenile onset diabetes mellitus, optic atrophy, cone-rod degeneration.

X-linked RP

1. Incontinentia pigmenti (Bloch-Sulzberger syndrome): Skin pigmentation in lines and whorls, alopecia, dental anomalies, optic atrophy, falciform folds, cataract, nystagmus, strabismus, conjunctival pigmentation, patchy mottling of retina.
2. Mucopolysaccharidosis II (Hunter's syndrome): Little corneal clouding, mild clinical course, mental retardation, some retinal arteriole narrowing; electroretinogram findings are subnormal.
3. Pelizaeus-Merzbacher Disease: Infantile progressive leukodystrophy, cerebellar ataxia, limb spasticity, mental retardation; pigmentary retinopathy with absent foveal reflex.

However, it is not known whether the pigment clumping contributes to the progressive loss of retinal function.

Epidemiology

The overall incidence of RP in the United States is in a ratio of 1:3500;[4] autosomal recessive occurs at a rate of 28–38 percent; autosomal dominant, 12–20 percent; and X-linked recessive, 1–5 percent.[4–9] Approximately half of the cases in the United States do not have a family history and are called "simplex RP," probably representing autosomal recessive RP. On careful searching, many sporadic cases are found to have other relatives who have RP, night blindness or blindness, or an unknown etiology. This process necessitates much investigation, but allows for more accurate genetic counseling.

Inheritance pattern

Autosomal dominant
Autosomal recessive
X-linked recessive
Sporadic—new mutational event or environmental cause

"Simplex" one member of a pedigree is affected. It has been postulated that 70 percent of the simplex cases are autosomal recessive.[10]

Family History

It is important to obtain a family pedigree.

WHO TO INTERVIEW

Mother, father, paternal and maternal grandparents, and siblings can be interviewed if available or accessible. Once an affected side of the family is ascertained, then it is important to ask about aunts, uncles, cousins and second cousins, and so forth. It is important to ask as many questions about as many family members in as many generations as possible.

Finally, it is important to ask if additional family members can be examined. If the family members cannot travel, suggest that retinal photographs be taken and be seen by an ophthalmologist in their community. Ask for the ophthalmic records of other family members be sent to you for review.

QUESTIONS

1. Are there any eye problems in the family?
2. For the affected family members, can the patient and other family drive an automobile? The level of vision required for the driving test is in the 20/40 to 20/60 range, depending on the locale in America. This information gives the examiner some idea as to the visual capability of various family members in the pedigree.
3. What is the occupation? This provides insight as to the visual needs and long-term capabilities of the patient and family members.
4. Do the affected family members have other associated conditions: deafness, mental retardation, neurological problems?
5. Is there consanguinity?

Clinical Course

The patient presents with poor vision and has usually been to other ophthalmologists or physicians for the diagnosis. The age of onset may vary from adolescence to young adult. Middle-aged adults can also present for the first time, also. It is at the time of the first visit that complete family history information should be obtained and recorded carefully.

Vision can vary from 20/50 levels to 20/200. The level of visual acuity depends on the age of presentation. There is usually a history of poor night vision from childhood, with a later onset of peripheral visual field loss.

Diagnosis

The patient with RP can present most commonly with some "bone spicules" or retinal pigment epithelial deposits over the four quadrants of the retina, most commonly found in the area of the equator to midperiphery. The retinal pigment epithelial deposits follow the vessels. There is a waxy pallor over the optic disc (this is found in the later course of the disease). This is usually due to gliosis overlying the optic disc (Fig. 17–1).

The majority of patients have cystoid changes in the macula.[11]

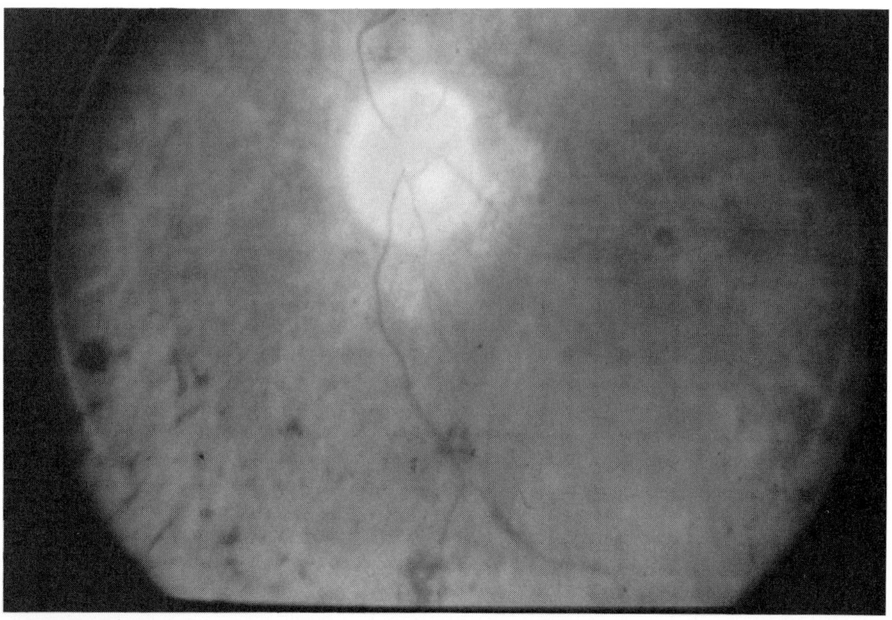

FIGURE 17–1

Retinitis pigmentosa.

Early presentation of the disease can be the abnormal golden or bronze sheen to the entire retinal surface, also called the "beaten metal or beaten bronze" appearance of the retina. Presumably, it is at this stage, that the retinal pigment epithelium is becoming abnormal. Late presentation of the disease usually manifests as diminished macular reflex, pale optic nerve, or pigment clumping over the entire equatorial region (Fig. 17–2).

Fluorescein Angiography

Fluorescein angiography will demonstrate cystoid changes in the macula with hyperfluorescence in late transit. It will be useful in the differentiation of other retinal diseases from RP.

Electroretinography

The electroretinogram is very useful in RP especially in patients with poor vision and almost normal-looking fundi. It allows the physician to make a more precise diagnosis.

In most cases of RP, the electroretinogram response is extinguished or "flatline." However, in early RP, and in autosomal recessive and dominant RP, small amplitudes may be recorded as compared to normal. In some cases, prolonged photopic b-wave

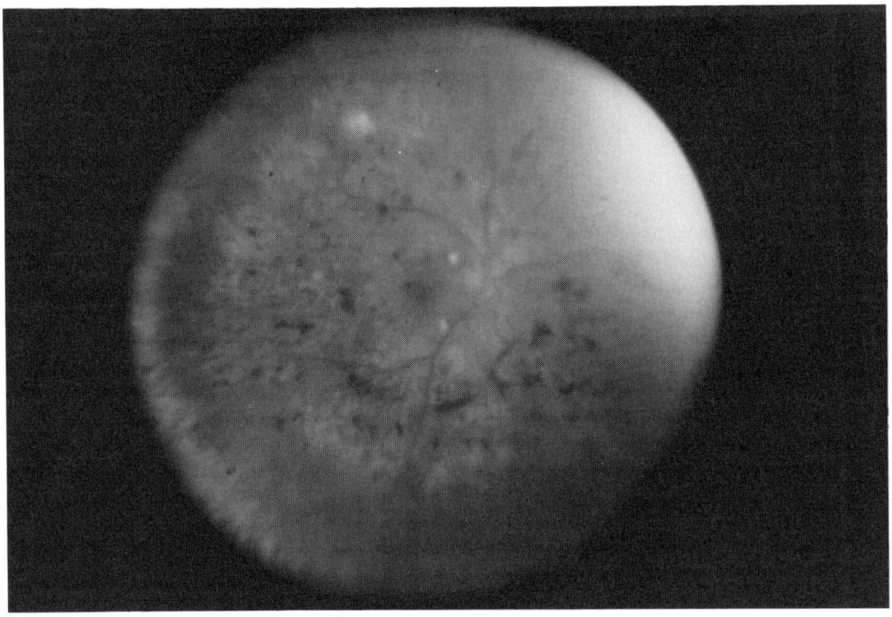

FIGURE 17–2

Wide-angle fundus photograph showing retinitis pigmentosa.

latencies can be seen.[12] Some autosomal dominant and recessive RP show a long, progressive course that may take many years and the degeneration of retinal function correspondingly occurs over a long period of time, as well.

Management

Careful evaluation of the retinal degeneration is necessary to ascertain the diagnosis of the exact type of RP.[13] This will help identify the inheritance pattern in cases where there is an inadequate family history. Oftentimes, electrophysiologic testing is most useful in early disease processes. Documentation of the visual field, electrophysiologic and/or psychophysical testing helps answer questions that arise as to how severe the condition is and how fast it is changing.

Counseling is directed on adaptation to narrowed visual fields, poor night vision, and low-vision aids. Advanced cases may need additional referral for vocational rehabilitation and mobility training. Such vocational rehabilitation services exist in every metropolitan center.

WILL MY PATIENT BECOME BLIND AND SHOULD I TELL HIM OR HER?

The course of the disease process may take up to 30 to 40 years. Consequently, it is not appropriate to tell the patient that he "will go blind." The varying time progression to severe visual loss is different for each patient. Hopelessly discouraging words are inaccurate and counterproductive in helping a patient with RP adapt to his or her circumstances.

SHOULD MY PATIENT HAVE CHILDREN?

It is important for the patient to obtain genetic counseling. Approximately three-fourths of patients with RP are not at risk to have children with the disease but will pass the gene in a carrier state mode if at all. It is important to obtain a blood sample since autosomal dominant RP has identifiable gene types: chromosome 3, rhodopsin-gene mutations; chromosome 6p, rds gene for peripherin; chromosome 8, pericentric variety; chromosome llq, rom-1 gene (subunit peripherin complex).

There are several guidelines for ophthalmic care of an RP patient: (1) provide the best corrective lenses for the best corrected vision, using optical aids as necessary and (2) examine for cataracts and glaucoma. With informed consent and good patient preoperative selection, patients with RP can do well with extracapsular cataract extraction and with posterior lens implants because these implants give them the largest possible visual field.[14]

Vitamin A and Autosomal Dominant Retinitis Pigmentosa

15,000 IU daily has been found to be beneficial in one study.[15,16] However, not every retinal specialist will agree on prescribing the vitamin A therapy which has known toxic side effects for their patients with RP.[15–25]

Retinitis Pigmentosa Sine Pigmento

RP sine pigmento is a rare condition that presents with normal fundus but on psychophysical testing, it is classic RP (i.e., nonrecordable electroretinogram). With the passage of time, there will be the appearance of bone spicules.

Leber's Congenital Amaurosis or Congenital Retinitis Pigmentosa

Leber's congenital amaurosis is seen at birth or in early infancy. The infant appears to be nonseeing. The electroretinogram is nonrecordable. The fundus examination may look to be normal by age 2; however, nystagmus may develop and later on, a pigmentary retinopathy is noted.[26,27]

Congenital RP I: Autosomal recessive disease that manifests at birth. Infant does not seem to see. Hypermetropia is present. The electroretinogram is nonrecordable, but the fundus looks normal.

Congenital RP II: Autosomal recessive disease. Infantile night blindness with vision 20/70–20/200 until midadulthood. Hypermetropia is present with visual field loss. Electroretinogram is nonrecordable to severely affected. Presents at age four. Early pigmentary retinopathy may be seen.

Congenital RP III: Autosomal recessive disease. There is pigmentary retinal degeneration with macular coloboma and occasionally keratoconus and skeletal abnormalities.

Congenital RP IV: Autosomal dominant disease. Acts like early onset progressive cone-rod degeneration (see below). Normal retina until the adult years, visual fields progressively contract, and patients become night blind.

Cone and Rod Disorders

Cone and rod disorders are classified by their electroretinogram response. For example, when cones mainly are affected, there is an absence of the photopic flicker. When the rod system is affected, the scotopic response is affected.

Rod Monochromatism

Rod monochromatism, also known as achromatopsia, is inherited in an autosomal recessive fashion. Patients may have full to partial expression of the disorder with visual acuity ranging from 20/60–20/200. There may be varying degrees of nystagmus.

Funduscopically, these patients have blonde fundi and minimal granularity of the macula. This condition may be confused with ocular albinism and the electroretinogram will be very helpful. (The electroretinogram is grossly abnormal in rod monochromatism and normal in ocular albinism until late in the course of the disease).

The VER will show abnormalities in ocular albinism whereas the VER is normal in the rod monochromatism.

There are two forms of rod monochromatism: complete and incomplete.

- Complete
    - Vision is 20/200
    - Achromatic color sense
    - Macular changes common
- Incomplete
    - Vision is 20/50–20/200
    - Color sense is abnormal but present
    - Macular changes rare

Both types have the same symptoms and electroretinogram findings

- Nystagmus
- Photophobia
- Electroretinogram: reduced photopic single flash
- Absent photoic flicker response
- Normal scotopic response

Cone Monochromatism

Cone monochromatism is extremely rare with only a ratio of 1: 1 million people having this entity. These patients have normal visual acuity so that they rarely present to the ophthalmologist's office. Achromatopsia or complete lack of color discrimination is present. The total cone population of the retina is intact but only with one color cone. Visual acuity is normal but there is no color discrimination. There is no nystagmus or photophobia. With the electroretinogram, there is normal flicker when done with white light.

Cone or Progressive Cone Dystrophy

With cone or progressive cone dystrophy there is a degenerative course over a period of years. There are no ocular signs at birth. In adult life, when the disease first presents, there is progressive loss of vision, variable (atypical) color vision defects, macular changes, and photophobia. Visual acuity usually is 20/200 range when these patients present to an ophthalmologist's office (Figs. 17–3 and 17–4).

Inheritance is found to be autosomal dominant or recessive.

The electroretinogram findings are (1) reduced photopic response to a single flash and (2) absent photopic flicker, but normal scotopic amplitudes.

Acquired cone dystrophy is usually most commonly associated with the bull's eye lesion in chloroquine toxicity. It is characterized by an uninvolved central area surrounded by a zone of retinal pigment epithelium alterations. This diagnosis is easily made once the patient's drug and medication history is obtained.

The electroretinogram findings can be reduced or normal.

Stargardt's Disease and Fundus Flavimaculatus

Stargardt's disease is characterized by progressive and symmetrical atrophy in a bull's eye pattern in the macula in young patients (Fig.

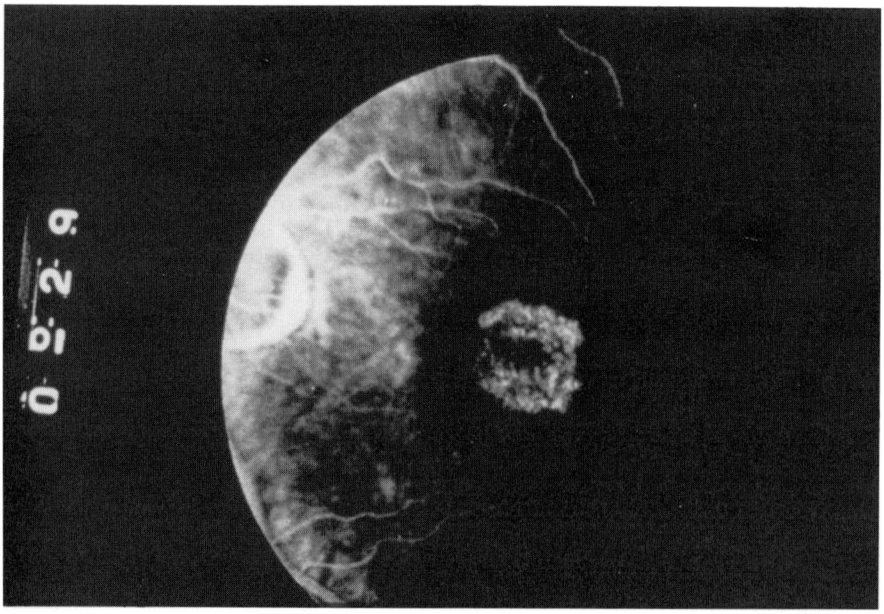

FIGURE 17–3

Cone dystrophy.

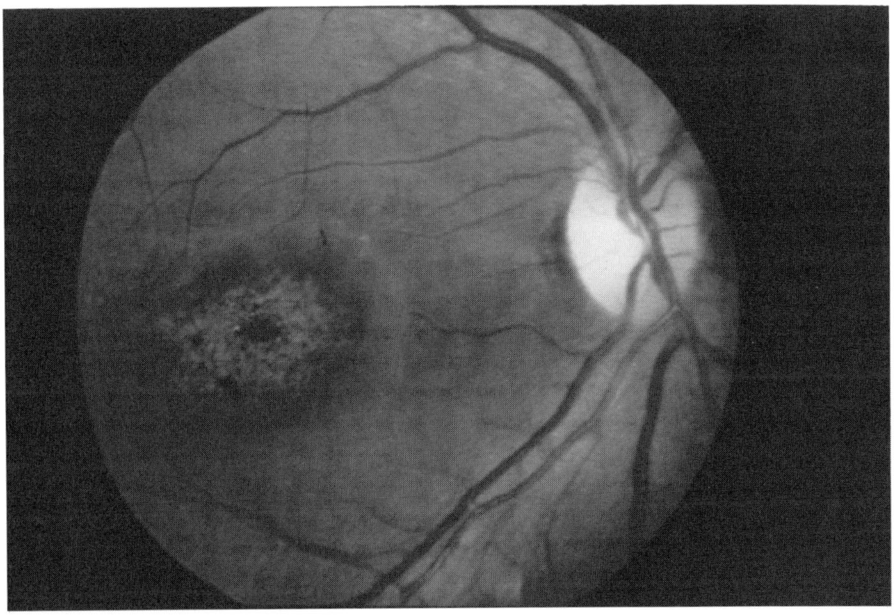

FIGURE 17–4

Fluorescein angiogram of cone dystrophy.

17–5). It is thought that Stargardt's disease and fundus flavimaculatus is part of the same spectrum of the disease process.

In fundus flavimaculatus, there are numerous yellow flecks in the periphery without necessarily the macular lesion (Figs. 17–6

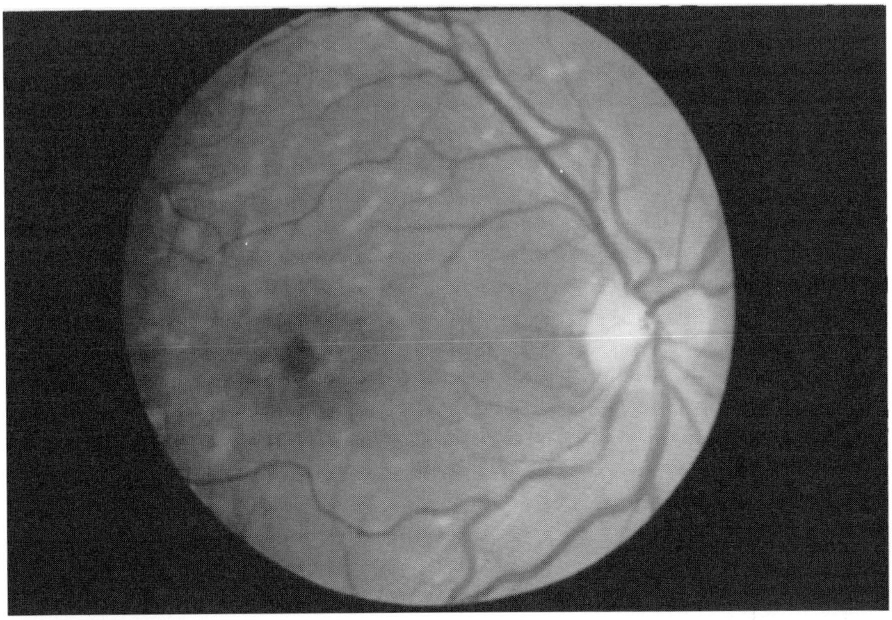

FIGURE 17–5

Stargardt's disease.

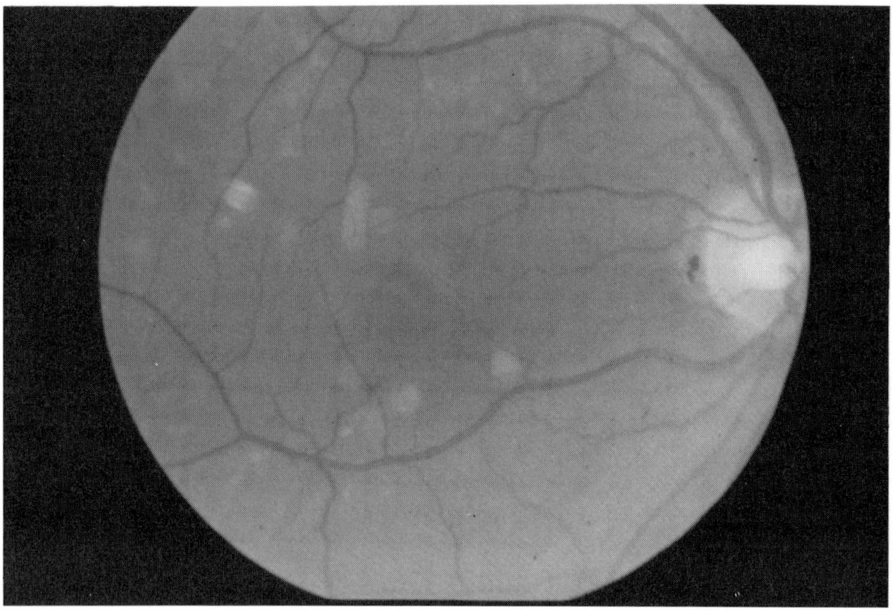

FIGURE 17–6

Fundus flavimaculatus.

and 17–7). Stargardt's disease is considered by many investigators to be a form of fundus flavimaculatus in which macular dystrophy predominates early in the disease.[28–30]

The heredity is autosomal recessive, although there have been dominant cases of Stargardt's disease reported.

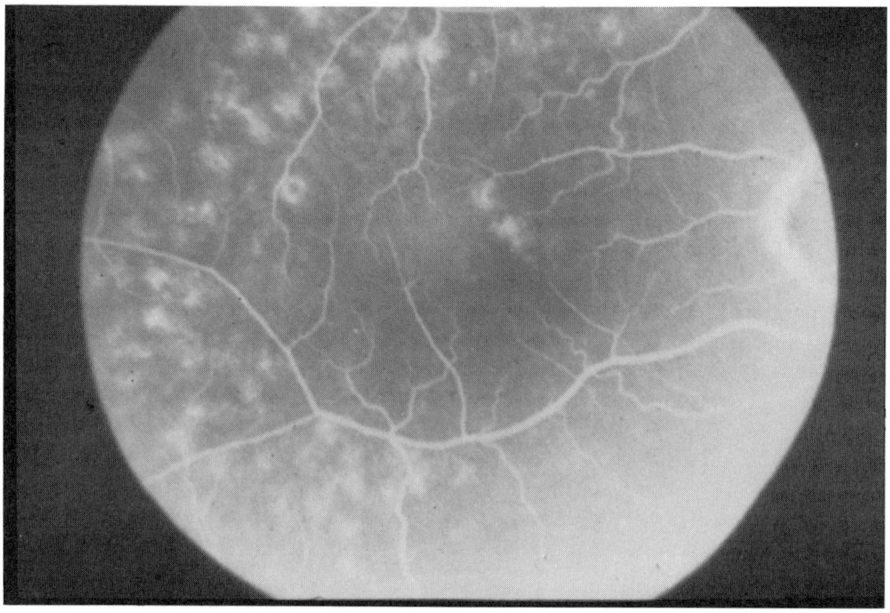

FIGURE 17–7

Fluorescein angiogram of fundus flavimaculatus.

Clinical findings are decreased central vision. The fundus may appear normal. First clinical funduscopic sign is the loss of the foveal reflex with the appearance of small macular yellow flecks which then coalesce to form a "bull's eye lesion." There is a central area of normal retina, surrounded by a zone of depigmented and pigment mottling. There may be diffuse pigmentary changes peripheral to the central area.

As the central lesion progresses, there may be the onset of small yellow flecks in the midperiphery. This is the classic appearance of fundus flavimaculatus.

Fluorescein Angiography

Fluorescein angiography can be used to detect macular lesions before they are seen clinically.

Electroretinogram

The electroretinogram is normal to slightly abnormal with reduced b-wave amplitudes.

Congenital Stationary Night Blindness with Normal and Abnormal Fundi

Congenital Stationary Night Blindness with Normal Fundi

Inheritance: Autosomal recessive, autosomal dominant, X-linked recessive.

This entity is different from RP because rod cone break in the dark adaptation curve shows only the cone response. This is not seen in RP.

Two ERG subtypes in congenital stationary night blindness with normal fundi:

1. No b-wave in photopic and scotopic conditions
2. Both a- and b-waves are reduced under all test conditions.

Also has abnormally low electro-oculogram light rise.

Congenital Stationary Night Blindness with Abnormal Fundi

Oguchi's disease

Inheritance: Autosomal recessive

The retina has peculiar silvery or metallic sheen and as a result the retinal vessels appear very dark by comparison. However, this sheen disappears after several hours of dark adaptation (Mitzuo's phenomenon).

Electroretinogram findings: Abnormal after 30 minutes of dark adaptation (decreased flicker response or absent b-wave), but after several hours, the electroretinogram returns to normal or near normal levels.

Fundus Albipunctatus

Inheritance: Autosomal recessive.

The retina shows multiple small white dots scattered all over the fundus.

The major diagnostic feature of this disease is the slow adaptation of the rods and cones. It can take longer than 1 hour for cones to attain normal thresholds and rods may be elevated for up to 2–3 hours before eventually attaining normal levels. The electroretinogram can return to normal over 2–3 hours.

Congenital Stationary Night Blindness with Myopia, Nystagmus and Decreased Visual Acuity

There is nystagmus, decreased vision, and night blindness, but the fundus appears normal.

The electroretinogram shows a normal a-wave, but an absent b-wave.

Best's Disease

Best's disease (vitelliruptive macular dystrophy or vitelliform macular dystrophy) is the only entity that is known to have normal electroretinogram, but abnormal electro-oculogram. The fundus changes are a central yellow "egg yolk" lesion that can begin as soft yellow eruptions clustered centrally around the fovea. Later, the "egg yolk" lesion may appear and later on, there can be a dispersion of the subretinal yellow lesions over the 1500 μ area of the macula to the posterior pole area. In the late stages, there is choroidal neovascularization and cicatricial scarring (Fig. 17–8).

Vision in the early stages can be in the 20/25–20/40 range with minimal impairment. Because the disease affects the macular area, the electroretinogram is often normal and the electro-oculogram is abnormal. In carrier states where the fundus is normal appearing, the electro-oculogram is abnormal.

Fluorescein Angiography

Fluorescein angiography demonstrates that the egg yolk lesions are nonfluorescent and the "scrambled or dispersed lesions" are hyperfluorescent.

Adult Foveomacular Dystrophy

Adult foveomacular dystrophy (pattern or butterfly dystrophy) is autosomal dominant.

The age of onset is 30–50 years and occurs in both eyes with mild visual blurring and metamorphopsia. The symptoms of metamorphopsia may be more pronounced in one eye although the

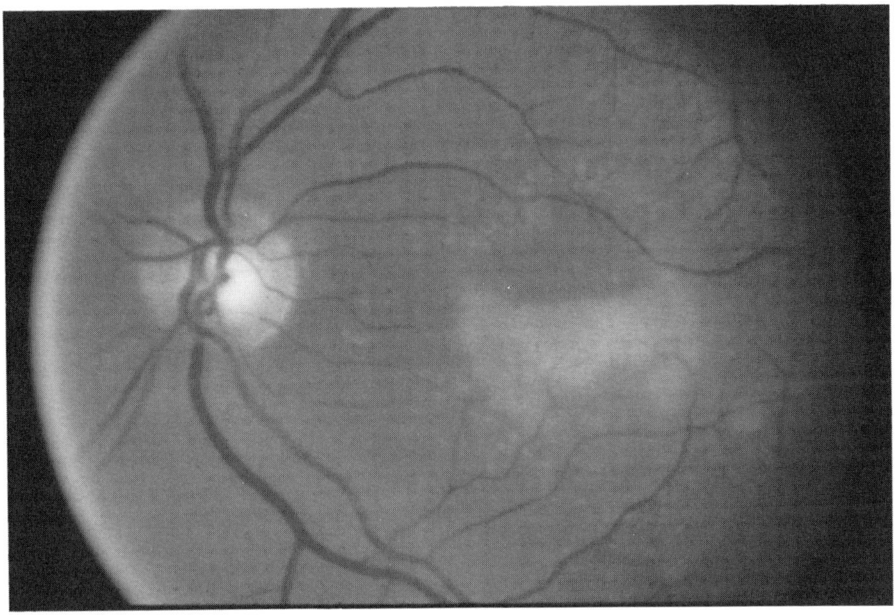

FIGURE 17-8
Best's disease.

lesions may be seen in both eyes. Clinically, there are symmetric, solitary, ⅓ to 1 disc diameter in size, round, oval or slightly elevated, and yellow subretinal lesions.

Fluorescein Angiography

Small irregular ring or hyperfluorescence surrounding a central nonfluorescent spot is seen on the angiogram. Some extrafoveal lesions show discrete staining, but others are either nonfluorescent or have a halo of fluorescence surrounding the lesions.

Pattern Dystrophy and Butterfly-shaped Pigment Dystrophy

Pattern dystrophy can be the pattern of pigmentation like a coarse-knotted fishnet, beginning in the macular area and extending in all directions for 4–5 disc diameters.

Gray or yellow pigment is organized in the shape of a butterfly in the macula, hence the term butterfly dystrophy.

Albinism

Classic or Complete Oculocutaneous Albinism

In classic or complete cutaneous albinism (tyrosinase negative-albinism) the patients have whitish blonde hair, have very pale skin with transilluminable irides and lack of fundus pigmentation. Macular hypoplasia is present (Fig. 17–9).

Tyrosinase-Positive Albinism

In tyrosinase-positive albinism, the patient may have some pigmentation and the skin is not as pale or as white as in oculocutaneous albinism. There is fundus pigmentation in the macula.

Ocular Albinism

In ocular albinism, the patients do not have any of the skin changes, but do show ocular changes similar to those patients with tyrosinase-positive albinism. This is an X-linked disorder and evaluation of the suspected female carrier may provide the diagnostic clues to make the diagnosis. The female carrier will show iris transillumination defects. In addition, the female carrier will show pigment granularity in the fundus periphery and will not have nystagmus and poor vision.

X-linked Juvenile Retinoschisis

X-linked juvenile retinoschisis is a disease that affects young males. Age of presentation is in the first and second decades of life.

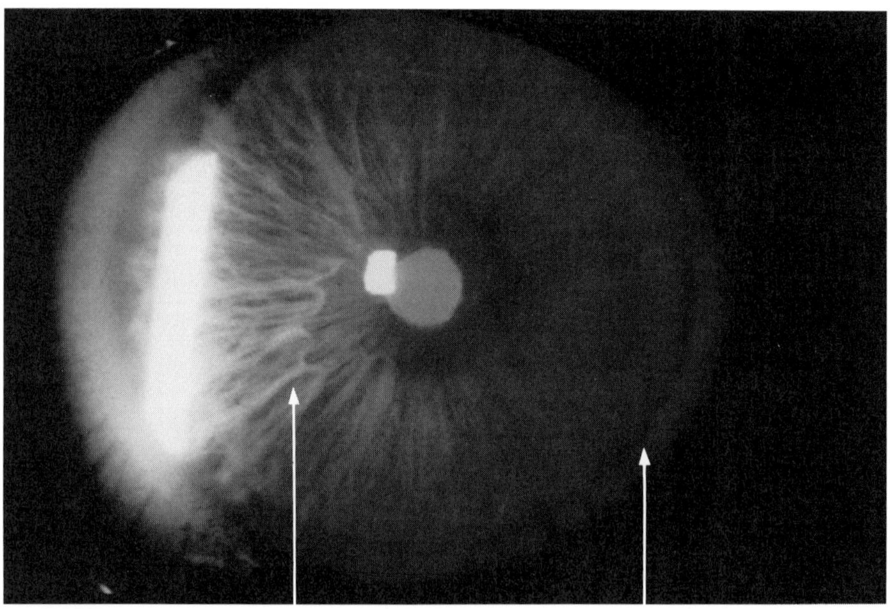

FIGURE 17–9

Albinism.

Typically, a young boy presents with poor vision in one eye and is found to have a vitreous hemorrhage.

The inheritance pattern is X-linked recessive. The mother is the carrier and often, in the carrier state, there is nothing seen. The mothers are usually asymptomatic, although there is one report of some macular changes in the carrier state.[31]

The physical findings in the affected patient are (1) foveal cysts, (2) outer retina hole, and (3) vitreous veils (Fig. 17–10). Usually the retinal vessels are pulled by the schisis cavity and there is a resultant vitreous hemorrhage. The schisis cavity is the splitting of the nerve fiber layer from the ganglion cell layer.

The prognosis for vision is that it will start at 20/40 level and progress in adult midlife to about 20/200 vision.

Fluorescein Angiography

There is no leakage at the site of the foveal cysts unlike those cases of petalloid macular edema. Areas of hyperfluorence can occur at the site of traction of the retinal vessels and schisis cavity.

Electroretinogram

There is an absent b-wave in the scotopic conditions. The electro-oculogram can be within the lower limits of normal and is not diagnostic.

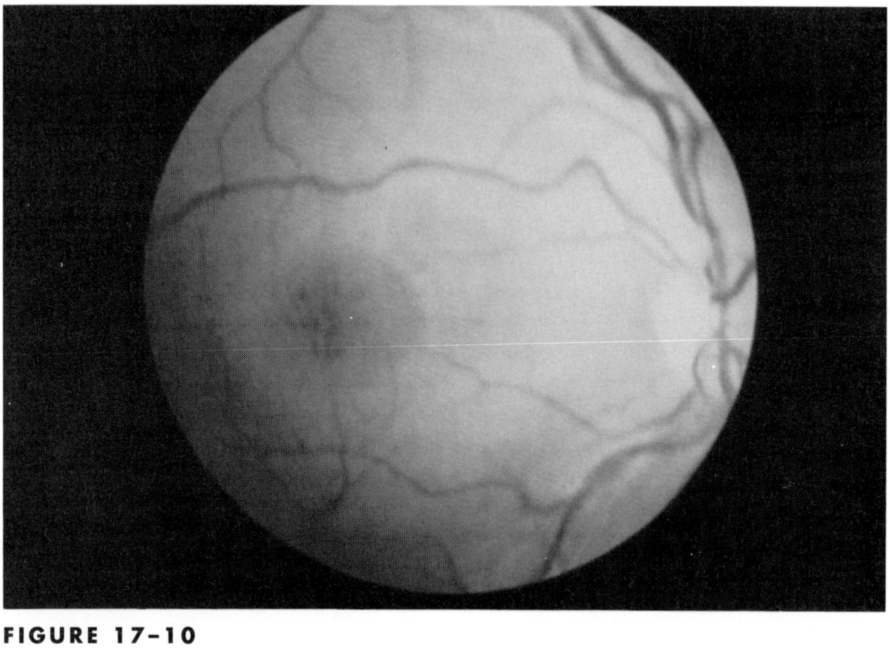

FIGURE 17–10

Juvenile X-linked retinoschisis.

Choroidal Dystrophies

Choroideremia is an X-linked recessive disease. The onset of symptoms is in the first or second decade and the major complaint is poor night vision. Physical examination shows salt and pepper pigment mottling in the equator and posterior pole. Carrier females show retinal pigment epithelial mottling in the midperiphery and macular area. However, the female carrier has normal retinal function throughout life (Fig. 17–11).

Electroretinogram

The electroretinogram findings are reduced or absent scotopic components.

Fluorescein Angiography

There is patchy loss of the choriocapillaris and choroidal vessels.

Gyrate Atrophy

Gyrate atrophy is autosomal recessive and an occasional dominant pedigree has been reported.

Symptoms appear in the second and third decades of life with poor night vision, constricted visual fields, and myopia.

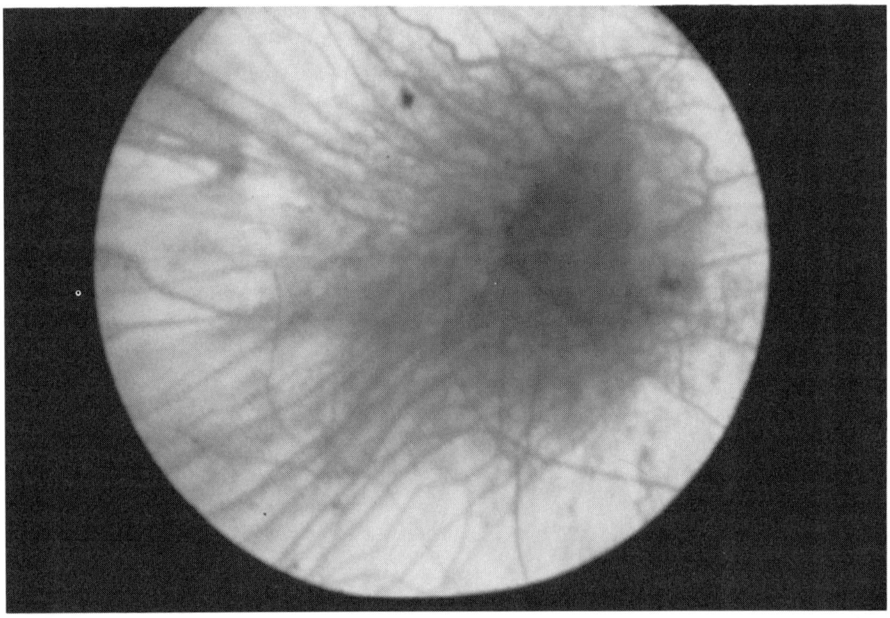

FIGURE 17–11

Choroideremia.

Physical examinations show thinning and transparency of the retinal pigment epithelium in the midperiphery. The underlying choroid appears sclerotic. Affected areas are separated from normal-appearing retina by scalloped borders which begin as isolated islands and merge to form a scalloped-edge rings. Due to the pigment accumulation, the scalloped borders have a darker appearance, thus increasing the contrast between the adjacent normal and abnormal retinal tissues (Fig. 17–12).

In the late stages of the disease, there is loss of the entire choroid and white sclera. In the very late stages, the periphery to posterior pole is affected, but there may be a remaining patch of choroid at the macula.

Patients have elevated levels of ornithine in the urine and plasma. There is the absence or near absence of the pyridoxine-dependent enzyme, ornithine aminotransferase, which is necessary for the breakdown of excess ornithine in humans.

Electroretinogram

Similar to choroideremia, but with a low-protein and low ornithine diet, there is a reduction of plasma ornithine and thus a consequent improvement in retinal function.

Fluorescein Angiography

There is a loss of choriocapillaries in the affected areas.

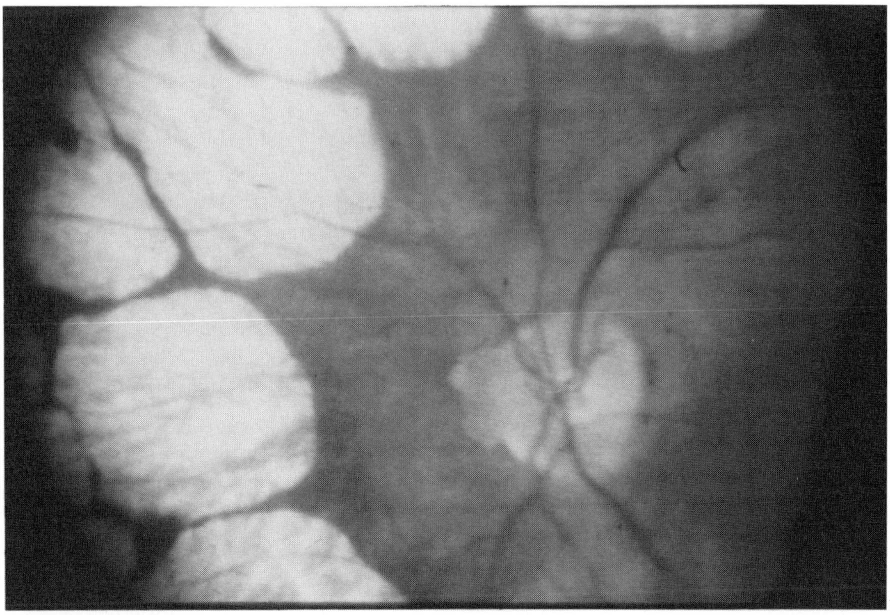

FIGURE 17–12

Gyrate atrophy.

Inherited Vitreous Degenerations

Wagner's Vitreoretinal Degeneration

Wagner's vitreoretinal degeneration is autosomal dominantly inherited. Clinically, these patients have an optically empty vitreous, a fibrillar anterior vitreous, cataract formation, and a generalized pigmentary degeneration of the retina with atrophy and sclerosis of the choroid and preretinal membranes. A late sequela is retinal detachment. The electroretinogram is similar as to that found in RP, i.e., nonrecordable.

If skeletal or facial anomolies are seen, this is known as Wagner-Stickler's syndrome.

Goldmann-Favre's Disease

Goldmann-Favre's disease is autosomal recessively inherited. Clinically, the patients complain of night blindness. The fundus examination shows an optically empty vitreous, vitreoretinal bands, pigmentary degeneration of the retina, and peripheral and central retinoschisis. In the late stages, there is the formation of preretinal membranes. The electroretinogram is extinguished.

REFERENCES

1. Heckenlively JR, Martin DA, Rosales TO: Telangiectasia and optic atrophy in cone-rod degenerations. Arch Ophthalmol 1981; *99:* 1983–1991

2. Arden GB, Carter RM, Hogg CR et al: Rod and cone activity in patients with dominantly inherited retinitis pigmentosa: comparisons between psychophysical and electroretinographic measurements. Br J Ophthalmol 1983; *67:* 405–418

3. Szamier RB, Berson EL, Klein R, Meyers S: Sex-linked retinitis pigmentosa: ultrastructure of photoreceptors and pigment epithelium. Invest Ophthalmol Vis Sci 1979; *18:* 145–160

4. Bunker CH, Berson EL, Bromley WC et al: The prevalence of retinitis pigmentosa in Maine. Am J Ophthalmol 1984; *97:* 357–365

5. Boughman JA, Conneally PM, Nance WE: Population genetic studies of retinitis pigmentosa. Am J Hum Genet 1980; *32:* 223–235

6. Boughman JA, Fishman GA: A genetic analysis of retinitis pigmentosa. Br J Ophthalmol 1983; *67:* 449–454

7. Heckenlively JR, Boughman JA, Friedman LH: Pedigree Analysis: the population perspective. p. 21. In Heckenlively JR, (ed): Retinitis Pigmentosa, Philadelphia, JB Lippincott Co, 1988, p. 21

8. Pearlman JT: Mathematical models of retinitis pigmentosa: a study of the rate of progress in the different genetic forms. Trans Am Ophthalmol Soc 1979; *77:* 643–656

9. Krill AE: Hereditary retinal and choroidal diseases. Vol II. Hagerstown, MD, Harper & Row, 1977, pp 481–482

10. Jay M: On the heredity of retinitis pigmentosa. Br J Ophthalmol 1982; *66:* 405–416

11. Fetkenhour CL, Choromokos E, Weinstein J, Shoch D: Cystoid macular edema in retinitis pigmentosa. Trans Am Acad Ophthalmol Otolaryngol 1977; *83:* 515–521

12. Berson EL, Gouras P, Hoff M: Temporal aspects of the electroretinogram. Arch Ophthalmol 1969; *81:* 207–210

13. Heckenlively JR, Silver J: Management and treatment of retinitis pigmentosa. Ch. 6. In Heckenlively JR (ed): Retinitis Pigmentosa. Philadelphia, JB Lippincott Co, 1988, ch 6

14. Bastek JV, Heckenlively JR, Straatsma BR: Cataract surgery in retinitis pigmentosa patients. Ophthalmol 1982; *89:* 880–884

15. Berson EL, Rosner B, Sandberg MA et al: A randomized trial of vitamin A and vitamin E supplementation for retinitis pigmentosa. Arch Ophthalmol 1993; *111:* 761–772

16. Massof RW, Finkelstein D: Supplemental vitamin A retards loss of ERG amplitude in retinitis pigmentosa. Arch Ophthalmol 1993: *111:* 751–754

17. Berson EL, Rosner B, Sandberg MA et al: Vitamin A supplementation for RP. Arch Ophthalmol 1993; *111:* 1456–1458

18. Massof RW, Finkelstein D: In reply. Arch Ophthalmol 1993; *111:* 1458–1459

19. Norton EWD: A randomized trial of vitamin A and vitamin E supplementation for retinitis pigmentosa. Letter to the editor. Arch Ophthalmol 1993; *111:* 1460

20. Marmor MF. Letter to the editor. Arch Ophthalmol 1993; *111:* 1460–1461

21. Clowes DD: Letter to the editor. Arch Ophthalmol 1993; *111:* 1461–1462

22. Gamel JW, Barr CC: Letter to the editor. Arch Ophthalmol 1993, *111:* 1462–1463

23. Fielder AR, Marshall J: Letter to the editor. Arch Ophthalmol 1993; *111:* 1463

24. Berson EL, Rosner B, Sandberg MA et al: In reply. Arch Ophthalmol 1993; *111:* 1463–1465

25. Felix JS, Laties M: In reply. Arch Ophthalmol 1993; *111:* 1465–1466

26. Foxman SG, Heckenlively JR, Bateman JB et al: Classification of congenital and early onset retinitis pigmentosa. Arch Ophthalmol 1985; *103:* 1502–1506

27. Sorsby A, Williams CE: Retinal aplasia as a clinical entity. Br Med J 1960; *30:* 293–297

28. Fishman GA: Fundus flavimaculatus. Arch Ophthalmol 1976; *94:* 2061–2067

29. Wu G, Weiter JJ, Hirose T: Autosomal dominant Stargardt's disease. Ophthalmol 1987; *94:* 112 (suppl.)

30. Lopez PF, Maumenee IH, de la Cruz Z, Green WR: Autosomal dominant fundus flavimaculatus: a clinicopathologic correlation. Ophthalmol 1990; *97:* 798–809

31. Wu G, Cotlier E, Brodie SE: A carrier state for juvenile X-linked retinoschisis. Ophthal Ped & Genet 1985; *5:* 13–18

CHAPTER EIGHTEEN

Toxic Retinopathy

CHLOROQUINE RETINOPATHY

Chloroquine and hydroxychloroquine are 4-aminoquinolone compounds, originally created for their antimalarial effects. These compounds form a complex with ferriprotoporphyrin IX, an intermediary product of hemoglobin ingestion by malarial parasites (plasmodia), which causes osmotic lysis of the parasites.[1]

In addition, these compounds are used in the treatment of rheumatoid arthritis, discoid lupus, and systemic lupus erythematosus. Chloroquine and hydroxychloroquine's anti-inflammatory properties are thought to be mediated by actions on intracellular DNA and lysosomal metabolism.[1]

Anatomy and Pathophysiology

The exact mechanism of choroquine toxicity is unclear. It has been thought that the binding of chloroquine to melanin interferes with the metabolism of the retinal pigment epithelium.[2,3] However, more recent studies have shown direct damage to the photoreceptors. The earliest pathologic findings show damage to the ganglion cells, followed by degeneration of the photoreceptors.[4,5] It is also thought that chloroquine produces toxic damage to the photoreceptors by interfering with protein synthesis of the photoreceptors.[6]

Epidemiology

A daily dose of 250 mg of chloroquine or 400 mg of hydroxychloroquine appears to be relatively safe.[7–9] Relatively low-weight patients may need a smaller daily dose.[7]

Diagnosis

Clinically, the patient reports decreased visual acuity, central and paracentral, and peripheral scotomata.

There is a loss of the foveal reflex and irregular and increased pigmentation of the macula. A ring of depigmentation surrounded by mild increased pigmentation usually develops, resembling a bull's eye. Arteriolar narrowing, vascular sheathing, and peripheral pigmentation may also develop (Fig. 18–1).

Color vision may be abnormal.[10] The electroretinogram shows a large a-wave or reduced b-wave and the electro-oculogram may be depressed. These findings may be present before the ophthalmoscopic findings. The electro-oculogram may revert to normal after cessation of the drug.[11] Dark adaptation remains normal even in the late stages, which is not the case in retinitis pigmentosa.[12]

Fluorescein Angiography

Early retinal pigment epithelial changes may be seen in the early transit.[13] However, some investigators find that fundus slides are more sensitive than fluorescein angiograms in detecting early retinopathy.[14]

Management

Prevention is the best treatment. After cessation of the drug, advanced chloroquine retinopathy can remain unchanged. Patients with early changes may develop improved visual acuity and lose

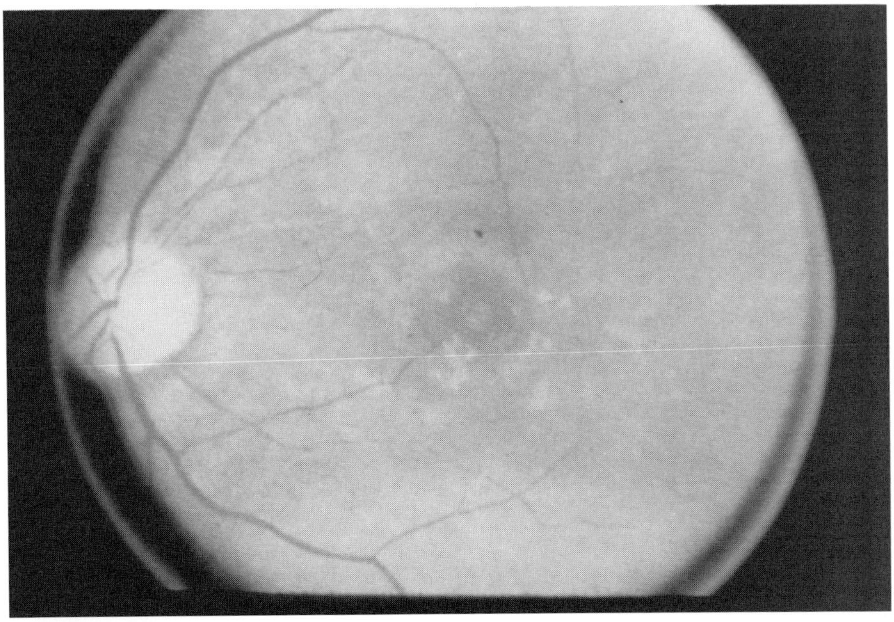

FIGURE 18–1

Chloroquine toxicity.

their scotomata if the drug is discontinued early enough.[15] But in advanced cases of chloroquine retinopathy, there is progression despite cessation of the drug.[16]

With the routine doses of 250 mg/day of chloroquine or 400 mg/day of hydroxychloroquine, the patients are seen every 6 months, and self-administration of the Amsler grid.[17] If there is change of the Amsler grid squares, the patients can be tested with perimetry with white and red test objects.

GENTAMICIN RETINOPATHY

Anatomy and Pathophysiology

It is thought that gentamicin causes direct neural toxicity. Gentamicin disrupts lysosomal enzymes, thus causing sequestration of unmetabolized substrates.[18] There may be direct disruption of oxidative phosphorylation in the mitochondria.[19]

Diagnosis

Clinically, the patient presents postoperatively after cataract or vitreal surgery where gentamicin is administered for endophthalmitis. The patient presents with profound visual loss and the retinal examination shows areas of necrotic white retina, localized retinal arteriolar occlusion, diffuse retinal hemorrhages, optic nerve atrophy, pigmentary degeneration of the retina, cherry-red spot, and a history of gentamicin injection intraoperatively. It mimicks that of acute central retinal artery obstruction, ophthalmic artery obstruction, or combined central retinal artery/central retinal vein obstruction.[20,21]

In some patients with gentamicin toxicity, there can be a peripheral retinal break seen after intraocular surgery, presumably from inadvertent intraocular perforation at the time of subconjunctival injection or subtenon's injection.

Fluorescein Angiography

Delay in retinal perfusion and nonfilling of macular vessels is prominent. Hyperfluorescence of the optic disc and large vessels in late transit is seen. Late complications documented on fluorescein angiography shows retinal pigment epithelial window defects reflecting retinal pigment epithelial degeneration as a late consequence of gentamicin toxicity.

In some cases, when the electroretinogram is extinguished, there is retinal vascular leakage on fluorescein angiogram.[20]

Electroretinography

In central retinal artery occlusion, there is a relatively normal a-wave on electroretinogram with minimal retinal vascular leakage. In ophthalmic artery occlusion, there is no cherry-red spot, however, there is an extinguished electroretinogram with compromised choroidal perfusion.

Management

Visual prognosis is poor in these eyes. Prevention is the best treatment: (1) It is best to avoid drawing up the antibiotics in unlabeled syringes ahead of time and (2) Label all syringes or color-code the syringes on the instrument tray. Treatment can be done by irrigation, aspiration, and vitrectomy. One should be aware that toxic reactions can occur within 5–10 minutes after intravitreal injection of high concentrations of antibiotics.[22]

MELLARIL (THIORIDAZINE HYDROCHLORIDE) RETINOPATHY

Anatomy and Pathophysiology

Histopathologic examination suggests that the initial site of damage is in the outer segment of the photoreceptors, which is then followed by degeneration of the retinal pigment epithelium and choriocapillaris.[23]

Diagnosis

Patients taking more than 700 mg a day of thioridazine hydrochloride (mellaril) are at risk for retinopathy. The patient complains of blurred vision, nyctalopia, dyschromatopsia. Initially the fundus appearance is normal, but a fine pigmentary stippling develops from the posterior pole to equator. Progression is heralded by large clumps of granular pigmentation that then become depigmented, resulting in multiple confluent nummular areas, typically posterior to the equator.[24,25]

Fluorescein Angiography

Retinal pigment epithelial window defects are seen in early transit. There is late hyperfluorescence corresponding to the window defects.

Treatment

With the cessation of the drug, the retinopathy is reversible in most cases.

NICOTINIC ACID AND EPINEPHRINE MACULOPATHY

Cystoid macular edema can occur with large doses of nicotinic acid to treat hypercholesterolemia. No leakage of fluorescein from the retinal or macular vessels is seen. There is marked improvement with the cessation of the drug.[26]

Topical epinephrine after intracapsular cataract extraction is associated with a reversible cystoid macular edema in 20–30 percent of the patients.[27,28] Fluorescein angiography shows petalloid hyperfluorescence seen in the mid- to late-transit films. (See Chapter 8.)

TAMOXIFEN RETINOPATHY

Tamoxifen is a nonsteroidal antiestrogen used in breast cancer treatment. After high-dose tamoxifen treatment, there have been cases of refractile intraretinal lesions with cystoid macular edema. Histopathologic examination shows nerve fiber layer and inner plexiform intracellular lesions, 3–35 μm in diameter, thought to be axonal degeneration.[29,30]

CRYSTALLINE RETINOPATHY

Crystalline retinopathy is also seen with canthaxanthine, a carotenoid that has been used as an oral tanning agent.[31] Six out of 51 patients developed a crystalline retinopathy after taking more than 100 capsules of canthaxanthine in less than 2 years.[32]

REFERENCES

1. Mackenzie AH: Pharmacologic actions of 4-aminoquinolone compounds. Am J Med 1983; *75:* 5–10

2. Bernstein HN, Ginsberg J: The pathology of chloroquine retinopathy. Arch Ophthamol 1964; *71:* 238–245

3. Rubin M, Slonicki A: A mechanism for the toxicity of chloroquine. Arthritis Rheum 1966; *9:* 537–542

4. Abraham R, Hendy RJ: Irreversible lysosomal damage induced by chloroquine in the retina of pigmented and nonpigmented laboratory animals. Exp Mol Pathol 1970; *12:* 185–200

5. Berson EL: Acute toxic effects of chloroquine on the cat retina. Invest Ophthalmol 1970; *9:* 618–628

6. Ivanina TA, Sakina NL, Lebedeva MN, Borovjagin VL: A study of the mechanisms of chloroquine retinopathy. Ophthal Res 1989; *21:* 272–277

7. Easterbrook M: Ocular effects and safety of antimalaria agents. Am J Med 1988; *85:* (suppl. 4A) 23–29

8. Tobin DR, Krohel GB, Rynes RI: Hydroxychloroquine a seven-year experience. Arch Ophthalmol 1982; *100:* 81–83

9. Finbloom DS, Silver K, Newsome DA, Gunkel R: Comparison of hydroxychloroquine and chloroquine use and the development of retinal toxicity. J Rhematol 1985; *12:* 692–694

10. Earnshaw ER, Miles DU, Stewart TW: Screening for chloroquine retinopathy. Br J Dermatol 1966; *78:* 669–675

11. Kolb H: Electro-oculogram findings in patients treated with antimalarial drugs. Br J Ophthalmol 1965; *49:* 573–590

12. Carr RE, Gouras P, Gunkel RD: Chloroquine retinopathy: early detection by retinal threshold test. Arch Ophthalmol 1966; *75:* 171–178

13. Kearns TP, Hollenhorst RW: Chloroquine retinopathy: evaluation by fluorescein fundus angiography. Arch Ophthalmol 1966; *76:* 378–384

14. Cruess AF, Schachat AP, Nicholl J, Ausburger JJ: Chloroquine retinopathy: is fluorescein angiography necessary. Ophthalmol 1985; *92:* 1127–1129

15. Nozik RA, Weinstock FJ, Vignos PJ Jr: Ocular complications of chloroquine: a series and case presentations with simple method for early detection of retinopathy. Am J Ophthalmol 1964; *58:* 774–778

16. Brinkley JR, DuBois EL, Ryan SJ: Long-term course of chloroquine retinopathy after cessation of medication. Am J Ophthalmol 1979; *88:* 1–11

17. Easterbrook M: Dose relationships in patients with early chloroquine retinopathy. J Rheumatol 1987; *14:* 472–475

18. D'Amico DJ, Caspers-Velu L, Shanks E et al: Comparative toxicity of intravitreal aminoglycoside antibiotics. Am J Ophthalmol 1985; *100:* 264–275

19. Vera-Roman J, Krishnakantha TP, Cuppage FE: Gentamicin nephrotoxicity in rats, I. Acute biochemical and ultrastructural effects. Lab Invest 1975; *33:* 412–417

20. Brown GC, Eagle RC, Shakin EP et al: Retinal toxicity of intravitreal gentamicin. Arch Ophthlamol 1990; *108:* 1740–1744

21. McDonald HR, Schatz H, Allen AW et al: Retinal toxicity secondary to intraocular gentamicin injection. Ophthalmol 1986; *93:* 871–877

22. Peyman GA: Discussion of retinal toxicity secondary to intraocular gentamicin injection. Ophthalmol 1986; *93:* 876–877

23. Miller FS, Bunt-Millam AH, Kalina RE: Clinical ultrastructural study of thioridazine retinopathy. Ophthalmol 1982; *89:* 1487–1488

24. Connell MM, Poley BJ, McFarlane JR: Chorioretinopathy associated with thioridazine therapy. Arch Ophthalmol 1964; *71:* 816–821

25. Scott AW: Retinal pigmentation in a patient receiving thioridazine. Arch Ophthalmol 1963; *70:* 775–778

26. Gass JDM: Nicotinic acid maculopathy. Am J Ophthalmol 1973; *76:* 500–510

27. Kolker AE, Becker B: Epinephrine maculopathy. Arch Ophthalmol 1968; *79:* 552–562

28. Thomas JV, Gragoudas ES, Blair NP, Lapus JV: Correlation of epinephrine use and macular edema in aphakic glaucomatous eyes. Arch Ophthalmol 1978; *96:* 625–628

29. Kaiser-Kupfer MI, Kupfer C, Rodrigues MM: Tamoxifen retinopathy: a clinicopathological report. Ophthalmol 1981; *88:* 89–93

30. McKeown CA, Swartz M, Blom J, Maggiano JM: Tamoxifen retinopathy. Br J Ophthalmol 1981; *65:* 177–179

31. Cortin P, Corriveau LA, Rousseau AP et al: Maculopathie en paillettes d'or. Can J Ophthalmol 1982; *17:* 103–106

32. Boudreault G, Cortin P, Corriveau LA et al: La retinopathie a la canthaxanthine: 1. Etude clinique de 51 consommateurs. Can J Ophthalmol 1983; *18:* 325–328

CHAPTER NINETEEN

Retinal Tumors

RETINOBLASTOMA

Epidemiology

Retinoblastoma occurs in 1/18,000 live births or 11 cases per million children under 5 years.[1,2]

Anatomy

The retinoblastoma locus in 13q 14 is the physical location of a large gene that codes for a 4.73 kilomessage. An intact gene appears to protect against malignancy. Both copies of the gene at the retinoblastoma locus must be destroyed, lost, mutated, or inactivated for the initiation of retinoblastoma. The function of the retinoblastoma gene is unknown.

Classification

The Reese-Ellsworth Classification of retinoblastomas is as follows:
Group I: Very favorable (Figs. 19–1 and 19–2)

A. Solitary tumor less than 4 disc diameter in size, at or behind the equator.

B. Multiple tumors none over 4 disc diameter in size, all at or behind the equator.

Group 2: Favorable (Figs. 19–3 and 19–4)

A. Solitary tumor 4–10 disc diameter in size, at or behind equator.

B. Multiple tumors 4–10 disc diameter in size, behind the equator.

Group 3: Doubtful (Figs. 19–5 and 19–6)

A. Any tumor anterior to the equator.

B. Solitary tumor larger than 10 disc diameter, behind equator.

Group 4: Unfavorable (Figs. 19–7 and 19–8)

A. Multiple tumors, some larger than 10 disc diameter in size.

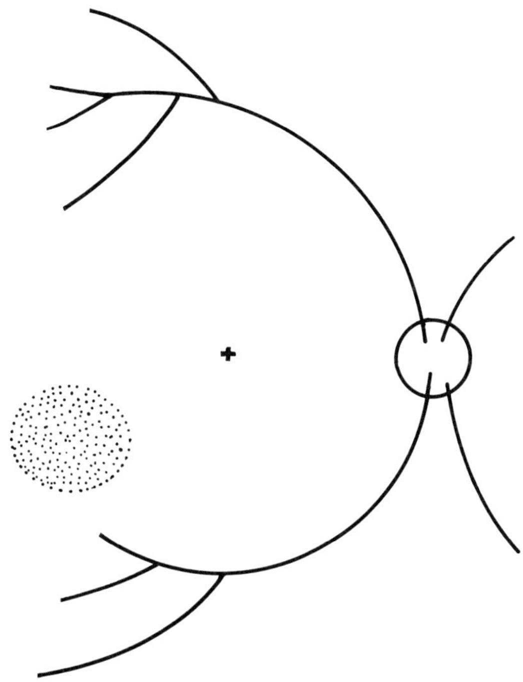

FIGURE 19–1

Group 1-A tumor according to the Reese-Ellsworth classification system.

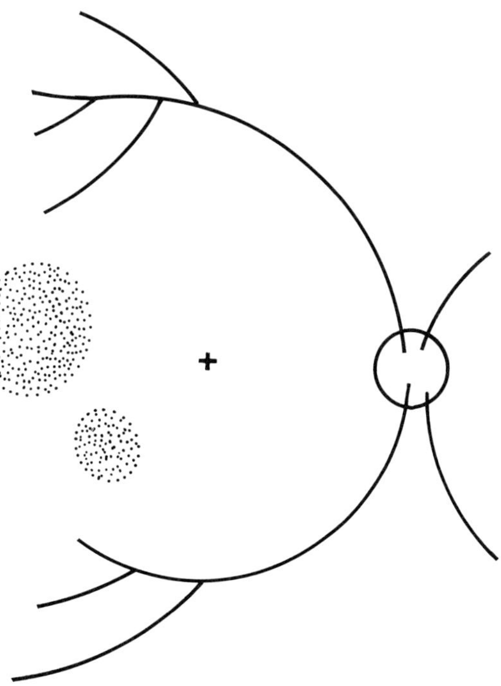

FIGURE 19–2

Group 1-B tumor according to the Reese-Ellsworth classification system.

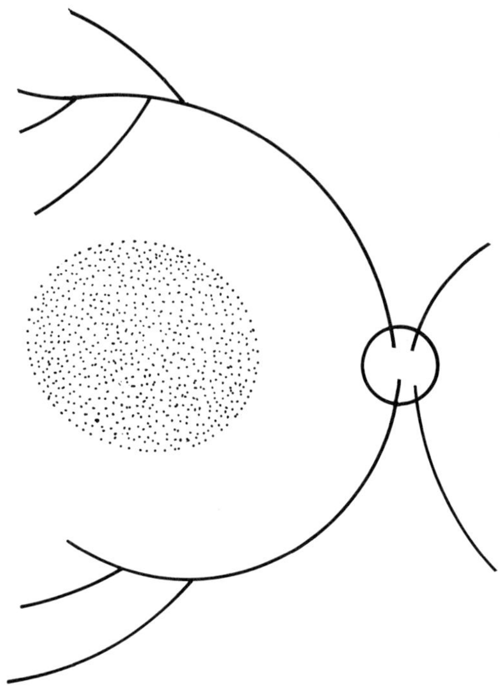

FIGURE 19–3

Group 2-A tumor according to the Reese-Ellsworth classification system.

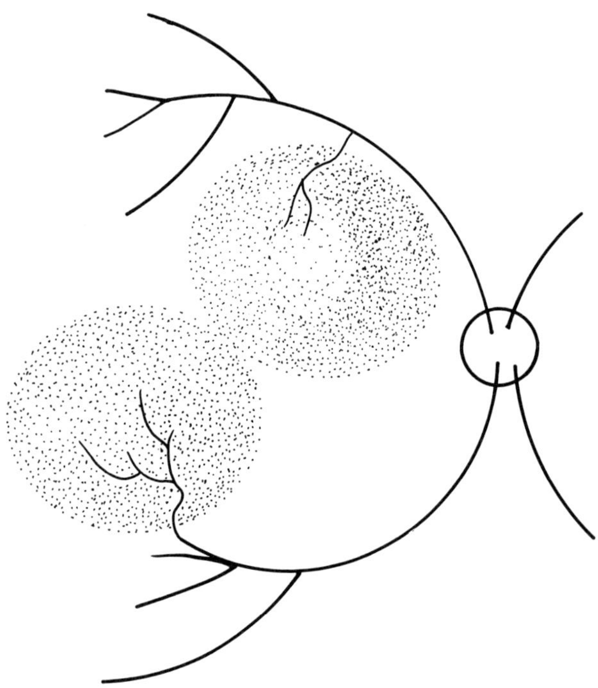

FIGURE 19–4

Group 2-B tumor according to the Reese-Ellsworth classification system.

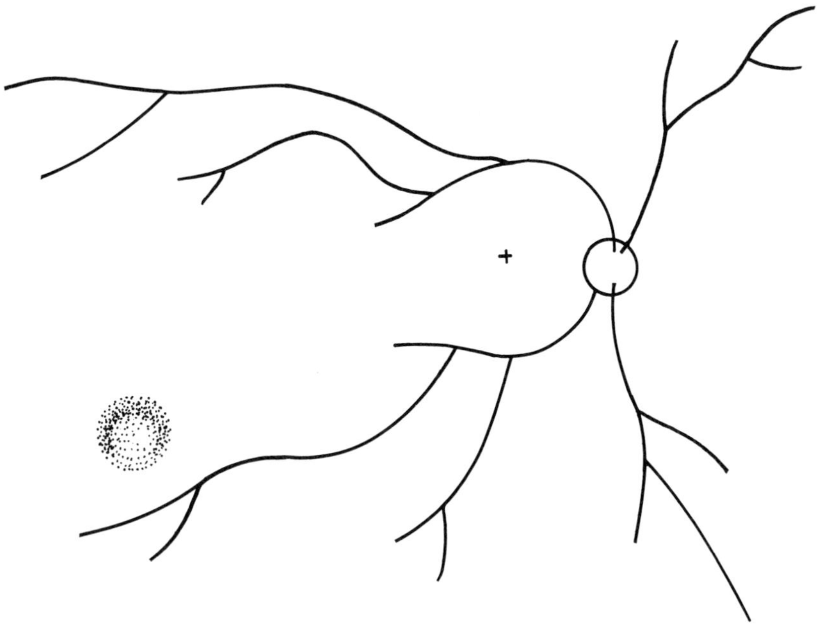

FIGURE 19–5

Group 3-A tumor according to the Reese-Ellsworth classification system.

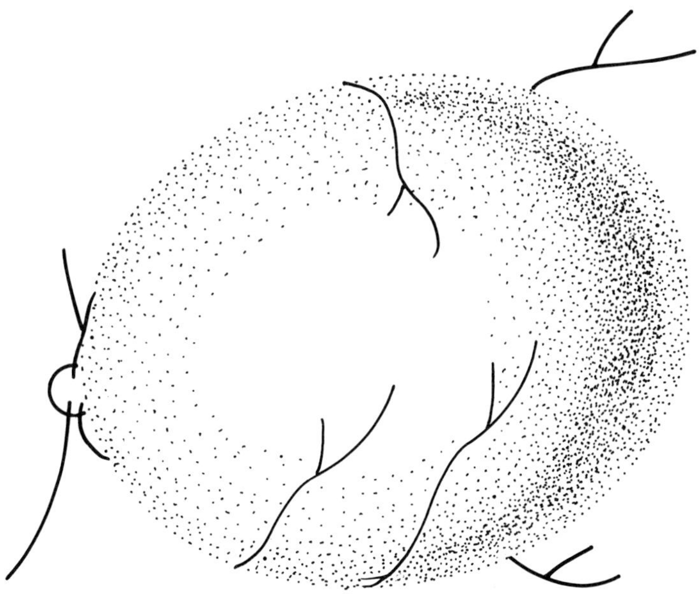

FIGURE 19–6

Group 3-B tumor according to the Reese-Ellsworth classification system.

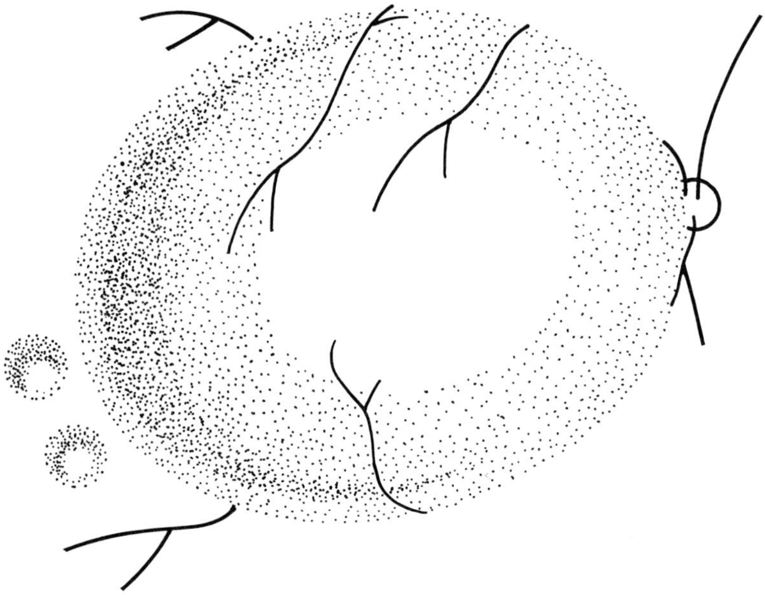

FIGURE 19–7

Group 4-A tumor according to the Reese-Ellsworth classification system.

B. Any lesion extending anteriorly to the ora serrata.

Group 5: Very unfavorable (Figs. 19–9 and 19–10)

A. Massive tumors involving over half the retina.

B. Vitreous seeding.

Examination

Usually the child is brought to the ophthalmologist for an examination. The child is examined by indirect ophthalmoscopy;

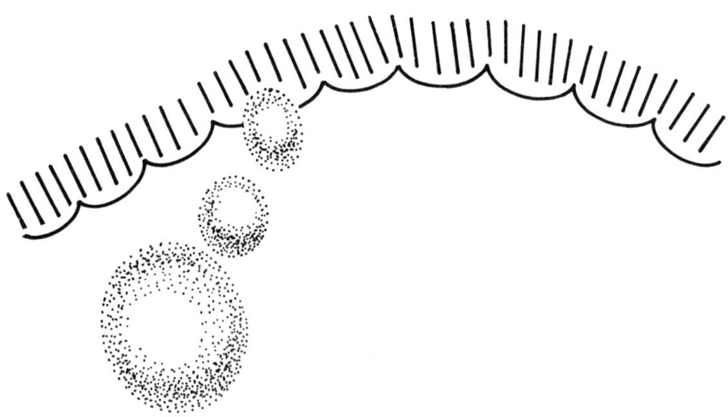

FIGURE 19–8

Group 4-B tumor according to the Reese-Ellsworth classification system.

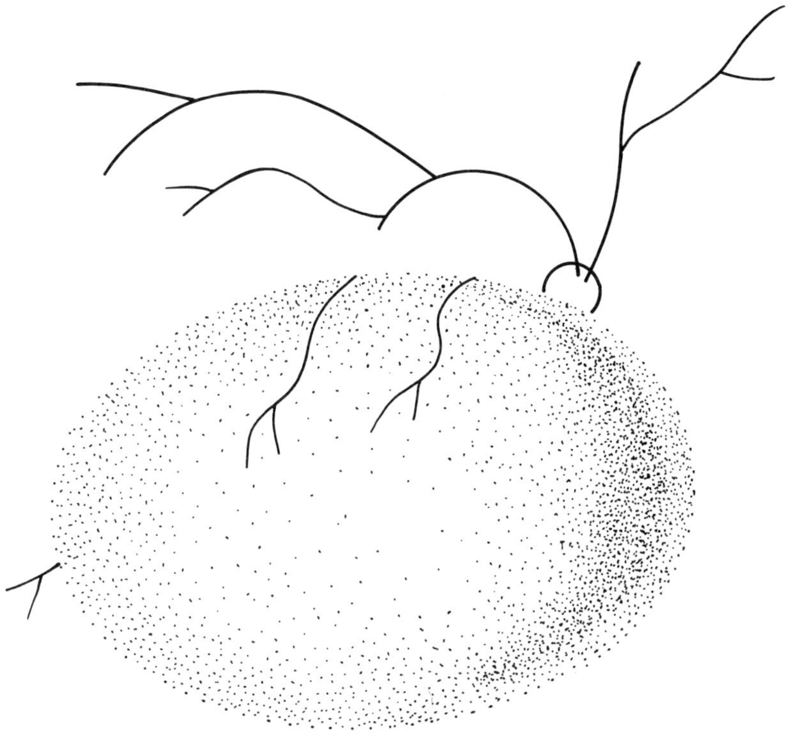

FIGURE 19–9

Group 5-A tumor according to the Reese-Ellsworth classification system.

however, an additional examination under anesthesia is necessary to identify all of the tumors. Intraoperatively, the child's fundus is usually drawn or photographed for classification and plans are then made at that time for further surgery or other treatment options.

Initial Signs and Symptoms

More than half of all retinoblastomas are diagnosed following observation of a white pupil or leukocoria (Fig. 19–11), by a family member or primary care physician. Strabismus is the initial symptom in one out of every five patients with retinoblastoma. Other signs and symptoms are red, painful eye with glaucoma, poor vision, and orbital cellulitis-like condition.[3] The median age of diagnosis for a child with unilateral retinoblastoma and a positive family history is 2.5 months, whereas the median age of diagnosis for a child with unilateral retinoblastoma without a family history is 27 months.[3] In a child with bilateral disease, the age of diagnosis is 4 months.[4] Ninety percent of all cases of retinoblastoma in the United States is diagnosed before age of 5.[5]

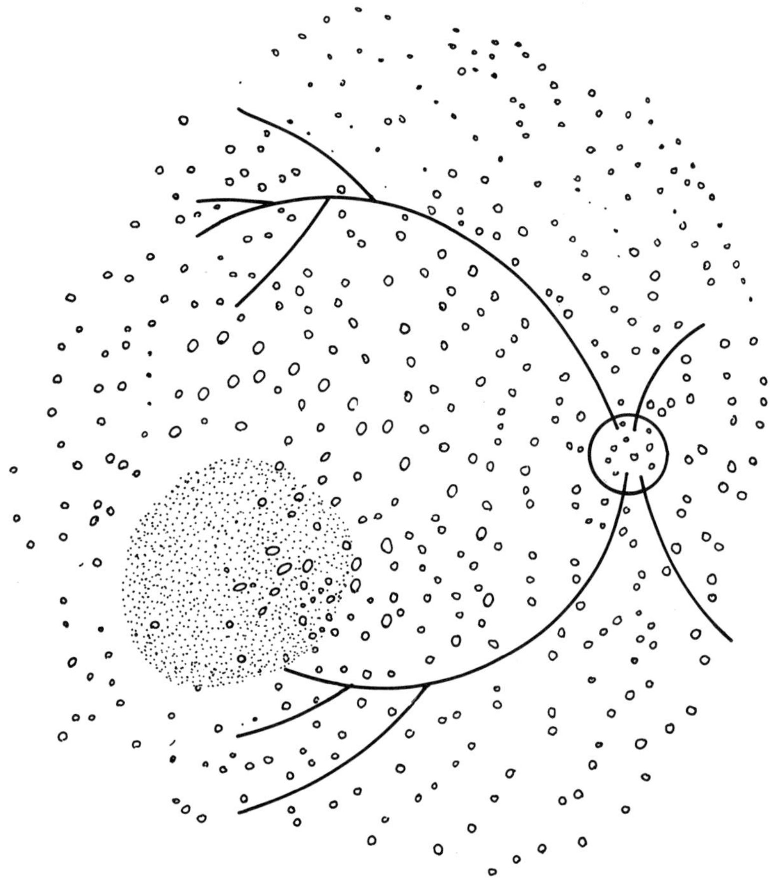

FIGURE 19–10

Group 5-B tumor according to the Reese-Ellsworth classification system.

Diagnosis

To confirm the diagnosis of retinoblastoma:

1. Computed tomography
2. Ultrasound
3. Magnetic resonance imaging

To ascertain if the tumor has metastasized:

1. Bone marrow aspiration from more than one site.
2. Lumbar puncture and cerebrospinal fluid analysis.

Genetic Counseling

Penetrance is the expression of the probability that an individual who inherits the mutation will indeed develop the tumor. The penetrance for the retinoblastoma gene is at least 80 percent.[6] Most

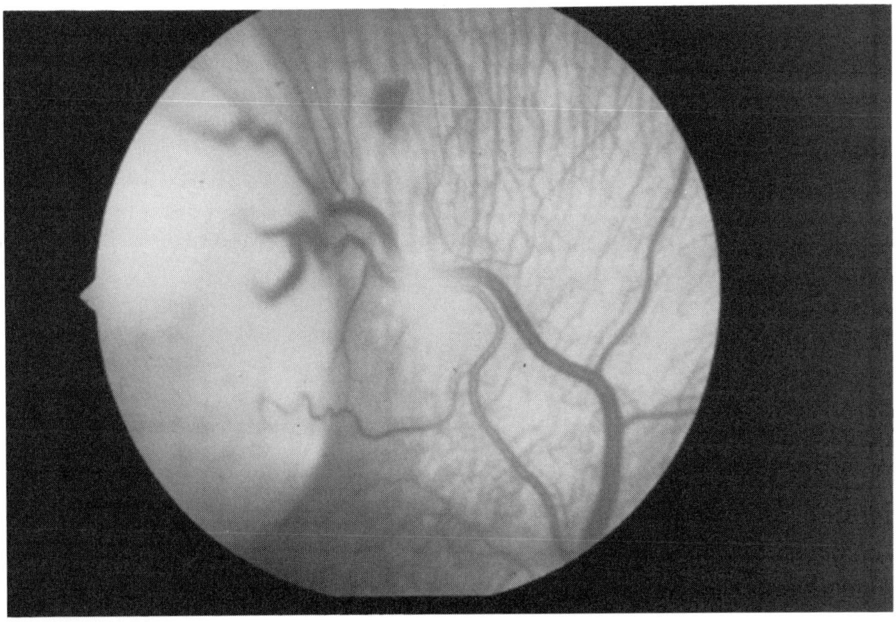

FIGURE 19-11

Retinoblastoma.

unilateral sporadic cases of retinoblastoma do not involve the germline and therefore are not hereditary. However, 10–15 percent of unilateral cases that develop tumors in only one eye are at risk and cannot be distinguished from the other unilateral cases. In the future, it will be possible, with the cloning of the retinoblastoma gene, to precisely identify the patient who carries the retinoblastoma gene and who is at risk for other malignant tumors.

Risk for Second Tumors

Patients with germline retinoblastoma mutation are genetically predisposed by their genotype to develop second malignancies: osteosarcoma, fibrosarcoma, and melanoma.[7]

Management

A multidisciplinary management team, including an ophthalmologist, oncologist, radiotherapist, and neuroradiologist, is now the routine. In the last 20 years, such a multidisciplinary approach occurs at ocular oncology centers where a concentration of this rare entity is seen. There are 200–300 new cases of retinblastoma seen each year in the United States.

Treatment

1. Enucleation: For eyes with no salvageable vision or when the optic nerve head cannot be seen.
2. Radiotherapy: External beam irradiation: Most common technique of salvaging the eye and vision (3500–4500 rads)
3. Cobalt plaque: If vitreous seeding is present, high radiation (35–40 Gy = 3500–4000 rads) to a local area. Very useful when local peripheral disease is too large or too extensive to treat with cryotherapy.
4. Cryotherapy: Local disease, anterior to the equator.
5. Photocoagulation: Small (less than 3–4 mm in diameter and 1–2 mm in thickness) posterior retinoblastomas, used relatively infrequently because of destruction of adjacent retina.

Retinal complications of above treatment modalities include retinal, choroidal, or vitreous hemorrhage, glial proliferation, posterior vitreous detachment, retinal detachment, and cataract.

DIFFERENTIAL DIAGNOSIS OF TUMORS

Phakomatoses ("mother-spot" in Greek) are a conglomeration of congenital retinal diseases with systemic manifestations.[8] Most but not all are hereditary in nature.

Ataxia Telangiectasia (Louis-Bar Syndrome)

Pathologically, the hamartoma site in ataxia telangiectasia is the capillaries. It is found in the cerebellum and conjunctiva.

Ataxia telangiectasia is autosomal recessive.

Clinical and pathognomonic findings are oculocutaneous and conjunctival telangiectasia and ocular motility disturbances.

Systemic findings are progressive cerebellar ataxia, dysarthria, drooling, dry, coarse skin and hair, rarely mental retardation.

Immunologic problems are deficiency of immunoglobulin A (IgA) thymus and lymph node abnormalities, prolonged skin homograft survival, recurrent infections usually sinopulmonary, decreased lymphocytes, and impaired lymphocyte transformation.

Associated malignancies are cerebellar or lymphoreticular malignancies, immunologic deficits, hypogammaglobulinemia, and infections.

Von Hippel-Lindau Disease (Retinocerebral Angiomatosis)

Pathologically, the site of hamartoma in von Hippel-Lindau disease is the blood vessels and stroma.[9] The site of involvement is the

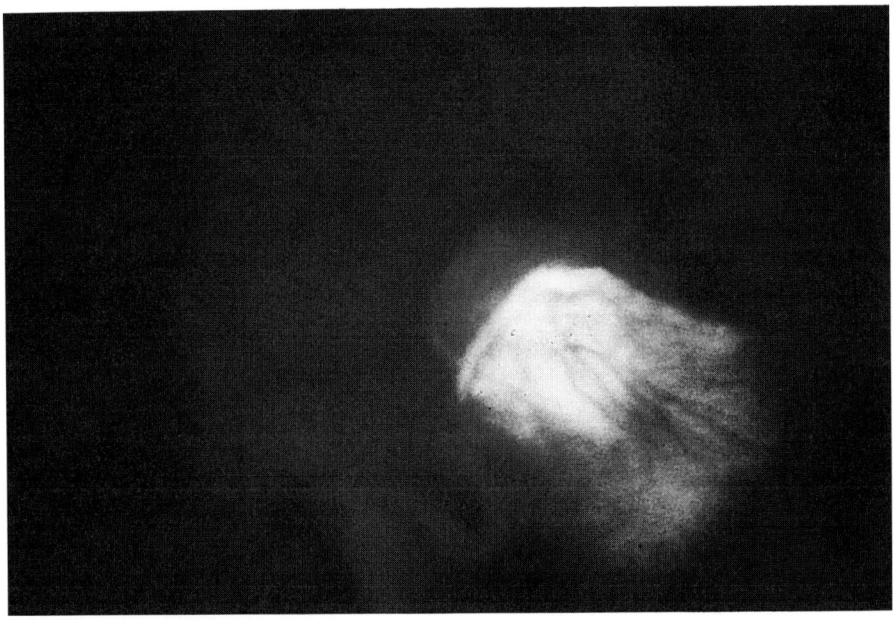

FIGURE 19–12

Retinocerebral angiomatosis.

retina, central nervous system, and the cerebellar system (Fig. 19–12). There are pancreas and kidney cysts. Infrequently, hypernephroma and pheochromocytoma occur.

When there is cerebellar involvement and medullar and spinal cord hemangioblastoma, the disease is called von Hippel-Lindau disease.

Von Hippel-Lindau disease is autosomal dominant and there is incomplete penetrance. The onset is early adulthood for ocular symptoms. The retinal hemangioblastoma can cause secondary hemorrhage and exudates from the abnormal blood vessels, then secondary retinal and chronic detachment, and consequently, rubeosis iridis and peripheral anterior synechiae. There are no associated systemic findings. Associated malignancies are cerebellar tumors and tumors of the central nervous system.

Tuberous Sclerosis

Pathologically, the hamartoma site in tuberous sclerosis is mixed glial tissue, found in the retina, brain, and viscera (Fig. 19–13).[8]

Tuberous sclerosis is autosomal dominant and usually occurs in persons younger than 20 years. It has the association with adenoma sebaceum. There is a white-ash leaf using Wood's light. There are giant drusen and the patient can present with "pseudopapilledema" of the optic nerve. The retina lesions are

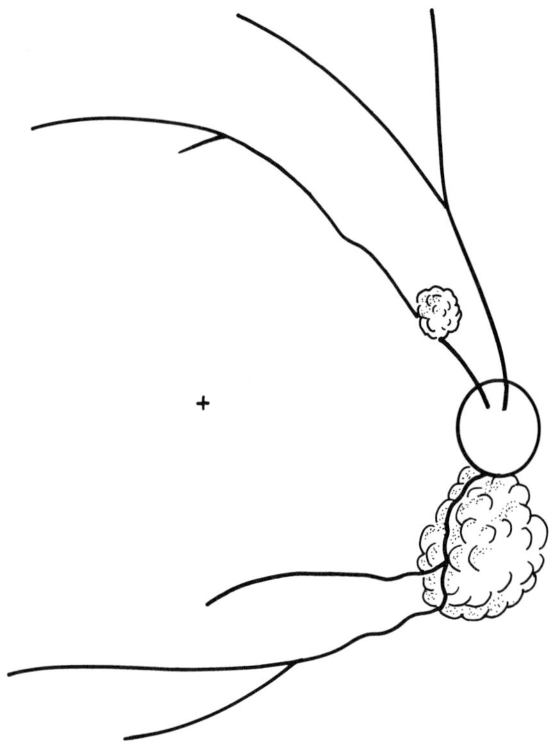

FIGURE 19–13
Tuberous sclerosis.

flat or raised. There are mulberry nodules (tapioca pudding lesions). Death occurs by 15 or 20 years of age.

Key systemic findings are severe mental retardation, seizures, and intracranial calcification of the third and fourth ventricles.

Associated malignancies are thyroid gland tumors, cardiac rhabdomyomas, and kidney and lung hamartomas.

OTHER PHAKOMATOSES

Neurofibromatosis

Pathologically, the hamartoma site in neurofibromatosis is the neural cell. The sites affected are the eye, gastrointestinal tract , and bone.[8] Neurofibromatosis is autosomal dominant and the onset of the disease occurs during puberty, pregnancy, and menopause. The skin findings are café au lait spots. Subcutaneous tumors are elephantiasis neurofibroma, fibroma molluscum, and plexiform neurofibroma. There is central nervous system involvement with gliomas of the cranial nerves I and II. Mental retardation also occurs.

Systemic involvement is bony hypertrophy, erosion lesions like osteitis fibrosa in the long and axial bones. Pheochromocytomas are rare. There are endocrinopathies and multiple congenital anomalies. There are also hamartomas of the gastrointestinal tract and other organs.

Key ocular findings are optic nerve gliomas, pulsating exophthalmos (absent greater wing of the sphenoid bone), and glaucoma. The eyelid shows plexiform neurofibromas, the orbit shows erosion of roof and wall. There are thickened nerves of the cornea or neurofibromas of the conjunctiva. There is associated mental retardation but no seizures.

Sturge-Weber Syndrome (Cutaneous Angiomatosis)

Pathologically, the site of hamartoma in Sturge-Weber syndrome is the cavernous hemangioma.[8] The eyelids, choroid, brain, and meninges are affected. The inheritance is unclear and the onset is usually congenital. The birthmark is a port-wine stain, often along the fifth cranial nerve. Glaucoma (the cause of glaucoma is thought to be faulty cleavage of the embryonic anterior chamber) and secondary retinal problems are found. Mental retardation is common. Seizures are common and intracranial calcification occurs in the meninges.

Eye findings include choroidal cavernous hemangioma, ipsilateral to facial nevus flammeus. Eyelids show cavernous hemangioma. The retina shows cavernous hemangioma of the choroid with associated microcystoid degeneration and subretinal serous fluid.

Arteriovenous Communication (Wyburn-Mason Syndrome)

Pathologically, the site of the hamartoma in arteriovenous malformation is the lack of capillaries.[8] The site affected is the retina and midbrain. The inheritance is possibly familial but unclear and the onset is early adulthood or adolescence. Clinical signs are pulsating exophthalmos, strabismus, gaze palsies, visual loss, retinal arteriovenous malformations, and facial nevi. There can be intracranial calcification.

Associated malignancies occur in the midbrain.

METASTASTIC DISEASE INVOLVING THE RETINA AND CHOROID

Metastatic choroidal lesions occur typically in the posterior pole. It is usually multifocal and bilateral. Visual acuity loss, visual field defects, and pain are the most common presenting complaints.[10]

For females, the most common metastatic tumor is the breast tumor, then bronchogenic and unknown primary tumors. In males, the most common are lung, unknown primary and kidney tumors and testicular, and prostate cancer.[10,11] Thus for females, the most common primary is breast cancer; in males, bronchogenic cancer.

Systemic Evaluation

Computed tomography scan of the brain is used to examine developing concurrent brain metastasis. Bone scan is used to look for lesions in the weight-bearing bones. A routine chest X-ray is also given.

Ophthalmic Examination

Dilated fundus examination is essential. Fluorescein angiography, although useful to detect tumor size, is not helpful in differentiating among other tumors. Metastic choroidal tumors hyperfluoresce early in the angiogram and become progressively hyperfluorescent in the late phases. Prominent early choroidal filling is seen in choroidal hemangiomas. Choroidal melanomas show a double circulation when these tumors have broken through Bruch's membrane.

Ultrasound

B-scan ultrasound shows the extent of the tumor, its width, depth, and height. The ultrasound can also vary in the presence of a retinal detachment in an eye where there is no view.

Treatment

Metastatic breast cancer is treated with radiotherapy or systemic therapy. During systemic therapy, a frequent observation is necessary to detect tumor progression or regression.[12,13]

For bronchogenic metastic disease, radiotherapy is usually used. In those instances where the choroidal metastasis is found before chemotherapy has been initiated, one can watch for a response. If no response, then the ocular tumor is usually treated with radiotherapy.

Ocular Toxicity or Complications of Radiation Therapy

Mild erythema is found. Ocular surface symptoms such as dry eye can be seen. Lacrilube ointment may be used as needed in those patients with dry eye.

Radiation Retinopathy

Radiation retinopathy usually occurs at 18 months to 2 years postradiation.[14] Radiation retinopathy manifests with dilated, tortuous vessels and with capillary telangiectasia as well as retinal neovascularization. Radiation cataract is also found.[15]

Congenital Hypertrophy of the Retinal Pigment Epithelium

These are focal nodular black subretinal lesions that extend anteriorly and usually through the thickness of the retina. There are no associated changes with the retinal pigment epithelium or retina. Usually vision is in the 20/20 or 20/25 range. Fluorescein angiography shows only some hyperfluorescence starting late in transit. Otherwise, these lesions are largely nonfluorescent.

Multiple and bilateral lesions of congenital hypertrophy of the retinal pigment epithelium have been associated with Gardner's syndrome.[16] Gardner's syndrome is an autosomal dominantly inherited disease characterized by intestinal polyposis.

Combined Hamartoma of the Retina and Retinal Pigment Epithelium

Combined hamartoma of the retina is seen in young adults with decreased vision at the level of 20/100 or better.[17] Dilated funduscopic examination reveals an ill-defined, slightly elevated partly pigmented tumor involving part of the optic nerve and adjacent retina. The tumor is composed of a fine granular distribution of pigment, giving it a gray appearance. There is usually a translucent membrane seen as well.

Fluorescein Angiography

In early transit, there is dilated, multiple, fine blood vessels within the tumor. In late transit, there is leakage of dye from these vessels.

UVEAL MELANOMA

See Chapter 20.

LEUKEMIA

The majority of patients with chronic leukemias have intraocular involvement at the time of death.[18,19]

Serous retinal detachment overlying choroidal infiltrates or choroidal masses have been seen.[18–21] Uveal infiltrates and intraretinal hemorrhages have also been observed. White-centered retinal hemorrhages are also seen. Vitreous hemorrhage is rare in this entity.

Vitreous infiltrates have been found in moribund patients.[22,23] The veins and arteries may develop a yellowish tinge because of the anemia,[19] and cotton wool spots.[24] Whole blood hyperviscosity may lead to venous occlusive disease, microaneurysm formation,[25,26] retinal hemorrhages,[27] and retinal neovascularization. Retinal neovascularization is associated with chronic myelogenous leukemia with peripheral capillary nonperfusion.[28–31]

LYMPHOMA

Retinal periphlebitis, vitritis, focal chorioretinitis, exudative retinal detachment, and necrotizing retinitis. It is thought that many of the previously published cases of Hodgkins lymphoma are really cases of viral retinitis.[32,33,34]

non-Hodgkins Lymphoma (Reticulum Cell Sarcoma)

In non-Hodgkins lymphoma retinal periphlebitis can be the initial presentation.[35–36] Retinal hemorrhages or cotton wool spots related to anemia or thrombocytopenia are common. Vitritis can also be present. In addition, in instances of longstanding uveitis of unknown etiology, reticulum cell sarcoma should be considered.

REFERENCES

1. Devesa SS: The incidence of retinoblastoma. Am J Ophthalmol 1975; *80:* 261–265
2. Pendergrass TW, Davis S: Incidence of retinoblastoma in the United States. Arch Ophthalmol 1980; *98:* 1204–1210
3. Haik BG, Siedlecki A, Ellsworth RM, Sturgis-Buckhout L: Documented delays in the diagnosis of retinoblastoma. Ann Ophthalmol 1985; *17:* 731–732
4. Abramson DH, Marks RF, Ellsworth RM et al: The management of unilateral retinoblastoma without primary enucleation. Arch Ophthalmol 1982; *100:* 1249–1252
5. Rubenfeld M, Abramson DH, Ellsworth RM, Kitchin FD: Unilateral vs bilateral retinoblastoma—correlations between age at diagnosis and stage of ocular disease. Ophthalmol 1986; *93:* 1016–1019
6. Rickman D, Murphree AL, Brecha N: Neurofilament immunoreactivity in retinoblastoma. Invest Ophthalmol Vis Sci 1987; *28:* 24
7. Abramson DH, Ellsworth RM, Kitchin FD, Tung G: Second nonocular tumors in retinoblastoma survivors—are they radiation induced? Ophthalmol 1984; *91:* 1351–1355
8. Font RL, Ferry AP: The phakomatoses. Int Ophthalmol Clin 1972; *12:* 1–50
9. Welch RB: Von Hippel-Lindau disease. The recognition and treatment of early angiomatosis retinae and the use of cryosurgery as an adjunct to therapy. Trans Am Ophthalmol Soc 1970; *68:* 367–424
10. Stephens RF, Shields JA: Diagnosis and management of cancer metastic to the uvea: a study of 70 cases. Ophthalmol 1979; *86:* 1336–1349

11. Ferry AP, Font RL: Carcinoma metastatic to the eye and orbit. I. A clinicopathological study of 227 cases. Arch Ophthalmol 1974; *92:* 276–286

12. Brinkley JR Jr: Response of a choroidal metastasis to multiple-drug chemotherapy. Cancer 1980; *45:* 1538–1539

13. Letson AD, Davidorf FH, Bruce RA Jr: Chemotherapy for treatment of choroidal metastases from breast carcinoma. Am J Ophthalmol 1982; *93:* 102–106

14. Brown GC, Shields JA, Sanborn G et al: Radiation retinopathy. Ophthalmol 1982; *89:* 1494–1501

15. Macfaul PA, Bedford MA: Ocular complications after therapeutic irradiation. Br J Ophthalmol 1970; *54:* 237–247

16. Blair NP, Trempe CL: Hypertrophy of the retinal pigment epithelium associated with Gardner's syndrome. Am J Ophthalmol 1980; *90:* 661–667

17. Gass JDM: An unusual hamartoma of the pigment epithelium and retina simulating choroidal melanoma and retinoblastoma. Trans Am Ophthalmol Soc 1973; *71:* 171–185

18. Kincaid MC, Green WR, Kelley JS: Acute ocular leukemia. Am J Ophthalmol 1979; *87:* 698–702

19. Kincaid MC, Green WR: Ocular and orbital involvement in leukemia. Surv Ophthalmol 1983; *27:* 211–232

20. Clayman HM, Flynn JT, Koch K, Israel C: Retinal pigment epithelial abnormalities in leukemic disease. Am J Ophthalmol 1972; *74:* 416–419

21. Rosenthal AR: Ocular manifestations of leukemia: a review. Ophthalmol 1983; *90:* 899–905

22. Swartz M, Schumann B: Acute leukemic infiltration of the vitreous diagnosed by pars plana aspiration. Am J Ophthalmol 1980; *90:* 326–330

23. Belmont JB, Michelson JB, Bordin GM: Ocular inflammation associated with chronic lymphocytic leukemia. J Ocul Ther Surg 1985; *4:* 125–129

24. Brown GC, Brown MM, Hiller T et al: Cotton wool spots. Retina 1985; *5:* 206–214

25. Duke JR, Wilkinson CP, Sigelman S: Retinal microaneurysms in leukemia. Br J Ophthalmol 1968; *52:* 368–374

26. Nelson CC, Hertzberg BS, Klintworth GK: A histopathologic study of 716 unselected eyes in patients with cancer at the time of death. Am J Ophthalmol 1983; *95:* 788–793

27. Mahneke A, Videbaek A: On changes in the optic fundus in leukemia: aetiology, diagnostic and prognostic role. Acta Ophthalmol 1964; *42:* 201–210

28. Frank RN, Ryan SJ Jr: Peripheral retinal neovascularization with chronic myelogenous leukemia. Arch Ophthalmol 1972; *87:* 585–589

29. Leveille AS, Morse PH: Platelet induced retinal neovascularization in leukemia. Am J Ophthalmol 1981; *91:* 640–643

30. Little HL: The role of abnormal hemorrheodynamics in the pathogenesis of diabetic retinopathy. Trans Am Ophthalmol Soc 1976; *74:* 573–636

31. Morse PH, McCready JL: Peripheral retinal neovascularization in chronic myelocytic leukemia. Am J Ophthalmol 1971; *72:* 975–978

32. Diddie KR, Schanzlin DJ, Mausolf FA et al: Necrotizing retinitis caused by opportunistic virus infection in patient with Hodgkin's disease. Am J Ophthalmol 1979; *88:* 668–673

33. Toy JL, Knowlden RP: Cytomegalovirus retinitis misdiagnosed as Hodgkin's lymphoma deposits. Br Med J 1978; *2:* 1398–1399

34. Barr CC, Joondeph HD: Retinal periphlebitis as the initial clinical finding in a patient with Hodgkin's disease. Retina 1983; *3:* 253–257

35. Freeman LN, Schachat AP, Knox DL et al: Clinical features, laboratory investigations and survival in ocular reticulum cell sarcoma. Ophthalmol 1987; *94:* 1631–1639

36. Brihaye-van Gerrtruyden M: Retinal lesions in Hodgkin's disease. Ann Ophthalmol 1956; *56:* 94–99

CHAPTER TWENTY

Choroidal Tumors

CHOROIDAL MELANOMA

Epidemiology

There are reported to be approximately 6 cases of choroidal melanoma per million per year.[1] Choroidal melanoma is the most common primary intraocular malignancy; it is the main primary intraocular disease that can be fatal in adults. The disease is most often diagnosed in the sixth decade of life. It is slightly more common in males.

Anatomy and Pathophysiology

Classically, the Callender classification consisted of six cell types: spindle A, spindle B, fascicular, epitheloid, mixed, and necrotic.[2]

Spindle A cells have small indistinct nucleoli and often have a prominent chromatin stripe, longitudinal fold in the nuclear membrane. Mitotic figures are uncommon.

Spindle B cells are slightly larger, with a larger nucleus and a single prominent round nucleolus. Mitotic figures are uncommon. When spindle B cells are arranged in cohesive units, seen on end, the nuclei are small and round. They appear as "fascicular."

Epitheloid cells are not cohesive, varying in cell, nuclear size, and shape. Nuclei are round with one or more prominent nucleoli. Mitotic figures are common.

There are recognized limitations of the Callender system: there are no histologic criteria to distinguish spindle A cell tumors from nevi. Second, there are no criteria for classification of a tumor composed of a mixture of spindle A and spindle B cells and no differentiation among the large group of tumors classified as mixed.

There is a 10-year mortality rate ranging from 11–19 percent in spindle A tumors, 21–36 percent in spindle B tumors, 63–79 percent in mixed cell tumors, and 72–100 percent in epitheloid tumors.[3–5]

Perhaps, the biggest problem is that the method involves the subjective evaluation of cell types and studies have shown that there may be variation among ophthalmic pathologists and laboratories.[6,7]

Clinical Course

Many patients with uveal melanomas present with retinal detachment. The exudative nature of the retinal detachment is not noted and the tumor is not seen. The typical presentation of a choroidal melanoma is a pigmented collar-button-shaped tumor, usually associated with an exudative retinal detachment (Fig. 20–1).

Small melanoma and large nevus can appear similar. A melanoma should be suspected if: (1) the thickness exceeds 3 mm, (2) orange pigment is seen over the tumor, (3) a serous detachment is present without drusen or choroidal neovascularization, and (4) fluorescein angiography shows multiple pinpoint subretinal leaks that progressively increase with late staining.

Fluorescein Angiography

Diagnostic accuracy of fluorescein angiography is limited.

Larger melanomas have an intrinsic tumor circulation, called "double circulation." Extensive leakage and hot spots are seen. The latter finding is due to point leaks in the retinal pigment epithelium

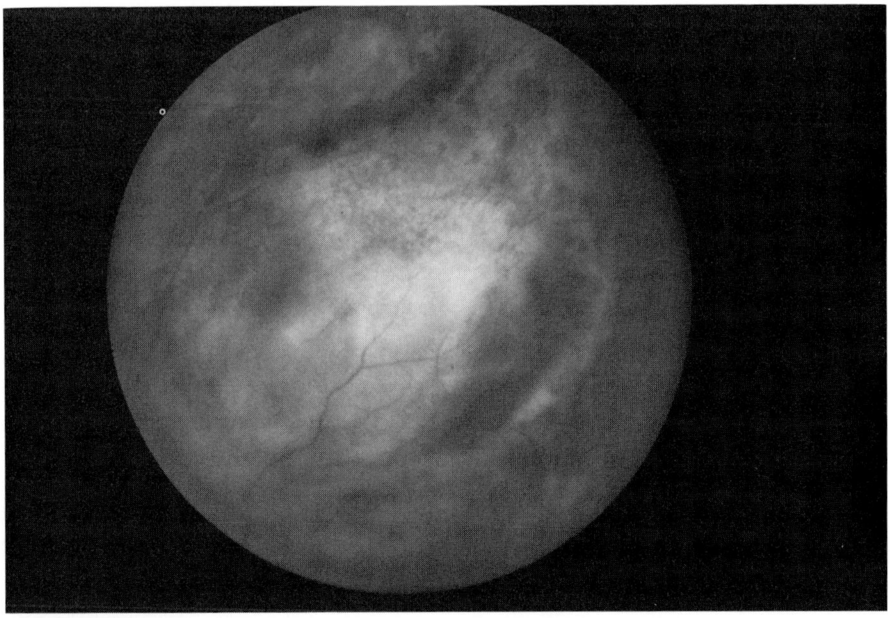

FIGURE 20–1

Malignant melanoma.

that stain late and show minimal enlargement during the course of the fluorescein angiogram.

Ultrasound

On B-scan, there is an acoustic quiet zone in the tumor, excavation of the choroid, and orbital shadowing. A quantitative A-scan shows medium-to-low reflectivity characteristics of melanoma.

Examination and Management

Examination with binocular indirect ophthalmoscopy is important in evaluating choroidal melanoma. In addition, gonioscopic examination for anterior extension of the tumor is necessary. In addition, during the Goldmann lens examination, the anterior mirror will reveal a view of the most anterior aspect of the retina as well.

It is during this examination that tumor size and extent are noted. Depending on the size, extent of the melanoma, and whether useful vision is present, treatment decisions can be made. Management techniques can be periodic observation, photocoagulation, radiotherapy, and enucleation.

Periodic observation is for small melanoma lesions of the posterior pole. Periodic fundus photographs and ultrasonography are used to document growth. Lesions less than 3 mm usually are not an immediate threat to the patient's survival.

Photocoagulation is a viable treatment modality for selected tumors that are less than 3 mm in thickness and that are located more than 3 mm from the fovea.

Radiotherapy is widely used for posterior uveal melanomas. The most commonly used isotopes are Co^{60}, Ru^{106}, Ir^{192}, I^{125}. The type of plaque chosen is usually coordinated with the radiation oncologist. Proton beam irradiation is also used for treatment. The type of radiotherapy available varies according to different ocular oncology centers in the country.

Enucleation is the traditional treatment, especially in cases where there is an advanced tumor which occupies most of the intraocular structure and produces secondary glaucoma.

Orbital exenteration is used in the rare instances of massive orbital extension in a blind, uncomfortable eye and in primary orbital extension.

Prognostic Factors

Extrascleral extension is a prognostic factor. The majority of patients with extrascleral extension die within 16 months after enucleation.[8]

Tumor size is another prognostic factor. Tumor size is defined as the largest tumor dimension, largest diameter in contact with the sclera, or a combination of largest diameter and height, area of the tumor base, and volume. Small tumors are those no larger than 10 mm in largest diameter and 2–3 mm in height. Medium size is considered to be no larger than 15 mm in diameter and 5 mm in height. The larger the tumor, the worse the survival rate.[8,9]

Location of anterior tumor margin is another prognostic factor. Ciliary body involvement is considered to be a poor prognostic sign. It is not clear why this is so, but perhaps the movement of the ciliary muscle causes the dislodging of tumor cells.[10]

Systemic Evaluation

Systemic evaluation is directed at frequent sites of metastatic involvement: liver, lung, bone, and subcutaneous tissues.[3,11]

Examination should include complete physical examination, with attention to skin and subcutaneous tissues, routine chest X-ray, and serum liver function studies (serum gamma-glutamyl transpeptidase, serum lactic dehydrogenase, serum glutamic-oxaloacetic transaminase).[12] If the liver function tests are abnormal, then an ultrasound or computed tomography scan of the liver is in order. Routinely, brain or hepatic imaging studies are not recommended. There are real risks of obtaining false positive results from imaging studies of the liver.[13]

DIFFERENTIAL DIAGNOSIS

Choroidal Hemangioma

Choroidal hemangioma is a rare, benign hamartoma. It occurs in two forms: discrete and diffuse. The latter is associated with the Sturge-Weber syndrome (see Chapter 19). The hemangioma is usually found posterior to the equator, temporal to the optic disc. Exudative retinal detachment can occur. Indistinct margins, dilated retinal or choroidal vessels can be seen contiguously. Macular changes can occur if there is an associated serous retinal detachment.

Fluorescein angiography shows irregular hyperfluorescence of the choroidal vessels within the tumor in the early, choroidal phase of the angiogram. In the arteriovenous phase of the angiogram, the fluorescence increases and the initial mottled pattern of fluorescence coalesces. In later transit, classically, there is multiloculated accumulation of the dye in the outer retina.

B-scan ultrasonography shows an elevated tumor with acoustic solidarity throughout the entire tumor. Choroidal excavation, a characteristic of choroidal melanoma, is not seen. On A-scan, there is high, consistent, internal reflectivity because of multiple vascular channels present throughout these tumors.

Light photocoagulation delivered in a scatter pattern has been found to be effective in treating these tumors that can cause a serous retinal detachment involving the fovea.[14]

Choroidal Nevus

Nevi are usually oval, flat, and nonelevated. They are sometimes slate gray with defined margins. They range in size from ⅓ disc diameter to several disc diameters. They are usually not more than 2 mm in thickness. Although very large nevi with elevations of 3 mm are hard to distinguish from small melanomas. However, the treatment can be periodic observation and fundus photos.

Drusen or retinal pigment epithelial changes are common.[15] However, large geographic areas of orange pigment may indicate malignant transformation of a suspicious nevus.[16] Serous detachments[17] and subretinal neovascularization rarely occur.[18]

Melanocytoma

Usually melanocytoma is jet black in color. Melanocytomas are found in the optic nerve area.

Metastatic Lesions to the Choroid

Metastases to the choroid rarely have intrinsic pigmentation although there can be overlying retinal pigment epithelial alterations. Frequently, multiple lesions are seen and are located in the posterior pole in the macular area.

Choroidal Osteoma

Choroidal osteomas are relatively flat lesions seen in young women. They occur in the area near the optic disc. They appear whitish and calcified, which can be documented on ultrasound.

COLLABORATIVE OCULAR MELANOMA STUDY

The Collaborative Ocular Melanoma Study was funded by the National Institute of Health in 1985 as a multicentered trial designed to evaluate treatments used to treat patients with choroidal melanoma. There is a medium tumor study: a randomized comparison of enucleation versus radiation with I^{125} plaques.

There is a large tumor study: a randomized comparison of standard enucleation versus enucleation preceded by external beam irradiation. The primary study outcome is survival. Secondary outcomes are years of metastasis-free survival, years of cancer-free survival, and years of useful vision. The results of these studies are still pending as of this writing.

REFERENCES

1. Scotto J, Fraumeni JF Jr, Lee JAH: Melanomas of the eye and other noncutaneous sites: epidemiologic aspects. JNCI 1976; *56:* 489–491

2. Callender GR: Malignant melanotic tumors of the eye: a study of histologic types in 111 cases. Trans Am Acad Ophthalmol Otolaryngol 1931; *36:* 131–142

3. Jensen OA: Malignant melanomas of the human uvea in Denmark, 1943–1952: a clinical histopathological and prognostic study. Acta Ophthalmol Suppl 1963; *75:* 1–220

4. Wilder HC, Paul EV: Malignant melanoma of the choroid and ciliary body: a study of 2535 cases. Mil Surg 1951: *109:* 370–378

5. Zimmerman LE, McLean IW, Foster WD: Does enucleation of the eye containing a malignant melanoma prevent or accelerate the dissemination of tumour cells. Br J Ophthalmol 1978; *62:* 420–425

6. Gamel JW, McLean IW: Quantitative analyses of the Callender classification of uveal melanoma cells. Arch Ophthalmol 1977; *95:* 686–691

7. Gass JDM: Problems in the differential diagnosis of choroidal nevi and malignant melanomas. Trans Am Acad Ophthalmol Otolaryngol 1977; *83:* 19–48

8. Shammas HF, Blodi FC: Prognostic factors in choroidal and ciliary body melanomas. Arch Ophthalmol 1977; *95:* 63–69

9. Jensen OA: Malignant melanomas of the human uvea: 25 year follow-up of cases in Denmark, 1943–1952. Acta Ophthalmol 1982; *60:* 161–182

10. McLean IW, Foster WD, Zimmerman LE: Prognostic factors in small malignant melanomas of choroid and ciliary body. Arch Ophthalmol 1977; *95:* 48–58

11. Char DH: Metastatic choroidal melanoma. Am J Ophthalmol 1978; *86:* 76–80

12. Murray JL, Lerner MP, Nordquist RE: Elevated gamma glutamyl transpeptidase levels in malignant melanoma. Cancer 1982; *49:* 1439–1443

13. Doiron MJ, Bernardino ME: A comparison of noninvasive imaging modalities in the melanoma patient. Cancer 1981; *47:* 2581–2584

14. Sanborn GE, Augsburger JJ, Shields JA: Treatment of circumscribed choroidal hemangiomas. Ophthalmol 1982: *89:* 1374–1380

15. Naumann G, Yanoff M, Zimmerman LE: Histogenesis of malignant melanomas of the uvea. I. Histopathologic characteristics of nevi of the choroid and ciliary body. Arch Ophthalmol 1966; *6:* 784–796

16. Smith LT, Irvine AR: Diagnostic significance of orange pigment accumulation over choroidal tumors. Mod Probl Ophthlmol 1974; *12:* 536–543

17. Pro M, Shields JA, Tomer TL: Serous detachment of the macula associated with presumed choroidal nevi. Arch Ophthalmol 1978; *96:* 1374–1377

18. Waltman DD, Gitter KA, Yannuzzi L, Schatz H: Choroidal neovascularization associated with choroidal nevi. Am J Ophthalmol 1978; *85:* 704–710

CHAPTER TWENTY-ONE

Choroidal Disorders

CHOROIDAL DETACHMENT

Choroidal detachment ensues when fluid collects between the uvea and the sclera. This accumulation of fluid has been recognized during surgery, early or late in the postoperative course.[1–5]

A special form of choroidal detachment may present suddenly with acute onset of intense pain, sudden blurring of vision, flat anterior chamber, and large "kissing" choroidals (Fig. 21–1).

Most choroidal detachments present as an episode of sharp ocular pain and prominent signs of ocular inflammation.

It is thought that intraocular hypotony precedes the accumulation of suprachoroidal fluid. The choroidal effusion results when there is a rapid transudation of fluid occurring across the capillary bed as a result of the pressure differential produced by hypotony and elevated episcleral venous pressure.[6]

Choroidal detachments can occur after scleral buckling surgery without drainage, usually in older patients with vortex vein compromise, cryotherapy, or diathermy.

Clinical Course

The patient presents with pain, shallow anterior chamber, and low-lying elevation of the peripheral retina. Ophthalmoscopically, the elevation can be shallow and between the peripheral retina and the equator.

Treatment

Clear corneal limbal paracentesis with blade directed at 6:00 meridian and reformation of anterior chamber is the form of treatment used. Radial posterior sclerotomies 4 mm from the limbus are performed. The sclerotomies are not sutured but the conjunctiva is closed with sutures.

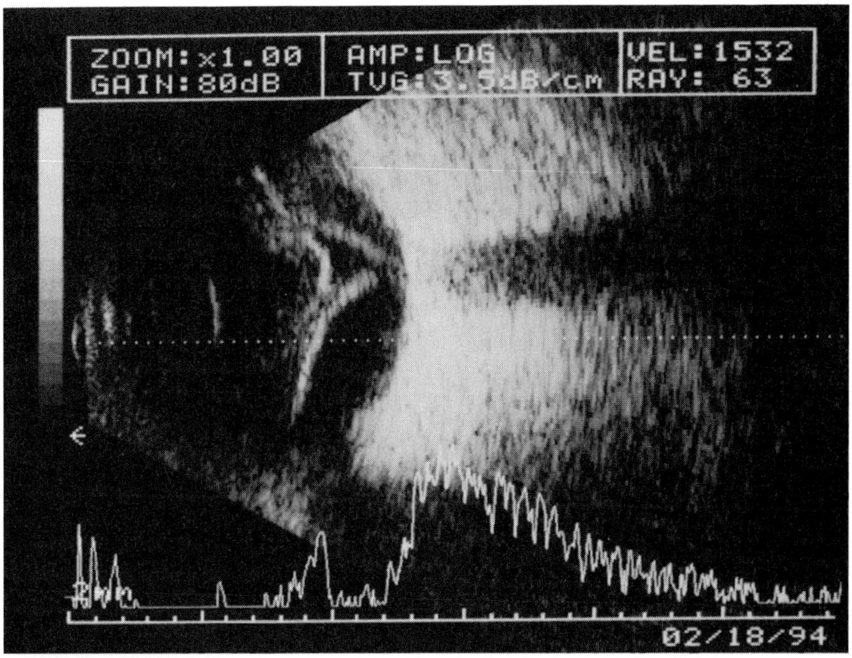

FIGURE 21-1

Ultrasound of "kissing" choroidals.

CHOROIDAL FOLDS

Anatomy and Pathophysiology

Choroidal folds are associated with those conditions that cause compression of the inner surface of the sclera, e.g., scleral thickening or shrinkage. Consequently, the inner portion of the choroid, Bruch's membrane, retinal pigment epithelium, and the outer retinal layers will be forming folds or buckling of the tissues.[7,8]

Clinically, acute choroidal folds cause disturbance in the visual acuity; however, longstanding idiopathic choroidal folds can have good visual acuity without symptoms.

Choroidal folds appear as alternating striae of orange and dark streaks that are seen most commonly in the posterior pole of the eye. These striae can also appear at a circumpapillar location.

Choroidal folds are seen in inflammation or uveitis, exophthalmos, Graves' disease, high hyperopia, hypotony, wound gape, tumor, choroidal osteoma, and rarely in age-related macular degeneration with subretinal blood. Choroidal folds can occur after scleral buckling and cataract surgery and surgery where there has been an episode of intraocular hypotony.

Fluorescein Angiography

Intense choroidal fluorescence occurs along the peaks of the choroidal and retinal pigment epithelial folds and produces a series of relatively hyperfluorescent streaks that are seen in the early arterial phase. The troughs of the folds are hypofluorescent, against a background of normal choroidal fluorescence.

In the folds are proliferative, metaplastic retinal pigment epithelial changes, drusen formation, and choroidal neovascularization.

Ultrasound

Ultrasound shows flattening or thickening of the posterior sclera and choroid in the areas of choroidal folds.

Treatment

The management of choroidal folds lies in finding and treating the cause. For example, after treatment for uveitis or postsurgical hypotony, there will be resolution of the fundus changes with a return of good vision.

UVEAL EFFUSION SYNDROME

Uveal effusion is a condition characterized by spontaneous serous detachment of the peripheral choroid and ciliary body in otherwise healthy middle-aged men.[9,10] Patients present with bullous nonrhegmatogenous retinal detachment that may precede ophthalmoscopic evidence of ciliochoroidal elevation.[11]

Nanophthalmos has been associated with this syndrome. Nanophthalmos is defined as between 14.5–20.5 mm (median 16.8 mm) and moderate to severe degrees of hyperopia.[12,13] Nanophthalmos is also associated with glaucoma and nonrhegmatogenous retinal detachment.

It is thought that there is a primary abnormality of the sclera such that there is a barrier to the transscleral outflow of protein from the suprachoroidal space and leads to vortex vein obstruction. An unusual picture of choroidal detachment ensues.

Pathology studies have shown that there is thickened sclera with increased glycosaminoglycanlike deposits between the scleral fibers.[14,15]

Drainage of the vortex veins is performed by surgically decompressing that part of the sclera that covers the exit of the vein. A scleral tunnel is made for an unroofing procedure or quadrantic lamellar sclerectomies and sclerostomies.[10,16]

There is resolution of the choroid detachment and subsequent return to good vision.

EXPULSIVE CHOROIDAL HEMORRHAGE

Sudden hemorrhage from the short posterior ciliary arteries from sudden lowering of intraocular pressure can cause an expulsive hemorrhage (see Chapter 26). A similar clinical setting can lead to a massive choroidal effusion. The treatment of expulsive choroidal hemorrhage is the same, i.e., rapid wound closure and posterior sclerotomies to decompress the eye. In the case of expulsive massive choroidal effusion, the visual prognosis is better than in expulsive choroidal hemorrhage.[1]

REFERENCES

1. Ruiz RS, Salmonsen PC: Expulsive choroidal effusion: a complication of intraocular surgery. Arch Ophthalmol 1976; *94:* 69–70

2. Girard LJ, Spak KE, Hawkins RS, Caldwell D: Expulsive hemorrhage during intraocular surgery. Trans Am Acad Ophthalmol Otolaryngol 1973; *77:* 119–125

3. Bellows AR, Chylack LT Jr, Epstein DL, Hutchinson BT: Choroidal effusion during glaucoma surgery in patients with prominent episcleral vessels. Arch Ophthalmol 1979; *97:* 493–497

4. Sawyers EM: Choroidal detachment immediately following cataract extraction. Arch Ophthalmol 1972; *88:* 632–634

5. McClure HL: Massive bilateral choroidal detachment occurring in an aphakic patient six years and nine months postoperatively. Am J Ophthalmol 1967; *63:* 295–297

6. Bellows AR, Chylack LT Jr, Hutchinson BT: Choroidal detachment. Clinical manifestation, therapy, mechanism of formation. Ophthalmol 1981; *88:* 1107–1115

7. Friberg TR: The etiology of choroidal fold. A biomechanical explanation. Graefes Arch Clin Exp Ophthalmol 1989; *227:* 459–464

8. Gass JDM: Stereoscopic Atlas of Macular Diseases, Diagnosis and Treatment. Vol. 1. St. Louis: The CV Mosby Co, 1987, p 222

9. Schepens CL, Brockhurst RJ: Uveal effusion: 1. Clinical picture. Arch Ophthalmol 1963; *70:* 189–201

10. Johnson MW, Gass JDM: Surgical management of the idiopathic uveal effusion syndrome. Ophthalmol 1990; *97:* 778–785

11. Gass JDM, Jallow S: Idiopathic serous detachment of the choroid, ciliary body, and retina (uveal effusion syndrome). Ophthalmol 1982; *89:* 1018–1032

12. Singh OS, Simmons RJ, Brockhurst RJ, Trempe CL: Nanophthalmos. A perspective on identification and therapy. Ophthalmology 1982; *89:* 1006–1010

13. Duke-Elder S: Normal and abnormal development. Congenital deformities. p. 488. In System of Ophthalmology. Vol. 3, pt 2. St Louis: The CV Mosby Co, 1964, pp 488–495

14. Trelstad RL, Silbermann NN, Brockhurst RJ: Nanophthalmic sclera. Ultrastructural, histochemical and biochemical observations. Arch Ophthalmol 1982; *100:* 1935–1938

15. Ward RC, Gragoudas ES, Pon DM, Albert DM: Abnormal scleral findings in uveal effusion syndrome. Am J Ophthalmol 1988; *106:* 139–146

16. Brockhurst RJ: Vortex vein decompression for nanophthalmic uveal effusion. Arch Ophthalmol 1989; *98:* 1987–1990

CHAPTER TWENTY-TWO

Vitreous Disorders

ANATOMY AND PHYSIOLOGY

The vitreous is a mesenchymal tissue that fills the posterior cavity of the eye, weighs 3.9 grams, and its volume is approximately 4.0 ml.[1] The water content is 98–99.7 percent. The density of the vitreous is 1.0053 and 1.0089.[2] The refractive index is 1.3345 and 1.3348 in man.[3,4] More than 90 percent of the visible light is transmitted through the normal vitreous in ultraviolet range. In phakic eyes, ultraviolet light is absorbed by the lens and little reaches the vitreous.

Embryologically, the vitreous develops in three stages: (1) primary or hyaloidal vitreous, (2) secondary or definitive vitreous, and (3) tertiary vitreous—zonule of Zinn. The primary vitreous forms when a space opens between the lens plate and the optic vesicle. In the fifth week (6.3 mm stage), vascularized mesoderm enters the optic fissure and in the sixth week, the hyaloid artery develops and reaches the posterior pole of the lens vesicle.

In the 11–12 mm stage, the embryonic cleft begins to close and secondary vitreous begins to appear at the margin of the retina. The secondary vitreous has finer network of filaments and fewer cells than the primary vitreous. The primary vitreous atrophies during this development.

By the seventh month, the hyaloid artery no longer carries blood and around the time of birth, it is reabsorbed. The embryonic remnant of the primary vitreous, called Cloquet's canal, is still visible during the first several decades of life.

The tertiary vitreous of the zonules begins to form in the fifth month (170 mm stage). However, the development of zonular fibers is not yet clearly understood.

Collagen and hyaluronic acid are the major structural molecules of the vitreous. In man, vitreous collagen is organized as thin fibrils 10–25 mm in diameter with cross striations.[5] These glycoproteins are the macromolecules or the "ground substance" of the vitreous.

There also exists low-molecular weight substances: sodium (Na), potassium (K), Chlorine (Cl), Calcium (Ca), phosphates and bicarbonate.[6]

Miscellaneous compounds are ascorbic acid, lactic acid, amino acids, lipids, oleate, linoleate, docosahexaenoate, palmitate, and stearate.[6]

AMYLOIDOSIS

Amyloidosis is the extracellular deposition of amyloid in various sites of the body. Amyloid has been found in the kidney, liver, heart, skin, gastrointestinal tract, nervous, endocrine, respiratory, hematopoietic systems, joints, and the eye.[7,8]

Vitreous opacities secondary to systemic amyloidosis were first recognized in 1953.[8] There can be opacities in the vitreous in one or both eyes. Bilateral involvement can be an early manifestation of the dominant form of familial amyloidosis, although rare cases of vitreous involvement in nonfamilial forms have been reported.[8–11]

Clinically, the patients are diagnosed late in the course of disease whereupon they may present with renal failure, dimentia, or arrhythmia and ophthalmic symptoms such as decreased lacrimation, vitreous veils, and internal ophthalmoplegia.[8–13]

The opacities appear anterior to retinal blood vessels. It has been described as a glass wool appearance.[13–14] When the vitreous opacity is visually significant, vitrectomy can be performed (Fig. 22–1).[12]

Pathologically, amyloidosis is a starlike structure with a dense, fibrillar center. The amyloid fibrils are 5–10 nm in diameter and are distinguished from the 10–15 nm vitreous fibrils when stained with amyloid stains.[15] The major amyloid component in immunocytologic studies is protein resembling prealbumin.[16]

ASTEROID HYALOSIS

The etiology of asteroid hyalosis is unclear. In general, asteroid hyalosis is a benign condition associated with small white or yellowish white spherical or disc-shaped opacities throughout the vitreous. Asteroid hyalosis is intimately associated with the vitreous gel and move with typical vitreous displacement during eye movements.

In 1921, Voerhoeff and more recent researchers thought this was due to calcium soaps.[17,18] In some studies, asteroid hyalosis has been found with higher incidence in diabetic patients than nondiabetic patients.[19–21]

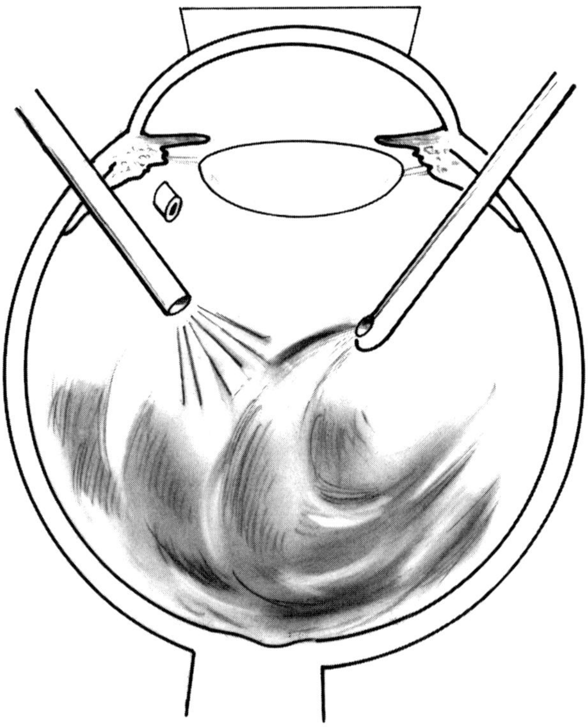

FIGURE 22–1
Diagram of a vitrectomy.

Clinically, the asteroid hyalosis may be very dense, but the patient will have 20/20 visual acuity. Ultrasound evaluation of the retina is sometimes necessary in very dense asteroid hyalosis.

Management

If the asteroid hyalosis is not visually disturbing, nothing needs to be done. Patients with dense asteroid hyalosis may have 20/20 vision. Vitrectomy in patients with asteroid hyalosis and diabetic traction retinal detachment is challenging because the view is compromised. In addition, the pars plana removal of the asteroid crystals can be difficult with the microvit because the calcium deposits dull the guillotine-cutting action.

TERSON'S SYNDROME

Terson's syndrome is the association of a vitreous hemorrhage with a subarachnoid hemorrhage. It is thought that the vitreous hemorrhage is caused by a sudden increase in venous pressure which ruptures epipapillary and peripapillary capillaries. This can occur in blunt or head trauma or with increased intracranial pressure.[22–27]

Visual acuity is in the 20/70 to count finger range. The dense vitreous hemorrhages need to be followed with serial ultrasounds and may need vitrectomy only if they do not resolve after 6 months to a year.[27]

The risk of visual loss is due to complications such as retinal holes and detachments, ghost cell glaucoma, and late cataract and late retinal detachments.

REFERENCES

1. Sebag J: Vitreous Structure. p. 1. In: The Vitreous. New York: Springer Verlag, 1989

2. Vissere-Heerema J: Ueber das spezifische Gewicht der bei der Operation bon Netz-hautablosungen gewonnenen Flussigkeit. Arch Augenheilk 1936; *109:* 543–561

3. Guggenheim I, Franceschetti A: Refraktometrische Untersuchungen des Glaskorpers bon Kaninichen und Mensch unter physiologischen und pathologischen Bedingungen. Arch Auenheilk 1928; *98:* 448–482

4. Paufique L, Fayet MT, Ravault M: Etude comparative du vitre humain normal et lyophilise. Ann Oculist 1959; *192:* 241–254

5. Snowden JM, Swann DA: Vitreous structure V. The morphology and thermal stability of vitreous coallagen fibers and comparison to articular cartilage (type II) collagen. Invest Ophthalmol Vis Sci 1980; *19:* 610–618

6. Sebag J: Biochemistry. p. 26. In: The Vitreous. New York: Springer Verlag, 1989

7. Cohen AS: Amyloidosis. p. 1417. In Wilson JD, Braunwald E, Isselbcher KJ, et al (eds): Harrison's Principles of Internal Medicine. 12th ed. New York: McGraw-Hill, Inc, 1991, pp 1417–1421

8. Kautarjian AD, DeJong RN: Familial primary amyloidosis with nervous system involvement. Neurology 1953; *3:* 399–409

9. Kaufman H: Primary familial amyloidosis. Arch Ophthalmol 1958; *60:* 1036–1043

10. Crawford JB: Cotton wool exudates in systemic amyloidosis. Arch Ophthalmol 1967; *78:* 214–216

11. Brownstein MH, Elliott R, Helwig EG: Ophthalmic aspects of amyloidosis. Am J Ophthalmol 1979; *69:* 423–430

12. Schwartz MF, Green WE, Michels RG et al: An unusual case of ocular involvement in primary systemic non-familial amyloidosis. Ophthalmol 1982; *89:* 394–401

13. Wong VG, McFarlin DE: Primary familial amyloidosis. Arch Ophthalmol 1967; *78:* 208–213

14. Spencer WH: Vitreous. p. 548. In Spencer WH (ed): Ophthalmic Pathology, An Atlas and Textbook. Philadelphia: WB Saunders, 1985

15. Streeten BA: Disorders of the Vitreous. p. 1381. In Garner A, GK Klintworth GK (eds): Pathobiology of Ocular Disease—a Dynamic Approach. Part B. New York: Marcel Decker, 1982

16. Sebag J: Pathobiology of the Vitreous. p. 142. In: The Vitreous. New York: Springer Verlag, 1989, p 142

17. Voerhoeff FH: Microscopic findings in case of asteroid hyalitis. Am J Ophthalmol 1921; *4:* 155–160

18. Rodman HI, Johnson FB, Zimmerman LH: New histopathological and histochemical observations concerning asteroid hyalitis. Arch Ophthalmol 1961; *66:* 552–560

19. Smith JL: Asteroid hyalitis—incidence of diabetes mellitus and hypercholesterolemia. JAMA 1958; *168:* 891–893

20. Bard LA: Asteroid hyalitis—relationship to diabetes and hypercholesterolemia. Am J Ophthalmol 1964; *58:* 239–242

21. Cockburn DM: Are vitreous asteroid bodies associated with diabetes mellitus? Am J Optom Physiol Opt 1985; *62:* 40–44

22. Terson A: De L'hemorrhage dans le corps vitre au cours de l'hemorrhage cerebrale. Clin Ophthalmol 1900; *6:* 309–315

23. Terson A: Le syndrome de l'hematome du corps vitre et de l'hemorrhagie intracranienne spontanes. Ann Ocul 1926; *163:* 666–673

24. Shaw HF, Landers MB, Sydnor CF: The significance of intraocular hemorrhages due to subarachnoid hemorrhage. Ann Ophthalmol 1977; *9:* 1403–1405

25. Khan SG, Frenkel M: Intravitreal hemorrhage associated with rapid increase in intracranial pressure (Terson's syndrome). Am J Ophthalmol 1975; *80:* 37–43

26. Shaw HF, Landers MB, Sydnor CF: Vitreous hemorrhages after intracranial hemorrhage. Am J Ophthalmol 1975; *80:* 207–213

27. Clarkson JG, Flynn HW Jr, Daily MJ: Vitrectomy in Terson's syndrome. Am J Ophthalmol 1980; *90:* 549–552

CHAPTER TWENTY-THREE

Retinal Detachment and Proliferative Vitreoretinopathy

RETINAL DETACHMENT

Epidemiology

The incidence of rhematogenous retinal detachment is 1/10,000 in the general population.[1] The prevalence of asymptomatic retinal holes in the general population is approximately 6 percent. The most common findings associated with a retinal detachment are lattice degeneration (40–55 percent), aphakia (30–40 percent), and direct ocular trauma (10 percent).

Pediatric detachments of the retina are rare. They comprise between 2.9 to 5.6 percent of all detachments.[2–4] They are usually associated with trauma, myopia, aphakia, and retinopathy of prematurity (in descending order of frequency).[2] The diagnosis of pediatric retinal detachments is made late because of the patient's failure to report symptoms. Consequently, one-half of the young patients present with total retinal detachments and one-third present with macular-off retinal detachments.

Aphakic and pseudophakic retinal detachments have approximately the same incidence; however, with the advent of extracapsular cataract surgery, the incidence is estimated to be 1.4 percent[5] to 3.6 percent.[6] After YAG laser capsulotomy, the incidence of retinal detachment is 1–3 percent.[7–10] With the current modern phacoemulsification techniques for cataract surgery, it is unclear about the future statistics for retinal detachment. In one series involving resident phacoemulsification cases, there is a 14.7 percent incidence of vitreous loss.[11]

Anatomy and Pathophysiology

Retinal detachments can be classified into four types: rhegmatogenous, traction, combined, and exudative.

1. Rhegmatogenous:
   This type of retinal detachment is due to a retinal break and the neurosensory retina separating from the retinal pigment epithelium with the potential space filling with fluid.
2. Traction:
   Tractional forces, such as a clot of blood inside the vitreous cavity which acts as a mechanical force serve to pull the retina from the pigment epithelium. This type of detachment is called a traction retinal detachment and occurs in patients with proliferative diabetic retinopathy, proliferative vitreoretinopathy, retinopathy of prematurity, and trauma where the presence of blood or scar tissue inside the vitreous cavity pulls the retina from the underlying pigment epithelium.
3. Combined rhegmatogenous and traction retinal detachment:
   There is both a retinal hole and a mechanical traction component in the retinal detachment.
4. Exudative:
   There is no retinal hole but there is the production of serous fluid under the retina such that the intact retina becomes detached from the pigment epithelium. The fluid can arise from existing neovascular membranes, leaking transudate, blood, or tumor growth. Inflammation of the choroid can cause leakage of serum proteins into the subretinal space. These detachments are usually due to diseases of the retinal pigment epithelium or the choroid.

Causes of exudative retinal detachments are as follows:

1. Harada's disease
2. Posterior scleritis
3. Collagen-vascular disease
4. Malignant hypertension
5. Toxemia in pregnancy
6. Malignant melanoma
7. Choroidal hemangioma
8. Metastatic lesions of the choroid
9. Central serous choroidopathy
10. Coats disease
11. Angiomatosis retinae

12. Idiopathic uveal effusion
13. Age-related macular degeneration: subretinal membranes that cause serous and hemorrhagic retinal detachments
14. Presumed ocular histoplasmosis syndrome

Classification of Retinal Breaks

1. Horseshoe-shaped retinal tear: Part of the vitreous is attached to one part of the retina, the flap of the horseshoe tear, pulling against the rest of the retina which is secured in place by the vitreous base. The opposing forces cause the separation of the retina from the retinal pigment epithelium. A retinal hole or tear ensues.
2. Lattice degeneration with or without holes: Retinal thinning occurs at these points of lattice degeneration. Holes can occur in the degenerative process. Vitreous traction can occur at this compromised area at times of trauma, intraocular surgery, and vigorous high-impact sports.
3. Aphakic or pseudophakic retinal holes: Usually these occur at the far periphery, near the ora serrata. They are usually round, small, difficult to see when an intraocular lens implant is in place. However, in eyes with total retinal detachments or where the detachment involves the superior 180 degrees, the holes are usually at or near 12:00.[12] Often, the surgeon must look intraoperatively and use cryotherapy to confirm suspicious areas of retinal holes.
4. Associated Conditions:
    1. Posterior vitreous detachment: In symptomatic patients with a posterior vitreous detachment, there is a 10.7–15.1 percent incidence of retinal holes.[13–16] As the vitreous becomes syneretic or changes its shape, the shearing forces can cause a retinal hole.[17]
    2. Myopia is associated with an increased incidence of retinal holes and detachment.[18–22] Severe myopia or pathologic myopia has a higher incidence of retinal detachments. The retina is thinned and attenuated over certain areas, that over time, there arises a retinal break. The retinal breaks can occur posteriorly near the vortex veins or anteriorly near areas of extensive lattice degeneration.
    3. Penetrating and blunt trauma are associated with retinal detachment due to the direct damage to the retina.[23,24]

PROLIFERATIVE VITREORETINOPATHY

Proliferative vitreoretinopathy is a feared complication of a rhegmatogenous retinal detachment. Five to 10 percent of all rhegmatogenous retinal detachments have proliferative vitreoretinopathy as its main complication.[25] Reattachment for these cases range from 14 percent to 84 percent.

In cases of proliferative vitreoretinopathy, where there is scar tissue on the retina, it is crucial to localize all of the retinal breaks and the areas of epiretinal membrane formation. Epiretinal membranes are scars or bands or sheets of tissue adherent to the surface of the retina causing mechanical traction. To reattach the retina, the surgeon aims to close all of the holes and remove all of the membranes. All of the modern surgical techniques have been aimed at these two goals (Fig. 23–1).

The grading scheme of proliferative vitreoretinopathy provides the ophthalmologist with an idea of the visual prognosis. Grades C-3 to D of proliferative vitreoretinopathy have the worst prognosis for vision and reattachment.

The Retina Society Classification for Proliferative Vitreoretinopathy

The Retina Society classifies retinal detachment with proliferative vitreoretinography as follows:[25]

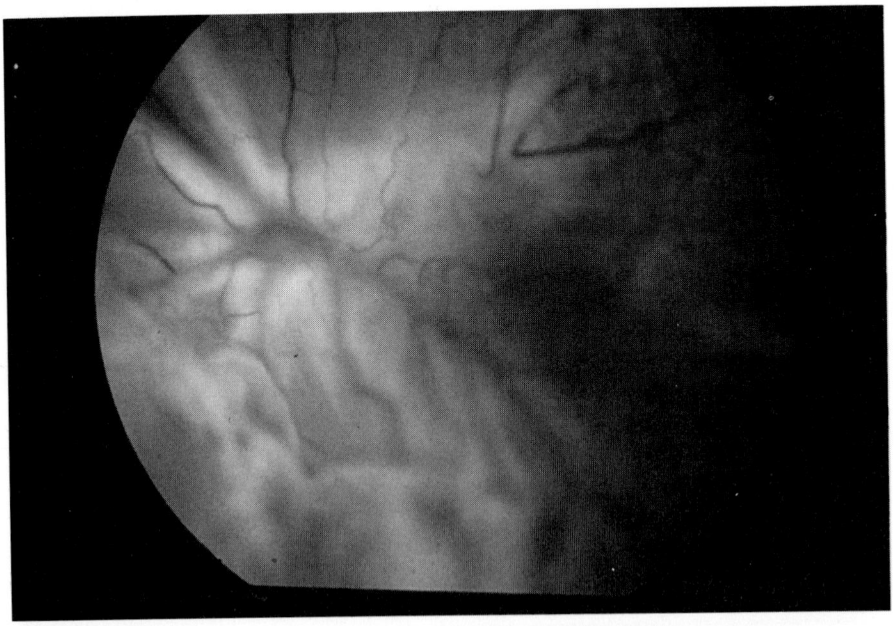

FIGURE 23–1

Proliferative vitreoretinopathy, grade D (Courtesy of Dr. Lory Snady-McCoy, Providence, Rhode Island).

Grade A: Minimal proliferative vitreoretinography; pigment clumps

Grade B: Moderate; surface wrinkling of inner retinal surface, rolled edge of a retinal break, retinal stiffness, vessel tortuosity.

Grade C: Marked; Full-thickness retinal folds

C-1: One quadrant

C-2: Two quadrants

C-3: Three quadrants

Grade D: Massive: Fixed retinal folds in four quadrants

D-1: Wide funnel shape

D-2: Narrow funnel shape

D-3: Closed funnel, optic nerve head not visible

Anterior Proliferative Vitreoretinopathy

A subtype of proliferative vitreoretinopathy is anterior proliferative vitreoretinopathy. This condition occurs anterior to the equator, usually occurring in eyes having proliferative vitreoretinopathy in the posterior pole. In addition, having membranes occurring behind the ciliary body, affects the ciliary processes and the ora serrata region.[26–29] These membranes are both preretinal and subretinal in nature causing traction of the retina and folds of the retina at the anterior aspect of the globe. Anterior proliferative vitreoretinopathy occurs in previously vitrectomized eyes where anterior vitreous surgery was inadequate.

Examination Techniques

The main principle is to find the retinal holes.

1. Indirect ophthalmoscopy: Lie the patient down. The examiner can be seated on a stool or standing so that there is proper viewing of 360 degrees of the retina. Perform scleral depression to look for pathology at the ora serrata.
2. Goldmann three-mirror examination to look for additional holes. At the same time, keep the following questions in mind:
    a. Is there pigment dust in the anterior chamber?—Schafer's sign.
    b. Is there pigment dust suggesting a longstanding retinal detachment or the early signs of proliferative vitreoretinography? (Grade A).
    c. Is there some white gliosis along the vessels? (Grade B)
    d. Is there shifting fluid? Think of exudative retinal detachment.
3. Vitreous examination with the Goldmann or 60 diopter

lenses at the slit lamp to evaluate the nature of the vitreous: Is it syneretic, is it gel-like?

4. Examine the macula: Look for degenerative changes, cystoid changes suggesting an older detachment. Use a 60 diopter, 78 diopter or 90 diopter or Hruby or Goldmann lenses.
5. Is there shifting fluid and no retinal hole? Think exudative retinal detachment.
6. Is there a localized area of retinal detachment but it does not extend to the ora serrata? Think of retinoschisis.

Surgical Management

The most important goal of rhegmatogenous retinal detachment surgery is to identify the retinal break(s) and then localize appropriately so as to support the retinal break on the scleral buckle. The next goal is to have the retina reattached before the patient leaves the operating room. This is usually accomplished by drainage of subretinal fluid. However, in some instances of nondrainage, the fluid can be left and during the postoperative period of observation, the fluid will naturally absorb and the retina will be reattached within 24–48 hours of the surgery.

In traction retinal detachment, the goal is to remove the traction intraoperatively. This can be done with pars plana vitrectomy techniques where the epiretinal membranes are removed under direct visualization with microinstruments. In cases where membrane dissection is difficult, surgeons have devised other modalities to aid in their surgery. Silicone oil and perfluorocarbon gas and liquids are used for the purpose of reattaching the retina with proliferative vitreoretinopathy.[30–34] Silicone oil and perfluorocarbon liquids have enabled surgeons to dissect preretinal membranes under direct visualization while the retina is stabilized by the intraoperative vitreous substitute. If perfluorocarbon liquid is used, it is usually removed at the end of the procedure and replaced by gas or silicone oil. If silicone oil is used, it is left in place for several weeks or even months for the retina to be stabilized before it is ever removed. In eyes with longstanding silicone oil, there have been corneal complications that necessitate the removal of the oil and corneal transplant procedures.

Gas tamponade has been a useful adjunct in the reattachment of the retina in severe cases of proliferative vitreoretinography.[35–38] With an intraocular gas bubble in place, the bubble flattens the retina by providing internal tamponade. If the gas bubble is larger than the retinal break, it prevents fluid from passing through the retinal break. Thus, the subretinal fluid can be reabsorbed through the retinal pigment epithelium and choroid.

Gas also prevents the recurrence of vitreous hemorrhage, which would, in turn, create the mechanical traction forces on the retina and again cause a new tractional detachment.

Following vitreous surgery, a gas bubble allows visualization of the retina in occasions of vitreous rebleeding. In addition, the gas bubble allows the retina surgeon to perform additional laser photocoagulation in the postoperative period if necessary.

Pneumatic Retinopexy

Pneumatic retinopexy has been used as a method of outpatient retinal detachment repair when there is a small localized retinal detachment in the superior 180 degrees of the retina, the retinal holes do not exceed more than one clock hour in size.[39] The surgeon localizes the retinal hole, performs cryopexy, and paracentesis by injecting a nonexpanding mixture of gas, usually perfluoropropane, C3F8 or SF6.

Postoperatively, patient positioning plays a key role in the success of the procedure. With physician instructions, the patient must either be face down or position the gas bubble such that it covers the hole, according to the specific anatomy of his/her case.

Indications

The patient has a small retinal detachment as described above and wants to have such a procedure as an outpatient. It is most commonly used in patients who medically cannot tolerate general anesthesia or who are very infirm and elderly where an outpatient procedure will suffice. It has been used with excellent success in motivated young, or middle-aged, healthy individuals who want to avoid surgery.

This technique is generally not used for multiple holes or holes in the inferior 180 degrees of the retina. It is not useful in cases with proliferative vitreoretinopathy or where the amount of subretinal fluid is massive, despite there being only one retinal hole or retinal tear.

Other contraindications are narrow or closed angles seen gonioscopically, cataract which precludes view of the retinal hole, and the patient's inability to be positioned in prone position secondary to neck or cervical disease.

The success rate of pneumatic retinopexy is approximately 85–90 percent,[39] whereas standard scleral buckle surgery is approximately the same.

Complications include additional retinal holes, proliferative vitreoretinopathy, macular pucker, vitreous floaters, uveitis, and subretinal pigment deposition. Surgery can be performed for these complications.

REFERENCES

1. Ashrafzadeh MT, Schepens CL, Elzeneneiny II et al: Aphakic and phakic retinal detachment I. Preoperative findings. Arch Ophthalmol 1973; *89:* 476–483

2. Winslow RL, Tasman W: Juvenile rhegmatogenous retinal detachment. Trans Am Acad Ophthalmol Otolaryngol 1978; *85:* 607–618

3. Tasman W: Retinal detachment in children. Trans Am Acad Ophthalmol Otolaryngol 1967; *71:* 455–459

4. Hilton GF, Norton EWD: Juvenile retinal detachment. Mod Probl Ophthalmol 1969; *8:* 325–341

5. Coonan P, Fung WE, Webster RG Jr et al: The incidence of retinal detachment following extracapsular cataract extraction: a ten-year study. Ophthalmol 1985; *92:* 1096–1101

6. Wilkinson CP, Anderson LS, Little JH: Retinal detachment following phacoemulsification. Ophthalmol 1978; *85:* 151–156

7. Van Westenbrugg JA, Gimbel HV, Souchek J, Chow D: Incidence of retinal detachment following Nd YAG capsulotomy after cataract surgery. J Cat Refract Surg 1992; *18:* 352–355

8. Smith PW, Stark WJ, Maumenee AE et al: Retinal detachment after extracapsular cataract extraction with posterior chamber intraocular lens. Ophthalmol 1987; *94:* 495–504

9. Dardenne M-U, Gerten GJ, Kokkas K, Kermani O: Retrospective study of retinal detachment following neodymium: YAG laser posterior capsulotomy. J Cat Refract Surg 1989; *15:* 676–680

10. Rickmann-Barger L, Florine CW, Larson RS, Lindstrom RL: Retinal detachment after neodymium: YAG laser posterior capsulotomy. Am J Ophthalmol 1989; *107:* 531–536

11. Allinson RW, Metrikin, Fante RC: Incidence of vitreous loss among third year residents performing phacoemulsification. Ophthalmol 1992; *99:* 726–730

12. Lincoff H, Gieser R: Finding the retinal hole. Arch Ophthalmol 1971; *85:* 565–569

13. Foos RY: Posterior vitreous detachment. Trans Am Acad Ophthalmol Otolaryngol 1972; *76:* 480–497

14. Linder B: Acute posterior vitreous detachment and its retinal complications. A clinical biomicroscopic study. Acta Ophthalmol 1966; *87:* (suppl.) 65–68

15. Jaffe NS: Complications of acute posterior vitreous detachment. Arch Ophthalmol 1968; *79:* 569–571

16. Tasman W: Posterior vitreous detachment and peripheral retinal breaks. Trans Am Acad Ophthalmol Otolaryngol 1968; *72:* 217–224

17. Schepens CL: Vitreous Changes in Retinal Detachment. p. 88. In Schepens CL, Neetens (eds): The Vitreous and Vitreoretinal Interface. New York: Springer Verlag, 1987; pp 88-90

18. Curtin BJ: Physiologic vs pathologic myopia: genetics vs environment. Ophthalmol 1979; *86:* 681–691

19. Curtin BJ, Iwamoto T, Renaldo DP: Normal and staphylomatous sclera of high myopia: an electron microscopic study. Arch Ophthalmol 1979; *97:* 912–915

20. Curtin BJ, Karlin DB: Axial length measurements and fundus changes of the myopic eye. Am J Ophthalmol 1971; *71:* 42–53

21. Curtin BJ: The pathogenesis of congenital myopia: a study of 66 cases. Arch Ophthalmol 1963; *69:* 166–173

22. Curtin BJ: The posterior staphyloma of pathologic myopia. Trans Am Acad Ophthalmol Soc 1977; *75:* 67–86

23. Freeman HM, Cox MS, Schepens CL: Traumatic retinal detachments. Int Ophthalmol Clin 1974; *14:* 151–170

24. Delori F, Pomerantzeff O, Cox MS: Deformation of the globe under high speed impact; its relation to contusion injuries. Invest Ophthalmol 1969; *8:* 290–301

25. The Retina Society Terminology Commitee: The classification of retinal detachment with proliferative vitreoretinopathy. Ophthalmol 1983; *90:* 121–125

26. Elner SG, Elner VM, Diaz-Rohena R et al: Anterior proliferative vitreoretinopathy. Clinicopathologic, light microscopic and ultrastructural findings. Ophthalmol 1988; *95:* 1349–1357

27. Elner SG, Elner VM, Freeman HM et al: The pathology of anterior (peripheral) proliferative vitreoretinopathy. Trans Am Ophthalmol Soc 1989; *86:* 330–351

28. Lewis H, Aaberg TM: Anterior proliferative vitreoretinopathy. Am J Ophthalmol 1988; *105:* 277–284

29. Aaberg TM: The management of anterior and posterior proliferative vitreoretinoapthy. XLV. Edward Jackson Memorial Lecture. Am J Ophthalmol 1988; *106:* 519–532

30. Scott JD: The treatment of massive vitreous retraction by the separation of pre-retinal membranes using liquid silicone. Mod Probl Ophthalmol 1975; *15:* 285–290

31. Grey RHB, Leaver PK: Silicone oil in the treatment of massive preretinal retraction: I. Results in 105 eyes. Br J Ophthalmol 1979; *63:* 355–360

32. Chang S, Ozmert E, Zimmerman NJ: Intraoperative perfluorocarbon liquids in the management of PVR. Am J Ophthalmol 1988; *106:* 668–674

33. Chang S, Lincoff H, Zimmerman NJ, Fuchs W: Giant retinal tears: surgical techniques and results using perfluorocarbon liquids. Arch Ophthalmol 1989; *107:* 761–766

34. Chang S, Reppucci V, Zimmerman NJ et al: Perfluorocarbon liquids in the management of traumatic retinal detachments. Ophthalmol 1989; *96:* 785–791

35. Lincoff H, Mardirossian J, Lincoff A: Intravitreal longevity of three perfluorocarbon gases. Arch Ophthalmol 1980; *98:* 1610–1611

36. Lincoff H, Coleman DJ, Kreissig I et al: The perfluorocarbon gases in the treatment of retinal detachment. Ophthalmol 1983; *90:* 546–551

37. Lincoff H, Kreissig I, Coleman DJ, Chang S: Use of an intraocular gas tamponade to find retinal breaks. Am J Ophthalmol 1983; *96:* 510–516

38. Lincoff H, Maisel JM, Lincoff A: Intravitreal disappearance rates of four perfluorocarbon gases. Arch Ophthalmol 1984; *102:* 928–929

39. Hilton GF, Grizzard WS: Pneumatic retinopexy: a two-step outpatient operation without conjunctival incision. Ophthalmol 1986; *93:* 626–641

CHAPTER TWENTY-FOUR

Nonpenetrating Trauma

Nonpenetrating trauma includes all injuries to the globe by blunt or direct force. The mechanism of action can occur in automobile accidents, work-related accidents, and sports-related injuries. Ocular trauma is the second common cause of visual loss after cataracts in the United States. There are approximately 2.4 million ocular injuries each year.[1]

CLINICAL COURSE

In nonpenetrating trauma, hyphema or anterior chamber bleeding is commonly seen. Usually, it is the iris root vessels that are the cause of bleeding. The patient presents with a mild decrease in visual acuity. There is a small amount of red blood cells layered in the six o'clock position. The hyphema may hide the traumatic iritis present. Cells and flare may be seen on careful slit-lamp examination.

A more serious hyphema can lead to corneal blood staining, ghost cell glaucoma secondary to blocked outflow from erythrocytes clogging the trabecular meshwork, chronic open-angle glaucoma from angle recession at the time of the blunt injury, or peripheral anterior synechiae formation. Rarely, central retinal artery occlusion can occur from elevated intraocular pressure.[2] These complications can occur 2–3 days after injury. A mild or small hyphema will resolve without long-term visual acuity impairment.

DIAGNOSIS

Initial examination entails careful history, description of the trauma to the eye, and the direction of the possible force towards the globe: anteroposterior or laterally. A contrecoup action involves the reverberation of the eye's inner contents and is more likely to cause a retinal detachment.

Visual acuity examination, intraocular pressure, gonioscopy to view for angle recession to verify the nature of the nonpenetrating injury, and absence of an intraocular foreign body. By slit-lamp biomicroscopy, the examiner needs to carefully evaluate the cornea and the anterior chamber, taking care to note the percentage of hyphema that is present. For example, if the layering of blood is one-third of the anterior chamber, a notation of 33 percent is helpful to follow daily progress in the medical chart.

Examination of the lens for cataract, blood, or fibrin is also necessary. Blood or fibrin on the lens leads to later cataract formation. In addition, the fibrin on the lens will lead to more aggressive topical steroid therapy.

Determination of the retinal status is important. When the view is obscured by anterior chamber blood, it is important to perform ultrasonography to ascertain the integrity of the retina.

MANAGEMENT

Daily management consists of atropine for cycloplegia, daily checking of visual acuity, corneal changes, and intraocular pressure. Rebleeding is a common complication of hyphema.[3] Recent studies have shown the usefulness of epsilon aminocaproic acid in reducing every 4 hours, up to 30 g/day, has led to the development of nausea, vomiting, dizziness, and postural hypotension in patients. A smaller dose of 50 mg/kg every 4 hrs for 5 days has decreased the side effects with similar effect on rebleeding.[7] Bedrest and corticosteroids have not been shown to definitively decrease the rate of rebleeding.[8] Usually hyphema treatment is directed at controlling the temporary elevation in intraocular pressure; however, when corneal staining occurs, consideration is then placed on the surgical removal of the anterior chamber hemorrhage.

Surgical removal of the blood can be accomplished with the irrigation-aspiration technique using two ports: in the first port, a butterfly needle infuses the saline into the anterior chamber and in the other port, at the limbus, the microvitreous cutter removes the blood by aspiration and cutting. Once the blood is removed, the infusion sites are then closed with 10-0 nylon suture, with the knot buried in the incision. The removal of the clot can also be accomplished through a trabeculectomy incision.[9]

COMMOTIO RETINAE

Commotio retinae or Berlin's edema is commonly seen following a contusive injury to the globe. The etiology of this entity is controversial. It is thought that the vitreous and retina interface undergoes trauma that causes subsequent extracellular edema[10] or glial swelling and photoreceptor cell damage.[11–13]

While vision can be decreased at initial presentation, visual acuity will return to normal in most cases within 4–6 weeks. On indirect ophthalmoscopy, there is a retinal whitening around the indirect ophthalmoscopy, and around the macula. The affected area can also appear at other parts of the posterior pole. However, the macula can develop atrophy with hyperpigmentation or macular cysts after such trauma (Fig. 24–1).

Examination

The commotio retinae is discernible with indirect ophthalmoscopy. Thorough evaluation of the vitreous with 60 diopter or Hruby lenses is useful in defining the vitreoretinal interface.

Management

Periodic monitoring for retinal hole formation or cystoid macular edema is necessary for patient care. This condition is usually self-limited and no treatment is necessary.

CHOROIDAL RUPTURE

A choroidal rupture is a tear in the choroid, Bruch's membrane, and retinal pigment epithelium.[14] Choroidal ruptures can occur at the

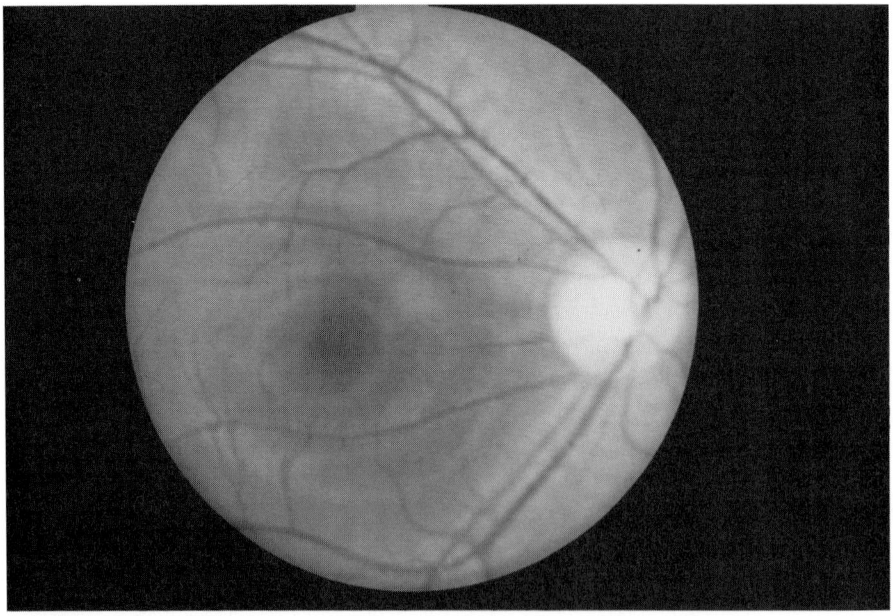

FIGURE 24–1

Berlin's edema in a 16-year-old male after being hit in the eye with a basketball.

ora serrata when the blunt trauma is directed in the anterior and lateral aspects of the globe. Posterior injuries can occur at the optic nerve, crescentic and oriented around the optic nerve. Subretinal, preretinal, or intraretinal hemorrhages may obscure the choroidal rupture.

The patient usually presents with decreased vision or a central scotoma if the macula is involved. This is most likely when the trauma is directly to the globe in the frontal anteroposterior fashion. There is a decrease of vision. The recovery of vision depends on the presence or absence of subretinal neovascular membranes in the area of choroidal rupture. Oftentimes, this area is associated with blood overlying the choroidal rupture.

Fluorescein Angiography

Fluorescein angiography delineates the presence of subretinal neovascular membranes in the center of the foveal avascular zone or macula. The area of subretinal neovascular membrane shows early choroidal hyperfluorescence, which in later transit develops into increasing density of hyperfluorescence.

Treatment

Usually this process is self-limited and the vision stabilizes. Laser photocoagulation is of limited benefit especially if the affected areas are near the fovea or the macula.[15]

PURTSCHER'S RETINOPATHY

Purtscher's retinopathy was originally used to describe retinal whitening, and hemorrhages and optic disc edema in a patient with a compression injury to the head.[16] A similar retinal picture has been seen with patients with severe compressive injury to the chest and the long bones.[17,18] A sudden increase in intrathoracic pressure is translated as an increase in venous pressure in the retinal venous system with consequent retinal exudation.

It has been postulated that retinal vascular injury with endothelial damage,[17,19] or complement-induced granulocyte aggregation[20] plays a role in this syndrome. In patients with pancreatitis and a Purtscher-like retinopathy, it has been postulated that the complement system is affected and there is an abnormality in retinal intravascular clotting.

Clinical findings are multiple hemorrhages of superficial retinal hemorrhages and retinal whitening surrounding the optic disc. The optic disc may present normally, but later develops an afferent pupillary defect and optic disc edema.

There is a rapid decrease in vision to the 20/200 level that may never fully resolve. There may be permanent central scotoma or partial visual loss.

Fluorescein Angiography

There is leakage of fluorescein in the region of the white retinal patches and retinal and disc edema. There is also venous staining and areas of capillary nonperfusion.[19]

Treatment

There is no treatment for this disease. For the patients with pancreatitis, the treatment of the underlying systemic disease leads to some resolution of the clinical retinal findings.

REFERENCES

1. National Society to Prevent Blindness: Fact Sheet. National Society to Prevent Blindness, New York, 1980

2. Radius RL, Finkelstein D: Central retinal artery occlusion (reversible) in sickle trait with glaucoma. Br J Ophthalmol 1976; *60:* 428–430

3. Thomas A, Parrish RK, Feuer WJ: Rebleeding after traumatic hyphema. Arch Ophthalmol 1986; *104:* 206–210

4. Crouch ER, Frankel M: Aminocaproic acid in the treatment of traumatic hyphema. Am J Ophthalmol 1976; *81:* 355–360

5. Kutner B, Fourman S, Brein K et al: Aminocaproic acid reduces the risk of secondary hemorrhage in patients with traumatic hyphema. Arch Ophthalmol 1987; *105:* 206–208

6. McGetrick JJ, Jampol LM, Goldberg MGF et al: Aminocaproic acid decreases secondary hemorrhage after traumatic hyphema. Arch Ophthalmol 1983; *101:* 1031–1033

7. Parrish CM, O'Day DM: Traumatic endophthalmitis. Int Ophthalmol Clin 1987; *27:* 112–119

8. Spoor TC, Hammer M, Belloso H: Traumatic hyphema: failure of steroids to alter its course. Arch Ophthalmol 1980; *98:* 116–119

9. Weiss JS, Parrish RK, Anderson DR: Surgical therapy of traumatic hyphema. Ophthalmic Surg 1983; *14:* 343–345

10. Gregor Z, Ryan SJ: Blood retinal barrier after blunt trauma to the eye. Graefe's Arch Clin Exp Ophthalmol 1982; *219:* 205–208

11. Blight R, Hart JCD: Histological changes in the internal retinal layers produced by concussive injuries to the globe. Trans Ophthalmol Soc UK 1978; *98:* 270–277

12. Bunt-Milam AH, Black RA, Bensinger RE: Breakdown of the outer blood retinal barrier in experimental commotio retinae. Exp Eye Res 1986; *43:* 397–412

13. Sipperley JO, Quigley HA, Gass JDM: Traumatic retinopathy in primates: the explanation of commotio retinae. Arch Ophthalmol 1978; *96:* 2267–2273

14. Aguilar JP, Green WR: Choroidal rupture. A histopathologic study of 47 cases. Retina 1984; *4:* 269–275

15. Fuller B, Gitter KA: Traumatic choroidal rupture with late serous detachment of the macula: report of successful argon laser treatment. Arch Ophthalmol 1973; *89:* 354–355

16. Purtscher O: Angiopathic retinae traumatica. Lymphorrhagien des augengrundes. Graefes Arch Clin Exp Ophthalmol 1912; *82:* 347–371

17. Kellen JS: Purtscher's retinopathy related to chest compression by safety belts: fluorescein angiographic findings. Am J Ophthalmol 1972; *74:* 278–283

18. Urbanek JH: Uber fettembolie des Auges. Graefes Arch Clin Exp Ophthalmol 1934; *131:* 147–173

19. Burton T: Unilateral Purtscher's retinopathy. Ophthalmol 1980; *87:* 1096–1105

20. Jacob HS, Craddock PR, Hammerschmidt DE, Moldow CF: Complement induced granulocyte aggregation: an unsuspected mechanism of disease. N Engl J Med 1980; *302:* 789–794

CHAPTER TWENTY-FIVE

Penetrating Trauma

After cataract surgery, ocular trauma is the most common cause of visual loss in America. Of 2.4 million eye injuries, 40,000 are left with significant visual loss. The National Society for the Prevention of Blindness estimates that there are 938,000 people with trauma-induced visual impairment in this country, of whom 75 percent are monocularly blind (20/200 or worse).[1]

Penetrating injuries can cause traumatic hyphema, dislocated lens, retinal detachment, intraocular foreign body, retinal dialysis, contusion necrosis, corneal scarring, cataract, vitreous hemorrhage, macular damage, and phthisis.

It is reported that the annual hospitalization costs for patients in the United States with penetrating ocular injuries alone costs approximately 120 million.[2]

DIAGNOSIS

It is important to take a good history from the patient. Although many victims of trauma are unable to provide a good history because of alcoholism, drug ingestion, shock, or neurologic problems associated with the traumatic event, it is important to establish clues about all sites of potential ocular damage.

The most important steps after the initial history are (1) vision, (2) gentle examination, (3) Fox shield, (4) antibiotics, and (5) tetanus antitoxin.

The visual acuity provides an important predictor for later visual potential. Even if Snellen visual acuity is not available at the emergency room, a near-vision card will suffice. In addition, because of the patient's condition, he or she may only be able to be tested with a near-vision card.

No light perception at presentation is an ominous sign. However, many of these patients with injuries of this severity are often intoxicated or have neurologic injuries preventing a coherent response. In these situations, check the visual acuity of the patient with the uninjured eye covered and with the indirect ophthalmoscope set at the maximum intensity (6 volts), with the light held at sufficient distance so that the patient cannot appreciate the heat of the light.

After the vision determination, examine the lid, adnexa, and globe gently so that there is no pressure on the globe. Any pressure on the globe will cause further prolapse of ocular contents which must be avoided.

Lid speculums and retractors should only be used with care so as not to prolapse the ocular contents. It may be best to perform this part of the examination in the operating room when all surgical instruments are prepared and available for the operative repair.

A small penetrating injury can be hidden in the angle and gonioscopy should be performed or at a later date after the initial attention is paid to the ruptured globe (Fig. 25–1).

Scleral rupture can be occult, hidden under the conjunctiva, Tenon's capsule, and/or the rectus muscles. Chemosis or conjunctival lid edema with or without subconjunctival hemorrhage is suggestive of such a rupture (Figs. 25–2 to 25–4). A ruptured globe has low intraocular pressure, but normal or elevated intraocular pressure does not rule out the possibility of a rupture.

Slit-lamp biomicroscopy of the anterior vitreous may demonstrate vitreous fibrils at the wound site. Ultrasound and computed tomography have been reported showing occult rupture with flattening of the posterior contour of the sclera (flat-tire sign).[3] In most situations, ultrasound will be performed in the operating or emergency room to evaluate the status of the retina. In cases of multiple, severe injuries to the orbit and globe, ultrasound may be performed in the operating room prior to the beginning of the operative repair, again with the principle of minimizing the risk of prolapsed ocular contents at the time of surgical repair.

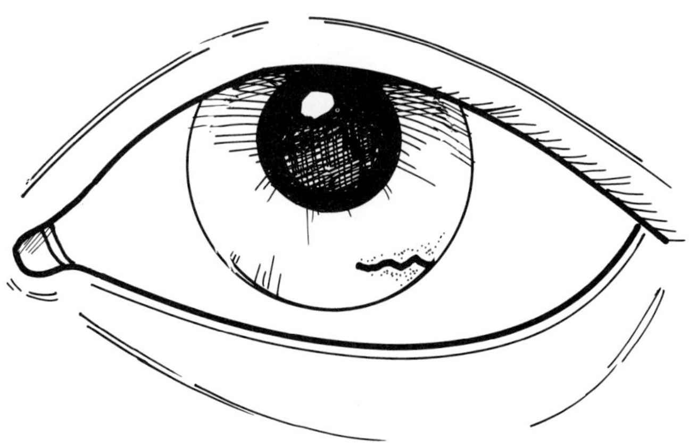

FIGURE 25–1

Small corneal laceration.

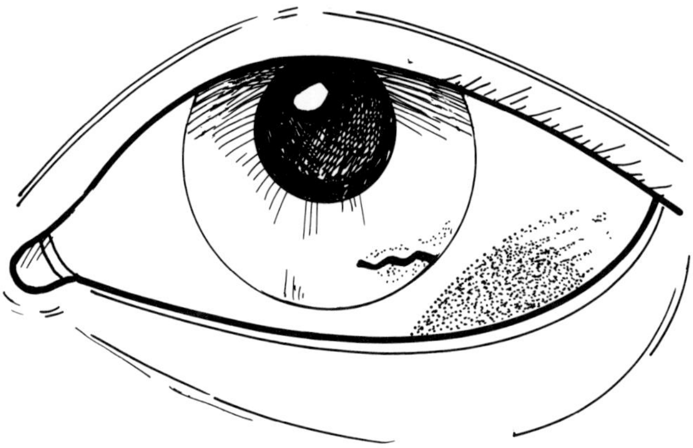

FIGURE 25–2

Small corneal laceration with subconjunctivial hemorrhage which may hide additional trauma to the globe.

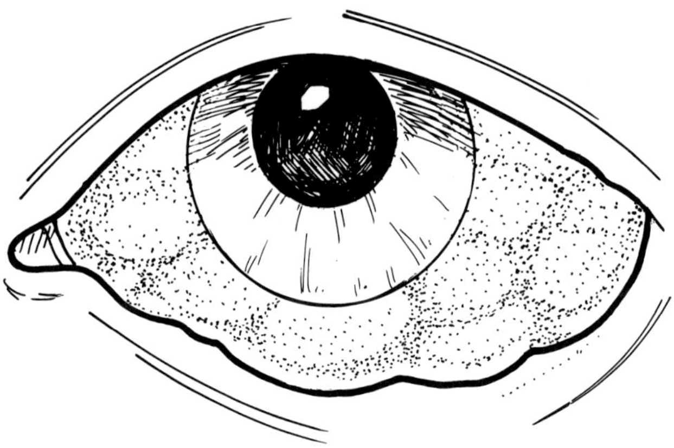

FIGURE 25–3

Severe conjunctival chemosis suggesting more severe trauma to the eye.

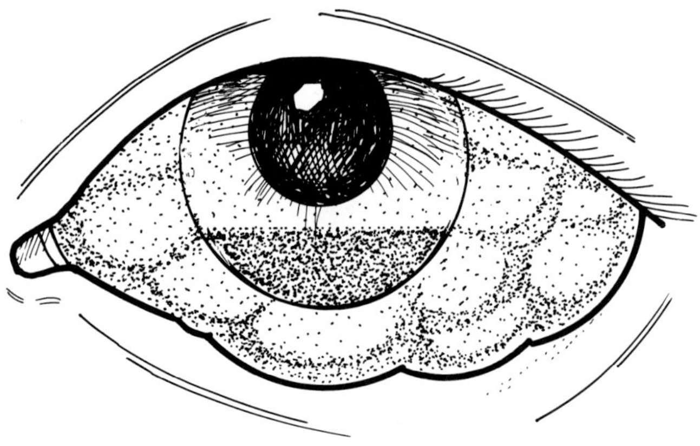

FIGURE 25–4

Hyphema suggests anterior chamber pathology. The severe conjunctival chemosis suggests trauma to the globe and retina.

The next step is the placement of the Fox shield which prevents further injury to the globe as the patient is transported from the emergency room to the operating room. Do not put any drops or ointment until the eye can be fully examined on the operating room table.

ANTIBIOTICS

Obtain cultures preoperatively and postoperatively. Send the cultures for Gram stain and start antibiotics. To cover gram-positive organisms, start with cephazolin 500 mg intravenously every 4 hours or another cephalosporin agent. To cover gram-negative organisms, one can consider gentamicin loading dose of 2 mg/kg, 80 mg every 8 hours if creatinine clearance is normal. If the patient is elderly, estimate for creatinine clearance as follows:

$$\text{Creatinine clearance} = \frac{(140 - \text{age}) \times \text{weight (kg)}}{72 \times \text{serum creatinine (mg/dl)}}$$

Topical antibiotics are used for gram-positive and gram-negative coverage. Subconjunctival injection of cephazolin 100 mg; gentamicin 40 mg/ml. Because of gentamicin-induced toxicity of the retina, it is possible to substitute vancomycin 25 mg instead.[4] Tetanus antitoxin should be given.

TRAUMATIC ENDOPHTHALMITIS

Traumatic endophthalmitis occurs in 2–7 percent of penetrating injuries.[5] Diagnosis of traumatic endophthalmitis is rare.[5] Ocular signs of traumatic endophthalmitis are similar to those with a postoperative infection. There is aqueous cell and flare and hypopyon. The aqueous cell and flare exceeds that expected from the injury.

One should obtain culture specimens, as with any endophthalmitis, with a vitreous aspiration.

Bacillus cereus causes up to 25 percent of traumatic endopthalmitis.[6,7] It usually is in the setting of a penetrating injury with a metallic foreign body occurring in an environment where soil contamination is likely. The course is rapid and severe characterized by profound orbital swelling and ring corneal ulcer.

Accepted management of endophthalmitis has included intravitreal injection of antibiotics: cefazolin (2.25 mg/0.1 ml) and gentamicin (200 µg/0.1 ml) or amikacin (400 µg/0.1).[4] However, *B. cereus* is resistant to penicillins and cephalosporins, thus, one has to consider vancomycin (1 mg/0.1 ml).[8] Others have advocated the use of clindamycin (450 ug/0.1 ml) for *B. cereus.*[6]

CORNEOSCLERAL LACERATION

Signs of global perforation can be subtle. However, the main characteristics are (1) decreased visual acuity, (2) hypotony which is measured by intraocular pressure, (3) shallowing or flattening of the anterior chamber, (4) alteration of pupil size, shape, or location, (5) obvious corneal or scleral laceration, (6) prolapse of the vitreous or iris or other intraocular contents, and (7) marked conjunctival chemosis.

Culture the eye preoperatively if there is no pressure placed on the globe. Place the Fox shield on the eye. Ultrasound the eye preoperatively only if there is no prolapse of intraocular contents.

Surgery

Determine the extent of the injury after the eye is prepared for surgery. Then determine if iris or vitreous incarceration is present. Suture the laceration. Reform the anterior chamber with balanced salt solution or hyaluronic acid or air.

If the iris is prolapsed from the wound, it can be reposited in most cases. We advise excision of the uveal tissue if it looks extremely necrotic or has been externalized for 24 hours or more. After reforming the anterior chamber, consider making a stab incision 90 degrees away from the prolapsed iris and insert a spatula sweeping the iris into place inside the anterior chamber.

Once that is done, perform a 360-degree conjunctival peritomy to investigate the extent of the corneal laceration and to ascertain if there is also a scleral laceration. Sharp dissection of conjunctiva and Tenon's capsule with sharp Westcott scissors is necessary to expose all four quadrants. It is during this dissection, that one must be looking for any prolapse of vitreous or retina to the wound.

Sometimes, a scleral laceration may continue under the muscles. It may be necessary to isolate the muscle with 6-0 vicryl and remove it from its insertion in order to perform the repair. If there is excessive loss of scleral tissue, it may be necessary to use a scleral patch graft.

When vitreous is extruding from the wound, it should be cut with Vannas scissors, with the scissors placed flush with the sclera. If there is extrusion of the retina, care should be taken to reposit the retina, avoiding excision or incarceration if possible.

In cases of vitreous hemorrhages and suspected scleral laceration posterior to the ora serrata, it will be difficult to identify the retinal laceration from looking inside the fundus with an indirect ophthalmoscope. Vitreous surgery should be performed in such cases (Fig. 25–5). There is considerable controversy about the proper timing of surgery. Some surgeons advocate operating in the

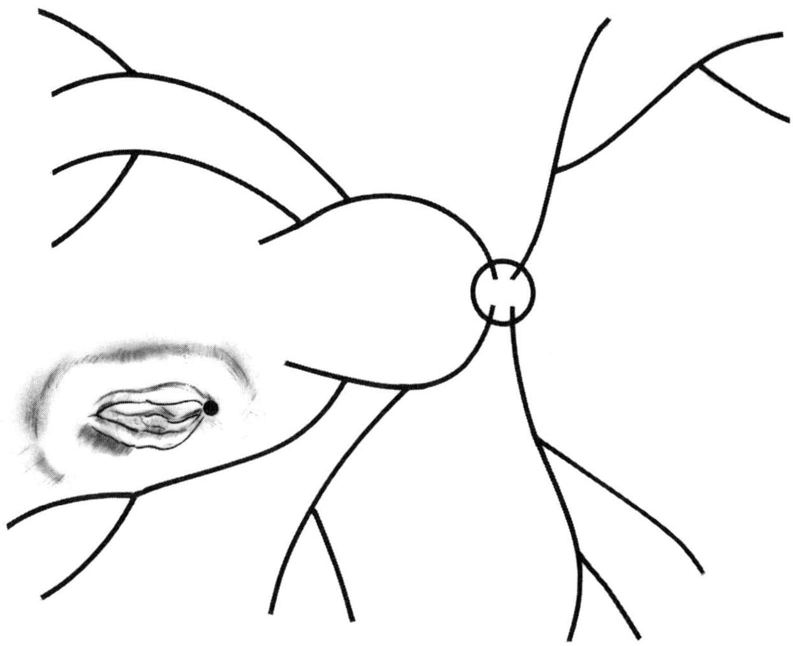

FIGURE 25-5

Foreign body on the retina with overlying vitreous reaction.

first 48–72 hours, others advocate delaying surgery up to 4–10 days after the initial injury.[9]

Another decision is the removal of the lens at the time of surgery. If the lens is subluxed or opacified, it will need to be removed so that the surgeon will have an adequate view of the posterior pole.

Prophylactic cryopexy should be avoided because cryopexy has been known to cause inflammation and thus promote the development of a retinal detachment or proliferative vitreoretinopathy.[10] However, some vitreoretinal surgery centers advocate a prophylactic scleral buckle at the time of primary repair.[11,12] However, with identifiable retinal detachments, scleral buckling is indicated. When retinal tears are identified, they should be treated with cryopexy for peripheral breaks or posterior endolaser for posterior breaks.

In addition, if there is a retinal detachment present, it is important to relieve all tangential and anteroposterior traction on the retinal break by vitreous surgical techniques of membrane peeling, delamination, or segmentation. When the traction cannot be relieved, a scleral buckle will be placed to support the break. Subretinal fluid can be drained through the existing retinal break. Long-acting SF6 or perfluoropropane can be injected to provide longer lasting internal tamponade to the detached retina.

COMPLICATIONS OF PENETRATING INJURY

Fibrotic membranes, fibrotic pupil secondary to glial membranes, occluded aphakic pupil, and macular pucker can develop.

Sympathetic ophthalmia is a bilateral inflammation of the uveal tract, characterized by ocular or diffuse infiltration with lymphocytes and epitheloid cells. Although its etiology is unknown, the majority of cases are associated with a penetrating injury and surgical penetration such as vitrectomy.[13] The inflammation occurs in the injured or exciting eye usually within 4–8 weeks. The sympathizing eye becomes involved simultaneously or shortly thereafter. The sympathizing eye remains injected with a persistent low-grade uveitis. The iris is thickened. The eye is unresponsive to light. There are associated nodules at the pupillary margin. Keratic precipitates can be seen, but these are nonspecific. Eventually phthisis bulbi may develop. Corticosteroids remains the treatment of choice for sympathetic ophthalmia.[14,15]

REFERENCES

1. The National Society for the Prevention of Blindness: Fact Sheet, National Society for the Prevention of Blindness, New York, 1980

2. Shanker B, Tielsch JM, Parver LM: Incidence of hospitalized ocular injury in Maryland. Invest Ophthalmol Vis Sci 1986; *27* (suppl.): 101

3. Sevel D, Krausz H, Ponder T, Centeno R: Value of computed tomography for the diagnosis of a ruptured eye. J Comput Assist Tomogr 1983; *7:* 870–875

4. Conway BP, Campochiaro PA: Macular infarction after endopthalmitis treated with vitrectomy and intravitreal gentamicin. Arch Ophthalmol 1986; *104:* 367–371

5. Brinton GS, Topping TM, Hyndiuk RA et al: Post traumatic endophthalmitis. Arch Ophthalmol 1984; *102:* 547–550

6. Schemmer GB, Driebe WT: Post traumatic *Bacillus cereus* endophthalmitis. Arch Ophthalmol 1987; *105:* 342–344

7. Parrish CM, O'Day DM: Traumatic endophthalmitis. Int Ophthalmol Clin 1987; *27:* 112–119

8. Pflugfelder SC, Pflugfelder ME, Fliesler SJ et al: Intravitreal vancomycin retinal toxicity, clearance, and interaction with gentamicin. Invest Ophthalmol Vis Sci 1986; 27:(suppl.) 88

9. Coleman DJ: Early vitrectomy in the management of the severely traumatized eye. Am J Ophthalmol 1982; *93:* 543–551

10. Campochiaro PA, Kaden IH, Vidaurri-Leal J, Glaser BM: Cryotherapy enhances intravitreal dispersion of viable retinal pigment epithelial cells. Arch Ophthalmol 1985; *103:* 434–436

11. Hutton WL, Fuller DG: Factors influencing final visual results in severely injured eyes. Am J Ophthalmol 1984; *97:* 715–722

12. Brinton GS, Aaberg TM, Reeser FH et al: Surgical results in ocular trauma involving the posterior segment. Am J Ophthalmol 1982; *94:* 271–278

13. Lewis ML, Gass JDM, Spencer WH: Sympathetic uveitis after trauma and vitrectomy. Arch Ophthalmol 1978; *96:* 263–267

14. Reynard M, Riffenburgh RS, Maes EF: Effect of corticosteroid treatment and enucleation of the visual prognosis of sympathetic ophthalmia. Am J Ophthalmol 1983; *96:* 290–294

15. Lubin JR, Albert DM, Weinstein M: Sixty-five years of sympathetic ophthalmia. A clinicopathologic review of 105 cases (1913–1978). Ophthalmol 1980; *87:* 109–121

CHAPTER TWENTY-SIX

Postcataract Complications

DISLOCATED LENSES INTO THE POSTERIOR SEGMENT

In the course of cataract surgery, there are certain moments when the delivery of the lens out of the lip of the wound is critical to the successful completion of the procedure. In intracapsular cataract surgery, the placement of the cryoprobe onto the lens and the motion of lifting the lens from the vitreous face are the critical points. It is usually at this juncture when the loss of the lens into the posterior pole occurs. Here, the cryoprobe breaks the anterior capsule of the cataract and the lens falls backward.

During extracapsular cataract surgery, the lens is gently rotated out of the capsular bag and delivered out into the scleral wound. It is at this point that the lens can be dislocated posteriorly. Another point of dislocation occurs with the forceful or inappropriate maneuvering of the can-opener incision in the capsule.

During phacoemulsification, the lens can dislocate during viscoelastic dissection of the lens from the capsule or dividing the nucleus with the phacoemulsification tip can force the lens posteriorly. The maneuvering of the lens inside the capsule during the midphase of phacoemulsification can cause the posterior movement of the lens. Lastly, high-infusion pressure, while in the phacoemulsification mode, can cause dislodgement of the lens posteriorly.

Risk factors for dislocated lens include (1) pseudoexfoliation of the lens capsule with risk of zonular weakening, (2) history of prior ocular trauma and zonular weakening, (3) large brunescent cataracts, and (4) syneretic vitreous in combination with weak zonular attachments makes phacoemulsification more difficult.

Dislocated intraocular lenses occur at the time of implantation. The lens can sit on the anterior vitreous face or dislocate onto the syneretic vitreous (Figs. 26–1 to 26–3).

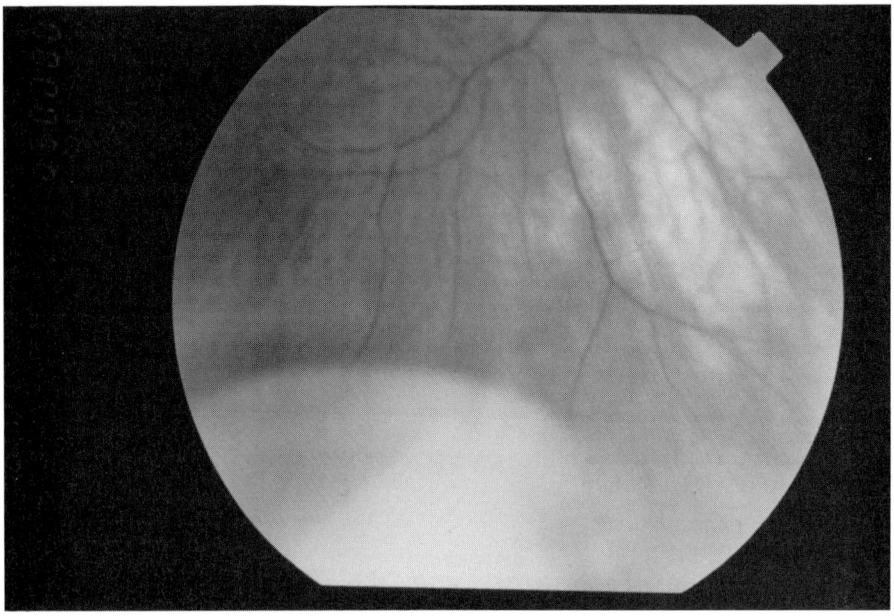

FIGURE 26–1

Dropped lens on retina.

Diagnosis and Management

The diagnosis of posterior dislocation of the lens happens at the operating table and the event can happen in a matter of seconds.[1–8] It is important not to retrieve the lens with the present cataract instruments.[1] This applies to the natural human lens as well as

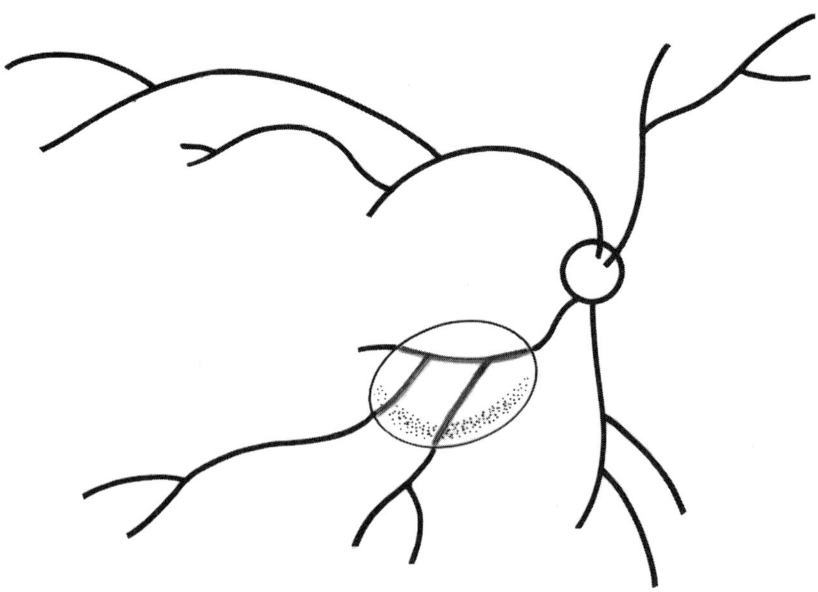

FIGURE 26–2

Diagram showing dropped lens on retina.

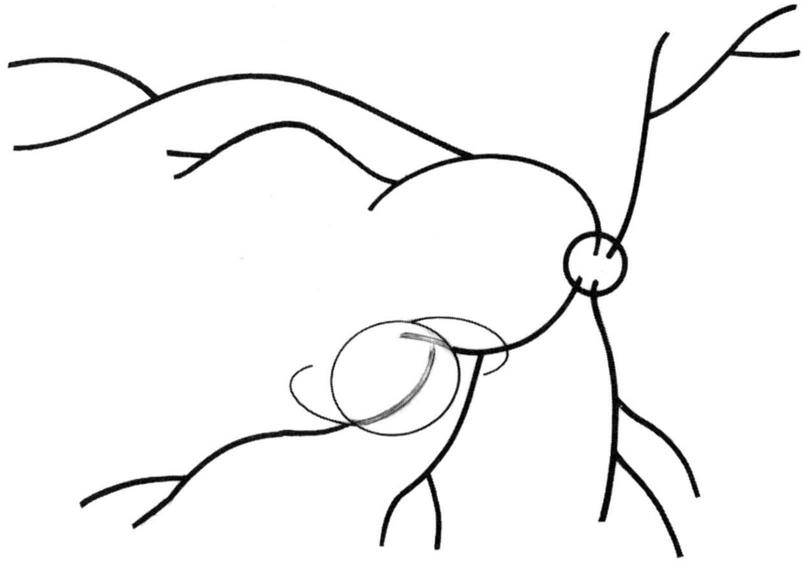

FIGURE 26–3

Diagram showing dropped intraocular lens on retina.

the intraocular lens. Perform an anterior vitrectomy and close the cataract wound securely. In cases of a scleral tunnel, suturing the wound is important since the vitrectomy surgeon will need to return the patient to the operating room for additional vitreous surgery.

The vitreous surgeon, with the pars plana vitrectomy, will use the lensectomy-fragmatome probe to aspirate the lens into the midvitreous. At that point, the lens will be aspirated, using the lightpipe to stabilize the lens as it is being aspirated. Indirect ophthalmoscopy can be used to inspect for retinal tears, dialysis, or giant retinal breaks. Appropriate retinal detachment techniques then will be used. Cryopexy or endolaser can be used to close peripheral breaks. In cases of retinal detachment, internal drainage may be necessary with air infusion and air/gas exchange at the end of the case.

The surgeon can also use perfluorocarbon liquid, which is denser in specific gravity than water, to float the lens or intraocular implant up into the midvitreous. If it is the human lens, aspiration is now the next step. If it is an intraocular implant, it can be brought up to the posterior capsular area by bimanual manipulation of foreign body forceps and placed into the sulcus or sutured in place.[10,11] Liquid perfluorocarbon can also be used for retinal detachment repair.[10,11]

VITREOUS HEMORRHAGE

Vitreous hemorrhage is rare after cataract surgery. When it occurs, there is usually only a small amount of blood and the view of the posterior pole is clear.

It is thought that the hyaloidoretinal adhesions that may be severed during cataract surgery play a role. There may be associated petechial hemorrhages indicating the site of ruptured vessels. Blood may leak from engorged vessels as a result of hypotension during cataract surgery. Always consider looking for a peripheral retinal tear whenever there is a nonclearing vitreous hemorrhage. Goldmann contact lens examination of the far retinal periphery is especially useful in the recently operated eye with a vitreous hemorrhage.

Diagnosis and Management

Indirect ophthalmoscopy with Goldmann contact lens examination is usually sufficient. Always consider retinal breaks when looking inside the posterior pole. In mild vitreous hemorrhages, follow-up examinations are important in monitoring the progression of the vitreous hemorrhage. In the rare cases of nonclearing and dense vitreous hemorrhage, ultrasonic evaluation is necessary to evaluate the integrity of the retina. In nonclearing vitreous hemorrhages, vitrectomy is performed. At this point, look for retinal breaks in the periphery and treat the retinal breaks with cryopexy or indirect laser.

CHOROIDAL HEMORRHAGE

Choroidal hemorrhage occurring after cataract surgery is especially common in the glaucoma patient.[13] The sudden decrease in intraocular pressure in elderly individuals with sclerotic choroidal vessels can result in minor choroidal hemorrhages that resolve within 4–6 weeks postoperatively with few untoward effects on final visual outcome. Rupture of the long or short posterior ciliary arteries into the suprachoroidal space can occur especially if these arteries are sclerotic and necrotic.[13] Those eyes that sustain large choroidal hemorrhages at the end of the cataract procedure will require posterior sclerotomies at the time of surgery and/or further vitreous surgery (Fig. 26–4).

Risk factors for choroidal hemorrhage include advanced age, glaucoma, history of age-related macular degeneration with large disciform scar, and history of uveitis.

Indications for immediate drainage of choroidal hemorrhage are (1) the forward movement of the vitreous and difficulty in controlling wound closure and (2) two large mounds of choroidal hemorrhage with the retina coming together in apposition ("kissing choroidals").

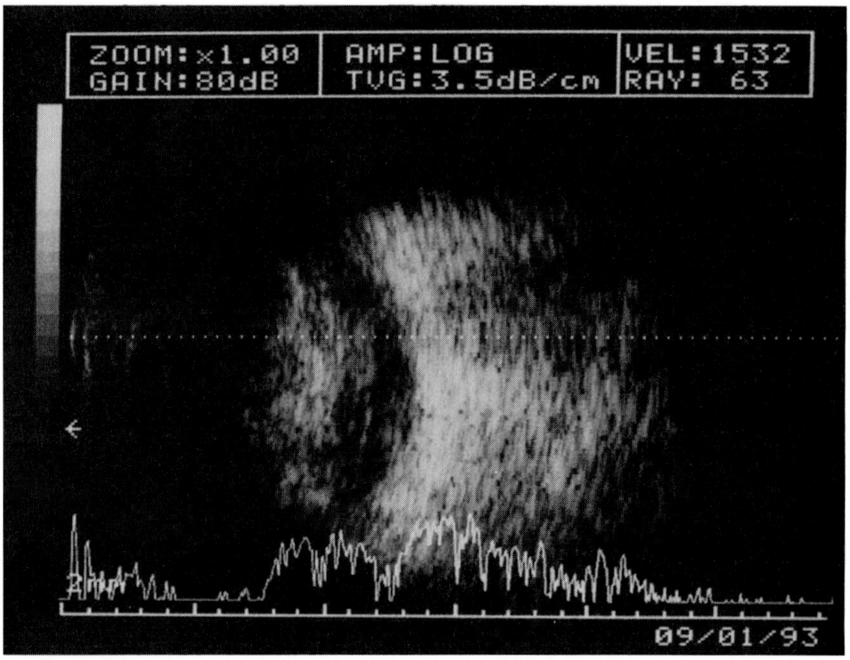

FIGURE 26-4

Choroidal hemorrhage on ultrasound.

Diagnosis and Management

In very shallow choroidal hemorrhages or hemorrhagic detachments, not approaching the posterior pole and with good visual acuity, biweekly or weekly follow-up examinations will enable close monitoring of the resolution of shallow choroidal hemorrhages. Postoperative topical steroid eyedrops are very helpful to decrease inflammation and the addition of oral steroids for 3–4 days can also be useful. The usual regimen is 100 mg of oral prednisone on the first day, followed by 80 mg then 60 mg on the subsequent 2 days. The initial dose can be smaller for the elderly, small body-weight, or diabetic elderly patients.

In large choroidal hemorrhages where immediate choroidal drainage is indicated, but is unsuccessful in decompressing the globe, additional vitreous surgery may be necessary. At the time of vitreous surgery, a limbal infusion of Balanced Saline Solution (BSS) while there is choroidal drainage in the equator of the four quadrants is performed. When the globe integrity is maintained, then pars plana vitrectomy is performed for removal of residual blood or repair of retinal detachment that has occurred with the choroidal hemorrhage.

EXPULSIVE CHOROIDAL HEMORRHAGE

The incidence of expulsive choroidal hemorrhage, a dreaded entity, is 0.19–0.25 percent.[13–15] It is defined as an extensive hemorrhage in the suprachoroidal space pushing the intraocular contents out of the eye or causing the retinal surfaces into near apposition.[16]

It occurs after cataract surgery, trabeculectomy, or penetrating keratoplasty when the globe undergoes sudden decompression of pressure.[17–19] When the pressure of the globe becomes firm, it becomes difficult to close the cataract wound and the lens-iris diaphragm pushes forward. The iris cannot be repositioned easily.

Closure of the wound as quickly as possible is necessary. Securely suture the wound with several interrupted sutures. It is important to decompress the eye.

Because the ocular media is now cloudy due to vitreous hemorrhage and corneal edema, follow up is necessary with ultrasound.

Oral prednisone is strongly recommended for 3–5 days (prednisione 100 mg orally on day 1, then 80 mg orally on day 2, 60 mg orally on day 3 [see above]). Monitor daily for improvement with ultrasound and indirect ophthalmoscopy.

Additional complications include glaucoma, uveitis, retinal detachment, and endopthalmitis.

Surgery

Vitrectomy can be done at a later date (1 week to 2 weeks postoperative) once the inflammation decreases. The surgical approach is similar to that of the choroidal hemorrhage (see above) with the use of perilimbal infusion of BSS or air and drainage of choroidals before proceeding to the repair of the retinal detachment with pars plana vitrectomy techniques.

REFERENCES

1. Smiddy WE, Flynn HW: Management of dislocated posterior chamber intraocular lenses. Ophthalmol 1991; *98:* 889–894

2. McCannel MA: A retrievable suture ideas for anterior uveal problems. Ophthalmic Surg 1976; *7:* 98–103

3. Sternberg P Jr, Michels RG: Treatment of dislocated posterior chamber intraocular lenses. Arch Ophthalmol 1986; *104:* 1391–1393

4. Brod RD, Flynn HW Jr, Clarkson JG, Blankenship GW: Management options for retinal detachment in the presence of posteriorly dislocated intraocular lens. Retina 1990; *10:* 50–56

5. Insler MS, Mani H, Peyman GA: A new surgical technique for dislocated posterior chamber intraocular lenses. Ophthal Surg 1988; *19:* 480-481

6. Campos RV, Chung KD, Oyakawa RT: Pars plana vitrectomy in the management of dislocated posterior chamber lenses. Am J Ophthalmol 1989; *108:* 529–534

7. Shapiro MJ, Resnick KI, Kim SH, Weinberg A: Management of dislocated crystalline lens with a perfluorocarbon liquid. Am J Ophthalmol 1991; *112:* 401–405

8. Liu KR, Peyman GA, Chen MS, Chang KB: Use of high density vitreous substitutes in the removal of posteriorly dislocated lenses or intraocular lenses. Ophthal Surg 1991; *22:* 503–507

9. Lambrou FH Jr, Stewart MW: Management of dislocated lens fragments during phacoemulsification. Ophthalmol 1992; *99:* 1260–1262

10. Chang S, Lincoff H, Zimmerman NJ, Fuchs W: Giant retinal tears. Surgical techniques and results using perfluorocarbon liquids. Arch Ophthalmol 1989; *107:* 761–766

11. Chang S, Repucci V, Zimmerman NJ et al: Perfluorocarbon liquids in the management of traumatic retinal detachment. Ophthalmol 1989; *96:* 785–792

12. Manshot WA: The pathology of expulsive hemorrhage. Am J Ophthalmol 1955; *40:* 15–24

13. Speaker MG, Guerriero PN, Met JA et al: A case control study of risk factors for intraoperative suprachoroidal expulsive hemorrhage. Ophthalmol 1991; *98:* 202–209

14. Holland G: Zur Klinik der expulsiven Blutung nach kataraktoperation. Klin Monatsbl Augenheilkd 1966; *149:* 859–864

15. Taylor DM: Expulsive hemorrhage. Trans Am Ophthalmol Soc 1974; *72:* 137–147

16. Welch JC, Spaeth CK, Benson WE: Massive suprachoroidal hemorrhage. Ophthalmol 1988; *95:* 1202–1206

17. Canton LB, Katz LJ, Spaeth G: Complications of surgery in glaucoma: suprachoroidal hemorrhage in glaucoma patients undergoing intraocular surgery. Ophthalmol 1985; *92:* 1266–1270

18. Fastenberg DM, Perry HD, Donnenfeld ED et al: Expulsive choroidal hemorrhage with scleral buckling surgery. Arch Ophthalmol 1991; *109:* 323

19. Brown SI, Tragakis MA: Wound dehiscence with keratoplasty. Am J Ophthalmol 1971; *72:* 115–119

INDEX

Note: Page numbers in *italic* refer to illustrations, page numbers followed by t refer to tables.

F

S